PAIN MANAGEMENT: NEW RESEARCH

PAIN MANAGEMENT: NEW RESEARCH

PAOLO S. GRECO AND FRANCESCO M. CONTI
Editors

Nova Biomedical Books
New York

NOTICE TO THE READER

The Publisher has taken reasonable care in the preparation of this book, but makes no expressed or implied warranty of any kind and assumes no responsibility for any errors or omissions. No liability is assumed for incidental or consequential damages in connection with or arising out of information contained in this book. The Publisher shall not be liable for any special, consequential, or exemplary damages resulting, in whole or in part, from the readers' use of, or reliance upon, this material.

Independent verification should be sought for any data, advice or recommendations contained in this book. In addition, no responsibility is assumed by the publisher for any injury and/or damage to persons or property arising from any methods, products, instructions, ideas or otherwise contained in this publication.

This publication is designed to provide accurate and authoritative information with regard to the subject matter covered herein. It is sold with the clear understanding that the Publisher is not engaged in rendering legal or any other professional services. If legal or any other expert assistance is required, the services of a competent person should be sought. FROM A DECLARATION OF PARTICIPANTS JOINTLY ADOPTED BY A COMMITTEE OF THE AMERICAN BAR ASSOCIATION AND A COMMITTEE OF PUBLISHERS.

Library of Congress Cataloging-in-Publication Data

Pain management : new research / Paolo S. Greco and Francesco M. Conti (editors).
     p. ; cm.
 Includes bibliographical references and index.
 ISBN 978-1-60456-767-0 (hardcover)
 1. Analgesia. 2. Pain--Treatment. I. Greco, Paolo S. II. Conti, Francesco M.
 [DNLM: 1. Pain--therapy. 2. Analgesia--methods. 3. Pain--psychology. WL 704 P14659554 2008]
  RB127.P332384 2008
  616'.0472--dc22
                              2008020867

Published by Nova Science Publishers, Inc. ✦ New York

Contents

Preface

Pain management (also called pain medicine) is the discipline concerned with the relief of pain. Acute pain, such as occurs with trauma, often has a reversible cause and may require only transient measures and correction of the underlying problem. In contrast, chronic pain often results from conditions that are difficult to diagnose and treat, and that may take a long time to reverse. Some examples include cancer, neuropathy, and referred pain. Often, pain pathways (nociceptors) are set up that continue to transmit the sensation of pain even though the underlying condition or injury that originally caused pain has been healed. In such situations, the pain itself is frequently managed separately from the underlying condition of which it is a symptom, or the goal of treatment is to manage the pain with no treatment of any underlying condition (e.g. if the underlying condition has resolved or if no identifiable source of the pain can be found. Pain management generally benefits from a multidisciplinary approach that includes pharmacologic measures (analgesics such as narcotics or NSAIDs and pain modifiers such as tricyclic antidepressants or anticonvulsants), non-pharmacologic measures (such as interventional procedures, physical therapy and physical exercise, application of ice and/or heat), and psychological measures (such as biofeedback and cognitive therapy). This new book presents the latest research in this growing field.

Chapter I - Panic disorder is characterized by a progression of panic symptom severity with repeated attacks. Repeated panic episodes evoke heightened anticipatory anxiety, phobic avoidance, and panic is typically associated with comorbid symptoms of depression. Due to the heterogeneity of the disorder, reliable neurochemical correlates attending panic have not been identified. However, variable neuropeptide interfacing with major and minor transmitter systems may modulate individual vulnerability to panic and account for variable panic profiles. The extensive colocalization of cholecystokinin (CCK) with other neurotransmitters, including dopamine (DA), enkephalin (ENK) and GABA, in specific central sites may influence various aspects of anxiety and panic. The behavioral correlates attending panic likely follow from variable neurochemical release and conditioning and sensitization. Clinicians maintain that panic attacks are spontaneous and fail to acknowledge the wealth of information implicating a role for stressful life events in panic. Conditioning and sensitization of both behavior (e.g., fear-motivated) and neurochemical events (e.g., DA and CCK) in response to uncontrollable stressors parallel the diverse heterogeneity of panic amongst clinical samples. Cholecystokinin-4, pentagastrin, lactate acid, and CO_2 induce panic attacks in both panic patients and healthy controls that are dependent on subjective history, expectancy measures and panic profiles. Panic disorder is associated with chronic illness, including Parkinson's disease and schizophrenia, and familial sick-role modeling exacerbates the course of the illness. The current review outlines the evidence supporting a conditioning/sensitization model for panic and accounts for the variable efficacies of pharmacological interventions.

Chapter II - Placebo treatments have proven effective to alleviate pain perception along with a variety of medical conditions. It is currently acknowledged that placebo effects can be induced by expectation of clinical improvement via specific brain mechanisms. Although research in this field has flourished over the last few years, the neurobiological mechanisms underlying placebo-induced clinical responses are not completely understood. This chapter focuses on the current evidence sustaining placebo responses in pain conditions. *In vivo* neurophysiological and functional neuroimaging studies currently shape our understanding of the neural changes associated with placebo effects. Converging evidence suggests that placebo analgesia is linked to the activation of the endogenous opioid network. Within this network, a pivotal role seems to be played by the rostral portion of the anterior cingulate cortex, an area characterized by high density of endogenous opioid receptors. The newborn neuroscience of placebo will likely prove useful in understanding how the context of beliefs and values influences brain processes related to perception and emotion in subjects with both psychological and physical dysfunctions. Further research on the placebo response is needed, both to shed more light on the complexity of mind-body interactions and to improve the efficacy of its applications to clinical practice.

Chapter III - Japanese traditional medicine that consists of *Acupuncture* and *Kampo* (Japanese herbal medicine), is widely used as a complementary and alternative medicine to cure and to care for patients in Japan. The origin of Japanese traditional medicine came from Chinese Medicine over 1500 years ago. However, it has evolved uniquely to develop different method, needles (e.g., smaller diameter), and adaptation of Herb, from those of Chinese Medicine.

We investigate the molecular mechanisms of Japanese traditional medicine especially the efficacy of *Acupuncture* in muscles. At first, the molecular evidence of the acupuncture stimulation in the muscle is explained. Then the clinical manipulation of *Acupuncture* and *Kampo* formulation are introduced.

Chapter IV - The solution calorimetry is a valuable instrument for the investigation of intermolecular interactions in condensed media. This chapter is the review of research carried out in this field during the last 50 years. The authors focused their attention on organic nonelectrolytes as solutes and on individual nonaqueous solvents. The peculiarity of water as a solvent (hydrophobic effect) was also considered.

It is assumed in this chapter that the term 'solution' distinct from 'mixing' means the transfer of a solute to a solvent at infinite dilution. It allows one to exclude the solute-solute interaction in the final state. Experimentally obtained enthalpies of solution were recalculated in the majority of cases to solvation enthalpies by subtraction of the vaporization enthalpies of the solutes. It allows one to exclude the solute-solute interaction in the initial state.

Resulted solvation enthalpies were analyzed using the traditional scheme which assumes that solvation enthalpy can be regarded as the sum of the cavity formation enthalpy and the interaction enthalpy. The former item reflects partial breaking of solvent-solvent interaction during the solvation.

The solute-solvent interaction enthalpy was regarded as the sum of the interaction enthalpies of specific and nonspecific types. Specific interactions are considered as localized donor-acceptor interactions. The examples of specific interactions are hydrogen bonding and charge transfer complex formation.

The attempts to correlate the nonspecific solvation enthalpies with the polarity and polarizability parameters of solute and solvent molecules was discussed. An attempt to estimate the contribution of polar interactions to the nonspecific solvation enthalpy.

The authors paid much attention to the methods of extraction of hydrogen bonding enthalpies from the solvation enthalpy data. The analysis of solvation enthalpies in the solvents associated via hydrogen bonding was performed by taking into consideration the cooperativity of hydrogen bonding formation. Combined use of solution calorimetry and IR spectral methods is especially productive in this case.

Chapter V - Although it has been well established that opioid analgesics relieve pain by acting on receptors in the central nervous system, research has suggested that similar analgesia can be achieved through peripheral opioid receptors. Basic science research has demonstrated that malignant or benign skin ulcers can expose peripheral sensory nerve terminals, while local inflammation within the ulcer up-regulates opioid receptors. Thus, one strategy to manage pain arising from these ulcers would be to apply topical opioid agonists, usually in the form of a gel. While systemic absorption likely varies with extent of ulceration, topical analgesics could reduce the need for systemic medications and the resultant adverse effects. However, research in the area has been slow; a few small randomized trials and case series suggest benefits from morphine gel. Whether it is a placebo effect or actual analgesia produced from peripheral receptors, many unfortunate patients suffer from difficult to treat ulcerative pain and may appear to benefit from a topical strategy. Larger studies are needed and, fortunately, are being conducted to help establish topical opioid therapy as a viable adjunct to systemic therapy in treating pain from ulcers.

Chapter VI - Non-specific abdominal pain is the commonest diagnosis for children presenting with abdominal pain to hospital. Chronic right iliac fossa (RIF) pain has been described in the adult population. The most common population subset to complain of this condition is women of childbearing age. This can be related to gynaecological or appendiceal pathology.

In children right iliac fossa or right lower quadrant pain lasting longer than one month is a common complaint. In many cases the symptoms resolve spontaneously. However a population exists where no pathology is identified and symptoms persist. Psychological pathology, stress or anxiety can manifest itself as functional abdominal pain syndrome. Children with functional abdominal pain are more likely to take time off school and to have parents of increased anxiety. Where psychological cause is not thought likely, routine investigations to exclude common conditions are performed.

In the acute setting the diagnosis that needs to be excluded is appendicitis. Acute appendicitis is a clinical diagnosis. This is not always accurate, and many surgeons use laparoscopy where doubt exists. In a series of 1,320 patients investigatory laparoscopy changed the diagnosis in 30% of cases. Chronic pain emanating from the pelvis or right iliac fossa is a vague symptom in which a definitive diagnosis remains elusive. There are multiple radiological and serological investigations at hand, although often these are inconclusive. Macroscopic assessment of the appendix at diagnostic laparoscopy is reliable and in the acute setting gynaecologists have a false negative rate of 0% in removing an inflamed appendix. This investigation has been used routinely in patients with chronic abdominal pain where other modalities have failed. Chronic pain emanating from the appendix can be due to one of two reasons, firstly chronic appendicitis/ recurrent appendicitis [12] and secondly appendiceal colic.

There is evidence to support the hypothesis that chronic appendicitis/ appendicael colic improves in children following appendicectomy. This chapter presents original scientific work followed by a literature review of chronic right iliac fossa pain in children to define the patient demographics, natural history of this condition and assess the value of laparoscopic appendicectomy in its treatment.

Chapter VII - One of the major attractions of laparoscopic surgery in children is the reduced pain experience. However minimally invasive surgery is not painless and a significant number of patients suffer discomfort in the first few hours following intervention. This chapter highlights the multifactorial nature of the pain and summarises the current management options available to children.

Chapter VIII - Pain control is an indisputable human act, but alone it doesn't enhance the postoperative recovery nor decrease the adverse effects. The failed organization of Acute Pain Services may be due to their no cost-utility, because of high costs that aren't followed by reduction of hospitalization and adverse effects. When analgesia is integrated in a multimodal perioperative program there is an enhancement of early and long term outcome. The authors achieved a pathway for abdominal aortic surgery, aimed to reduce the postoperative pain and perioperative stress. The team work chose: transversal left subcostal incision, continuous epidural thoracic analgesia [48 hours], immediate transfer to the surgical ward, opiates-free perioperative analgesia, early feeding and deambulation. This pathway resulted from interaction between surgeons, anesthesiologists and nurses, aiming to improve not only best postoperative comfort, but also outcome and early resumption of daily living. For instance, although opiates are excellent analgesic drugs, we chose an opiates-free analgesia, in order to avoid nausea, vomiting and delay bowel movement, critical feature in this kind of surgery. From 2000 to 2007 the authors treated on this program more than 600 non selected patients. During the postoperative time they obtained a good pain control (Visual Analogical Scale: 0-2) without adverse effects analgesic therapy related. Conversely, this technique helped the postoperative rehabilitation; in particular postoperative morbidity was low, without any respiratory complication. Almost all patients had deambulation and took food on the day of surgery. The median hospital stay was 3 days. The authors observed an excellent recovery of the quality of life at sixth month and twelfth month postoperatively [Short Form 36]. An optimum analgesic strategy integrated with mini-invasive surgery and rehabilitative perioperative program improves short and long term outcome, reducing perioperative length of stay and costs.

Chapter IX - Surgical incision results in both peripheral and central changes in sensory processes. Postoperative pain features involve pain associated with mechanical stimulations, like mobilization and cough, and also hypersensitivity to light touch in tissues surrounding the wound, even in areas distant from the incision. Current research, both in animal models and in patients, indicate that the presence and the extent of punctate mechanical hyperalgesia in uninjured tissues surrounding the wound (*secondary mechanical hyperalgesia*) is a clinical expression of the changes occurring in the nervous system after injury, reflecting a state of central nervous system sensitization which manifests as an increase in the responsiveness of the sensory system. This mechanical hyperalgesia expressing central hyperexcitability is important for several reasons. First, hyperalgesia participates to the postoperative pain experience and might enhance pain for some patients. Second, severe and undertreated postoperative pain seems to contribute to the risk of developing persistent postsurgical pain.

Several analgesic drugs and techniques which are commonly used during the perioperative period are able to modulate peri-incisional mechanical hyperalgesia, either to enhance it (i.e. systemic opioids) or to decrease it (ketamine, intrathecal clonidine, intraoperative neuraxial analgesia). Interestingly, a reduction of the area of mechanical hyperalgesia surrounding the incision positively correlates with lesser risk for the patient to develop persistent pain after major abdominal surgery. Further studies are mandatory to assess the development of peri-incisional hyperalgesia in other procedures such as orthopedic and spinal surgeries. Clinical trials are also ongoing to evaluate the preventive antihyperalgesic effects of novel drugs like gabapentin, pregabalin and selective COX-2 inhibitors which are currently proposed as perioperative analgesic adjuvants.

Chapter X - Neonatal pain has become a much discussed topic. Premature births are more and more frequent and consequently many more babies need long periods of intensive care; but most manoeuvres performed in neonatal intensive care units are stressful or painful. This paper wants to promote the awareness that not only physical pain, but also the lack of a comfortable baby-centred environment can be the cause of suffering. This awareness rises from recent data about neonatal suffering and neonatal pain treatment.

A distinction should be made between pain and suffering: the former is due to a physical harm, while the latter (which may also be provoked by pain) results from harm done to a person's desires. This difference explains why the struggle against pain cannot be overcome without the full recognition of babies' personhood, i.e. being subjects capable of desires and fears: we cannot only administer analgesics, but we must also promote the integral wellbeing of premature babies. Pain and suffering are still poorly understood in neonatal age. The authors argue that this has multiple causes: a) bad definition of pain and difficulty in recognizing it; b) lack of concern about newborns' suffering; c) lack of legal consequences for provoking unnecessary pain; d) diffidence towards newborns' vitality which leads to diffidence of their personhood; e) lack of empathy toward the preverbal patient. An ethical approach towards neonatal pain should consider the right of the babies to analgesia and relief to be as mandatory as it is in adults. An ethical treatment of pain should start from recognizing newborns' personhood and their need to be soothed, comforted and respected during painful treatment. Recent studies show that this approach not only respects newborns' personality, but also increases the analgesic effect of the resources we employ against pain.

Chapter XI - The pain of labour is a central part of women's experience of childbirth. Many factors are considered influential in determining women's experience of and her satisfaction with childbirth. Women's expectations of the duration and level of pain suffered, quality of her care-giver support, and involvement in labour decision making are the most commonly reported factors[1].

Significantly, there have been more clinical trials of pharmacological pain relief during labour and childbirth than of any other intervention in the perinatal field[2] however to what degree this evidence is available or discussed with pregnant women before labour is unclear.

Chapter XII - Over the past 27 years, investigations have benefited our understanding of pain in the rapidly developing newborn. Researchers now understand that the infant's gestational age, gender, pain history and the quality of care provided by the infant's parents and healthcare professionals greatly influence the infant's pain response. Of the many factors investigated, maternal caregiving, long considered important to promoting infant development, is now beginning to emerge as an important study variable within the infant pain field. The purposes of this paper are to summarize findings of two maternal pain caregiving interventions (breastfeeding and maternal skin-to-skin contact) during infancy and to comment on issues related to their clinical implementation. The authors also discuss the benefits of enhanced inclusion of maternal caregiving as a direct study variable to further the comprehensive assessment and treatment of newborn (NB) pain. Currently, few newborn pain studies examine maternal caregiving effects during the NB period. There is some evidence that maternal behavior before and after a painful event results in less cry intensity and duration, easy recovery and self-regulation in full term infants. Most of those studies focused on older infants, they measured the infant's global rather than individual responses to intramuscular injection pain and only one examined pain recovery. Also evident, is the lack of investigation on maternal behavior on the behavioral and physiological response of the premature infant during the first month of life although studies have been conducted that include maternal skin-to-skin contact and breastfeeding to promote neonatal acute pain relieve during minor acute pain events. These particular forms of maternal caregiving have been recommended by international groups and associations to reduce infant pain reactivity and to facilitate recovery after pain event. However, no published data exists on the efficacy of both interventions with longer or repeated painful procedures. There is also a dearth of study on the effectiveness of combining maternal skin-to-skin with other pain treatments in the clinical setting. Moreover, there is a dearth of investigation that considers the perceptions of health professionals, the experiences and the mental health status of mothers for both interventions. While knowledge gaps exist in this still evolving field, clinicians must have access to existing research for judicious clinical application. Conceptual frameworks from knowledge transfer theory and collaborative interdisciplinary research may help facilitate the clinical use of these maternal non-pharmacological interventions for adequate neonatal pain relieve in many countries.

Chapter XIII – Background: The gap between scientific knowledge and clinical practice is a major challenge in neonatal pain management. The aim of this study was to describe the perceptions of physicians and nurses regarding the treatment of procedural pain in neonates two years after they had been exposed to new pain-management strategies, and how their perceptions changed over the period.

Materials and methods: The study population consisted of physicians and nurses in two neonatal intensive care units in southern Norway. A multifaceted approach to changing practice was evaluated. It comprised the establishment of multiprofessional groups, the active support of leaders and the senior neonatologists at both study-sites, facilitation, education, and the introduction of evidence-based guidelines and procedures for blood collection. Data were collected before (2003) and after (2005) the intervention, with a questionnaire. Ten commonly performed procedures were assessed. The response rates were 79% and 73%, respectively.

Results: Although the answers of both the nurses and physicians indicated a slight increase in the use of pharmacological agents, they also displayed a persisting significant difference between what clinicians believe to be the current and optimal treatment for procedural pain. Only the nurses' answers indicated a change in their views about procedure painfulness, the current use of comfort measures, and the optimal treatment of pain. These changes have not diminished the differences between the views of nurses and physicians concerning procedure painfulness and the treatment of procedural pain.

Conclusions: Despite the use of a multifaceted intervention to support evidence-based practice, pharmacological agents and comfort measures appear to be underutilized in the treatment of procedural pain in neonates. Pharmacological treatments for procedural pain might have improved, but the overall results point clearly to difficulties in applying evidence to practice.

Chapter XIV - Pain may afflict humans anytime, anywhere. There are usually considerable delays before relief, for example, time to find a doctor, expert, or pharmacist, or, time for the analgesic to take effect. To quickly overcome the pain is the goal sought by researchers for a very long time. The authors recently published a new analgesic method, acute mechanical pressure stimulation of the sciatic nerves, which resulted in relief of pain within a few minutes. The method is generally useful, and has been tested on pain from many diseases seen in emergency clinics as well as pain from various dental, renal, and tumor pathologies. The technique is simple, can be applied at home, immediately upon the onset of pain. No side effects have yet been observed in more than 600 subjects tested at 10 hospitals and universities. This chapter discusses more aspects of this new analgesic method.

In: Pain Management: New Research
Editors: P. S. Greco, F. M. Conti

Chapter I

The Myth of Panic Spontaneity: Consideration of Behavioral and Neurochemical Sensitization

Andrea L.O. Hebb[1], Gregory J. Anger[1], Fuschia Sirois[3], Paul D. Mendella[4] and Robert M. Zacharko[2]

[1]Dalhousie University, Department of Pharmacology, Halifax, Nova Scotia, Canada
[2]Carleton University, Institute of Neuroscience, Ottawa, Ontario, Canada
[3]University of Windsor, Ontario, Canada
[4]University of Ottawa, Ontario, Canada

Abstract

Panic disorder is characterized by a progression of panic symptom severity with repeated attacks. Repeated panic episodes evoke heightened anticipatory anxiety, phobic avoidance, and panic is typically associated with comorbid symptoms of depression. Due to the heterogeneity of the disorder, reliable neurochemical correlates attending panic have not been identified. However, variable neuropeptide interfacing with major and minor transmitter systems may modulate individual vulnerability to panic and account for variable panic profiles. The extensive colocalization of cholecystokinin (CCK) with other neurotransmitters, including dopamine (DA), enkephalin (ENK) and GABA, in specific central sites may influence various aspects of anxiety and panic. The behavioral correlates attending panic likely follow from variable neurochemical release and conditioning and sensitization. Clinicians maintain that panic attacks are spontaneous and fail to acknowledge the wealth of information implicating a role for stressful life events in panic. Conditioning and sensitization of both behavior (e.g., fear-motivated) and neurochemical events (e.g., DA and CCK) in response to uncontrollable stressors parallel the diverse heterogeneity of panic amongst clinical samples. Cholecystokinin-4, pentagastrin, lactate acid, and CO_2 induce panic attacks in both panic patients and healthy controls that are dependent on subjective history, expectancy measures and panic profiles. Panic disorder is associated with chronic illness, including Parkinson's disease and schizophrenia and familial sick-role modeling exacerbates the course of the illness.

The current review outlines the evidence supporting a conditioning/sensitization model for panic and accounts for the variable efficacies of pharmacological interventions.

Introduction

Panic disorder is characterized by the repeated occurrence of panic attacks. During a panic attack, fear, shortness of breath, dizziness, heart palpitations, chest pain, sweating, faintness, paresthesia, nausea and cognitive symptoms including depersonalization and fear of losing control are typically reported (Gardner, 1996; Shioiri et al., 1996; Weissman et al., 1995). Panic disorder is invariably associated with anticipatory anxiety (Cox et al., 1993; Kenardy et al., 1992; McNally, 1992; Zeitlin and McNally, 1993), anxiety sensitivity (McNally, 1992) and is characterized by phobic avoidance (Shioiri et al., 1996). Indeed, agoraphobic behavior routinely accompanies panic disorder and is more prevalent among females (Grant et al., 2006; Lepine and Lellouch, 1995; Wittchen and Essau, 1993). In any event, panic disorder with or without agoraphobia ordinarily persists for protracted periods and is accompanied by social and occupational impairments (Massion et al., 1993; Sherbourne et al., 1996; Skodol et al., 1995; Wittchen and Essau, 1993), health risks (Chignon, et al., 1993; Paradis et al., 1993; Raj and Sheehan, 1990; Wittchen and Essau, 1993; Yeragani et al., 1990) and comorbid psychiatric disturbances including changes in cognitive function (Clark et al., 1996; Ludewig et al., 2005), major depression (Andreoli et al., 1992; Breier et al., 1984; Grunhaus et al., 1988; Keller et al., 1993; Laberge et al., 1992; Leckman et al., 1983; Maier et al., 1995; Raskin et al., 1982; Reich et al., 1993; Roy-Byrne et al., 1992; Rush et al., 2005; Weissman et al., 1993), schizophrenia (Argyle, 1990; Goodwin et al., 2002; Heun and Maier, 1995) and substance abuse (Kushner et al., 1996; Maier et al., 1993; O'Brien et al., 2005; Pallanti and Mazzi, 1992; Stewart, 1992).

Current neurochemical descriptors of panic are suggestive rather than persuasive and animal models of panic are provisional (Blanchard et al., 2003; Charney 2003). Inferences concerning central correlates of panic have been derived from behavioral and neurochemical alterations attending systemic cholecystokinin (CCK) administration among nonhuman subjects in paradigms that simulate anxiety (Frankland et al., 1996; Harro and Vasar, 1991; Rex et al., 1994; Rodgers and Johnson, 1995). The panic properties of systemic CCK (Abelson et al., 1994; Bradwejn et al., 1990; de Leeuw et al., 1996; Koszycki et al., 1996; van Megen et al., 1996) prompt suggestion that brain stem and spinal respiratory and cardiopulmonary CCK sites contribute to panic (Bystritsky and Shapiro, 1992; Gardner, 1996; Lara et al., 2003; Ley, 1996). Panic attacks have been posited to occur in the absence of demonstrable precipitants (e.g., Kasdorf et al., 1988), despite evidence that stressful life events precede panic (Faravelli, 1985; Jordan et al., 1991; Kenardy et al., 1992; La Via et al., 1996; Ley, 1996; McNally and Lukach, 1992; Nutt and Glue, 1991; Raskin et al., 1982; Rosenbaum, 1990; Roy-Byrne et al., 1986; Scocco et al., 2006; Servant et al., 1993; Southwick et al., 1995). This observation is appealing, although the distribution, severity and controllability of stressful life events have received poor clinical documentation. In any event, the proposal that panic or the symptoms of panic are influenced by a stressor-CCK interface is intriguing. In fact, evidence implicating CCK and panic is convincing and a

DA/CCK link to the disorder has been derived from neurochemical and behavioral evidence with nonhuman experimentation (Berg and Davis, 1984; Claustre et al., 1986; Coco et al., 1992; D'Aquila et al., 1994; Fadda et al., 1978; Lane, 1992; McBlane and Handley, 1994). Embedded in this matrix are issues pertaining to validity and generalizability of nonhuman experimentation and operational definition of psychological dysfunction.

Dopamine-CCK colocalization has been detected in DA neurons of the VTA, substantia nigra, prefrontal cortex, medial aspects of the nucleus accumbens and the central amygdaloid nucleus (Bunney, 1987; Hokfelt et al., 1980; Hokfelt et al., 1994; Lundberg and Hokfelt, 1983). Identification of same vesicle DA/CCK (Studler et al., 1984) is consistent with speculation that DA and CCK co-release contributes to psychological disturbance (Hokfelt et al., 1980). Cholecystokinin-derived inhibition (Fuxe et al., 1981) and facilitation (Crawley et al., 1985; Crawley et al., 1995; Hommer and Skirboll, 1981; Vaccarino and Rankin, 1989) of DA release is associated with mesocorticolimbic and nigrostriatal CCK_1 (Phillips et al., 1993) and CCK_2 receptors, respectively (Marshall et al., 1991) (Jackson and Westlind-Danielson, 1994). At the very least, the variable influence of CCK on central DA should provide species-specific behavioral correlates of anxiety.

It will be recalled that stressful life events may precede panicin-vulnerable individuals (Faravelli, 1985; Jordan et al., 1991; Kenardy et al., 1992; La Via et al., 1996; Ley, 1996; McNally and Lukach, 1992; Nutt and Glue, 1991; Raskin et al., 1982; Rosenbaum, 1990; Roy-Byrne et al., 1986; Scocco et al., 2006; Servant et al. 1993; Southwick et al., 1995). Accordingly, the responsivity of DA and CCK to aversive life events may influence the severity of panic symptoms. Mild stressors promote mesocorticolimbic DA (Cabib et al., 1988; Deutch et al., 1985; Imperato et al., 1989; Keefe et al., 1990; Saavedra, 1982; Watanabe, 1984) and CCK release (Harro et al., 1996; Siegel et al., 1987; Pavlasevic et al., 1993) in rats, while variations of stressor intensity favor mesocorticolimbic diazepam-binding inhibitor (Ferrarese et al., 1991), corticotropin-releasing factor (Anderson et al., 1993; Chappell et al., 1986; Nemeroff, 1992) or β-carbolinerelease (e.g., β-CCE and β-CCM) (Alho et al., 1985; Claustre et al., 1986; Guidotti et al., 1983; Novas et al., 1988; Roth et al., 1988) in sites responsive to stressor associated alterations of DA and CCK. Taken together, diverse anxiogenic agents are released by stressors and the proposal that panic occurs in response to innocuous events is neither parsimonious nor appealing (Wolpe and Rowan, 1988). The present review suggests that conditioning and sensitization of anxiety may promote gradients of psychological dysfunction that eventuate in panic. Such an analysis suggests that life events are appraised soon after panic and rumination defines situational variables and provides a framework concerning the risk value of environmental events.

Animal models of conditioning/sensitization focus on long-term neurochemical alterations attending psychostimulant administration and the influence of transmitter variations on locomotor activity and stereotypy (Kalivas et al., 1993; Post et al., 1992). For example, re-exposure of animals to a mild stressor or neutral psychostimulant challenge following a chronic, low dose psychostimulant schedule increases activity and extracellular DA availability (Antelman et al., 1980; Cassens et al., 1980; Pierce and Kalivas, 1995). In addition, acute, mild footshock elicits protracted variations of locomotor activity as well as DA and CCK concentrations reminiscent of acute psychostimulant challenge (Antelman et al., 1980). Among animals exposed to graded levels of footshock (Siegel et al., 1987), restraint, systemic saline administration (Rosen et al., 1992), predator-associated olfactory cues (Pavlasevic et al., 1993) or decapitation of conspecifics (Harro et al., 1996), enhanced CCK release is detectable from the prefrontal cortex, amygdala, hippocampus, nucleus accumbens and mesencephalon. However, isolation (Brodin et al., 1994), elevated plus maze exposure (Pratt and Brett, 1995) or 2 min of footshock (1 mA, 1 pulse/5sec, 600-ms pulse duration, Siegel et al., 1987) fail to alter hippocampal, amygdaloid or hypothalamic CCK concentrations, respectively. Evidently, CCK availability in specific central sites is influenced by stressor severity as well as the nature of the stressor employed. Chronic, low dose psychostimulant challenge alters CCK concentration and mRNA expression in the prefrontal cortex, hippocampus (Fukamauchi, 1996), VTA and the medial, caudal aspects of the nucleus accumbens (Hurd et al., 1992) in rats, which can be detected for several weeks following the last injection. Psychostimulant-associated sensitization of activity and stereotypy also favors behavioral cross-sensitization with footshock (Antelman et al., 1980; Leyton and Stewart, 1990; Robinson et al., 1985; 1988). Consistent with such demonstration, the stress of social isolation and footshock (500 μA) enhances acoustic startle to acute amphetamine (1.0 mg/kg and 3.0mg/kg) in mice (Kokkinidis and MacNeill, 1982). Taken together, these data are suggestive of shared sensitized neurochemical substrates in nonhuman (Post et al., 1992; Robinson, 1988) and human subjects (Strakowski et al., 1996) that persist for periods exceeding 12 months (Robinson et al., 1991).

Although locomotor activity and stereotypy are not indices of anxiety, the neural mechanisms underlying behavioral sensitization affected by stressors and psychostimulants are relevant to panic induction. In this respect, emergence and aggravation of panic symptoms may be occasioned by the conditioned pairing of anxiogenic agents, including CCK, and stressful life experience(s). Site-specific central CCK release may be influenced by the nature and severity of the stressor (Lachuer et al., 1991; Sudo and Miki, 1993) and the sensitivity of the brain sites examined (Siegel et al., 1987). Such variables may define vulnerability to panicogenic environmental events. Exacerbation of panic symptoms might be occasioned by recurrent stressors, panic experience and/or cues associated with such stimuli. In this regard, panic profiles may parallel nonhuman instances of sensitization while psychological disorders, including depression may outline the variable contributions of experiential and organismic factors (Jones et al., 1992), including gender susceptibility (Beatty and Holzer, 1978; Blanchard et al., 1995; Camp and Robinson, 1988; Grilo et al., 1996; Heinsbroek et al., 1990; Robinson et al., 1980; Robinson et al., 1982; Wittchen and Essau, 1993) as well as environmental context and conditioning (Grillon et al., 1994; Kuribara, 1996; Post et al., 1980; Schnur et al., 1994; Stewart and Vezina, 1988; Vezina et al., 1989) to the expression of pathological states. Parametric analyses reveal variability in the induction, persistence and magnitude of effects relative to the behavior examined and the brain sites involved.

Behavioral sensitization induced by stressors appears to be influenced by mesolimbic (Di Chiara, 1993; Ding and Mocchetti, 1992; Fukamauchi, 1996; Higgins et al., 1994; Hurd et al., 1992; Kalivas et al., 1992; Kihara et al., 1993; Phillips et al., 1993; Suzuki et al., 1993), mesocortical (Clarke et al., 1988; Eichler and Antelman, 1979; Kalivas et al., 1993; Kopchia et al., 1992; Robinson and Berridge, 1993) and nigrostriatal (Bunney and Aghajanian, 1976; Ziegler et al., 1991) DA activity. Moreover, CCK appears to modulate mesolimbic and nigrostriatal DA-dependent locomotion and stereotypy, respectively (Crawley et al., 1995). Systemic administration of a CCK_1 receptor antagonist decreases amphetamine-induced locomotion in rats that have been chronically treated with amphetamine (Wunderlich et al., 2000). Furthermore, injection of PD-140548, a selective CCK_1 receptor antagonist, directily in the nucleus accumbens has been shown to attenuate amphetamine-induced locomotion only in animals that had been exposed to chronic amphetamine treatment or chronic restraint stress (Wunderlich et al., 2004). In view of the observation that stressors and acute and chronic psychostimulant administration influence DA (Antelman et al., 1980; Cassens et al., 1980 Pierce and Kalivas, 1995) and CCK turnover (Fukamauchi, 1996; Hurd et al., 1992; Pavlasevic et al., 1993; Pratt and Brett, 1995; Siegel et al., 1987) and both DA (Pitchot et al., 1992; Roy-Byrne et al., 1986) and CCK (Brambilla et al., 1993; Lydiard et al., 1992) alterations appear in panic patients, it is suggested that neurotransmitter sensitization may contribute to panic symptoms.

A sensitization/conditioning account of panic is appealing because (a) protracted anxiety has been associated with central DA variations in nonhuman (Wedzony et al., 1996; Yoshioka et al., 1996) and human subjects (Kellner et al., 1975; Menza et al., 1993; Rasmussen, 1994; Stein et al., 1990), (b) CCK/DA colocalization is prevalent in mesocorticolimbic sites associated with arousal, reward, learning/conditioning (Crawley and Corwin, 1994), (c) anxiety among nonhuman subjects is readily induced by CCK administration in animal models of anxiety including the elevated plus maze (Harro et al., 1993) and (d) stressor-associated environmental cues influence behavioral (Davis, 1989; Inoue et al., 1994; Servatius et al., 1995) and neurochemical change (Coco et al., 1992; Ida et al., 1988) among nonhuman subjects reminiscent of the anticipatory anxiety associated with panic disorder. The current review attempts to determine whether there is sufficient evidence to suggest that panic symptoms follow from conditioning of central DA/CCK activity induced by anxiety provoking conditions. A synthesis of such information is not meant to characterize the human disorder but rather to evaluate a limited subset of symptoms, including but not limited to, anticipatory anxiety.

Central Dopamine Turnover: Prelude to Anxiety and Emergence of Panic Disorder

Investigations of the pathophysiology of panic have focused on the serotonergic (5-HT), noradrenergic (NE), and the GABA-benzodiazepine systems (see Bremner et al., 1996; Charney et al., 1983; Charney and Heninger, 1986; Charney et al., 1989; Guthrie et al., 1993; Hoehn-Saric, 1982; Nutt, 1989; Nutt, 1990; Uhde et al., 1989 for review) among other neurotransmitters. Nevertheless, several lines of evidence suggest that DA may be involved in anxiety (Pitchot et al., 1990; 1991) and panic (Pitchot et al., 1992; Roy-Byrne et al., 1986). In the former instance, the paucity of information for DA in clinical anxiety is paralleled by a comparable lack of evidence for DA in anxiety among nonhuman subjects. Nevertheless, mild stressors, that provoke mesocorticolimbic DA turnover, have demonstrable anxiogenic effects in the elevated plus maze (Cole et al., 1995; D'Aquila et al., 1994; McBlane and Handley, 1994) and fear potentiated startle (Servatius et al., 1995) in rats. Such paradigm-associated anxiety, which is responsive to acute benzodiazepine administration, increased DA concentrations in the frontal and pyriform cortices, nucleus accumbens, septum, medial hypothalamus and amygdala (Berg and Davis, 1984; Claustre et al., 1986; Coco et al., 1992; Fadda et al., 1978; Lane, 1992). In the latter instance, plasma and cerebrospinal homovanillic acid (HVA) concentrations, a DA metabolite, fail to discriminate panic and control subjects (Eriksson et al., 1991; Johnson et al., 1994; Roy-Byrne et al., 1986). The lack of a neurochemical panic index is not without precedent since NE alterations, for example, have likewise failed to discriminate panic and non-panic subjects (see Charney et al., 1990 for review; Lepola et al., 1989). Some laboratories have identified DA perturbations among panic patients with increased anxiety on the Spielberger State Anxiety scale, augmented panic frequency in the 12 months preceding clinical interview and reduced symptom free periods relative to other panic patients (Roy-Byrne et al., 1986; Pitchot et al., 1992). Unfortunately, evidence for central DA and laboratory induced panic remains obscure. Laboratories that have assessed peripheral DA metabolites among normal subjects during laboratory exercises have failed to produce anxiety comparable to panic (Zemishlany and Davidson, 1996). Indeed, there is no *a priori* reason to suspect that innocuous laboratory challenges will induce panic in patients with the disorder (Leyton et al., 1996). Still, contrived laboratory situations provoke panic in some panic patients (see Grillon et al., 1994 for discussion) suggesting that some individuals are more vulnerable than others to the impact of specific environmental encounters. It would be of considerable advantage to secure measures of central DA prior to, during and following panic induction in a laboratory situation.

Panic is well documented among Parkinsonian patients and individuals with schizophrenia. Despite the neurodegenerative nature of Parkinson's disease and the veiling of central neurochemisty by therapeutic interventions, panic in Parkinson's disease and schizophrenia provides subtle evidence for the involvement of DA in the phenomenology of panic-like states. It is interesting that divergent alterations in DA associated with Parkinson's disease and schizophrenia are associated with the elicitation of panic-like symptoms. While mesocorticolimbic contribution to behavioral sensitization following stressor encounter (Hamamura and Fibiger, 1993; Eichler and Antelman, 1979; Kalivas et al., 1988; Kalivas and Stewart, 1991) has received extensive documentation, nigrostriatal DA/CCK alterations may also alter sensitivity to stressors.

Nigrostriatal Dopamine and Cholecystokinin: Anxiety and Panic-Like Behavior in Parkinson's Disease

Parkinson's disease is characterized by insidious nigrostriatal DA and CCK depletion (Agid and Javoy-Agid, 1985; Bruno et al., 1985; Fernandez et al., 1992; Kontur et al., 1994; White et al., 1992; Piolti et al., 1992). In addition to tremor, inertia, rigidity, bradykinesia, akinesia, flexed posture and gait disturbance, Parkinsonian patients experience mild depression and irritability as well as memory and attentional perturbations (Mahurin et al., 1993; Pirozzolo et al., 1988; Rafal et al., 1984; Taylor et al., 1986; Vogel, 1982; White et al.,

1992). L-dopa ordinarily ameliorates Parkinsonian associated motoric impediments but is ineffective in alleviating affective and cognitive symptoms of the disorder (White et al., 1992). Advanced Parkinsonian stages reduce the efficacy of l-dopa in alleviating motoric disturbance and not surprisingly symptom free intervals (Riley and Lang, 1993). Parkinsonian patients experiencing daily on/off episodes and report increased instances of anxiety and depression during l-dopa off stages (Lezak, 1983; Menza et al., 1993; Siemers et al., 1993; White et al., 1992), prompting increased l-dopa therapy (Vazquez et al., 1993). Alleviation of mood disturbance and anxiety at this juncture may be attributable to the l-dopa dose employed (Maricle et al., 1995) or perhaps patient appraisal of restored motor function (Menza et al., 1990). It should be considered that approximately 40% of l-dopa treated Parkinsonian patients (>4 years, Factor et al., 1995; Kulkarni et al., 1992; Oyebode et al., 1986) exhibit a DA mesocorticolimbic-associated psychosis (Carey et al., 1995; Rich et al., 1995). Protracted l-dopa treatment, therapeutic dose increases and episodic instances of pharmacological insensitivity to peripheral DA loading have been linked to the emergence of panic-like symptoms (2.6 ± 1.4 panic attacks per day) among Parkinsonian patients (Menza et al., 1993; Vazquez et al., 1993). Nevertheless, panic frequency comparison between Parkinsonian and panic patients is obscured in the latter instance by investigations that fail to provide definitive panic statistics. Despite such difficulties, Parkinsonian panic (a) represents a relatively severe version of the disorder, (b) is distributed equally among male (45%) and female subjects (55%) (Vazquez et al., 1993) and (c) only emerges during latter stages of the disease (60-70 years of age). In contrast, panic patients are most likely to experience a panic episode when they are middle-aged, rarely following 65, and the disorder is more prevalent among females (Grant et al., 2006). Nigrostriatal degeneration may contribute to the paresthesias, burning sensations and discomfort emanating from the feet, chest or face immediately prior to panic (Vazquez et al., 1993). Although a Parkinsonian focus on specific symptoms preceding panic has not been verified, such vigilance would parallel the documented physiological monitoring characteristic of panic subjects (Schmidt et al., 1997). In this respect, distraction of Parkinsonian patients from antecedent neuromuscular perturbations attenuates panic (Vazquez et al., 1993).

It is unlikely that estrogen availability can account for panic among Parkinsonian patients. While panic frequency and severity could be reduced in female relative to male Parkinsonian patients owing to menopause onset, such predictions have not been verified. In fact, estrogen replacement has been associated with the alleviation (Chung et al., 1995) and the exacerbation (Price and Heil, 1988) of panic symptoms in panic patients. Panic episodes characterized by pre-panic palpitation, chest discomfort, tightness of jaw, teeth grinding and muscle ache were attenuated by estrogen. In contrast, panic episodes lacking such a prominent motor profile are exacerbated by estrogen. In Parkinsonian patients, l-dopa fluctuations and panic are often coupled to mood alterations such as depression. Increased estrogen levels in female rats have been associated with an increase in the rewarding value of brain stimulation from the medial forebrain bundle (Bless et al., 1997). Taken together, the demonstration that (a) estrogen alleviates l-dopa nigrostriatal perturbations, (b) l-dopa fluctuations are associated with cognitive alterations including depression and psychosis (e.g., mesocorticolimbic DA alterations) and (c) the demonstration that l-dopa motoric fluctuations and depression are associated with the development of panic among

Parkinsonian patients preclude an estrogen-based argument. In effect, an estrogen hypothesis defining emergence, maintenance and exacerbation of panic in Parkinson's disease cannot readily account for the available data. In addition, the nature of the somatic experience per se does not appear to be relevant to the induction of panic. Rather, it seems that the intensity of the cognitive experience, regardless of the symptom cluster anticipated, may be sufficient to elicit panic. Such an interpretation suggests that panic emerges following rumination over perceptually defined salient cues in diverse pathological states. In effect, panic among cardiac patients (Beitman et al., 1993), depressed subjects (Andreoli et al., 1992; Breier et al., 1984; Grunhaus et al., 1988; Keller et al., 1993; Laberge et al., 1992; Leckman et al., 1983; Maier et al., 1995; Raskin et al., 1982; Reich et al., 1993; Roy-Byrne et al., 1992; Weissman et al., 1993) or individuals with myasthenia gravis (Paradis et al., 1993) is not surprising. Clearly, conspicuous neurochemical variations attending Parkinson's disease contribute to the emergence of somatic complaints and favor vigilance during treatment resistant intervals. In effect, fluctuations in Parkinsonian symptoms, coupled with pervasive, anticipatory stressors, may promote panic among treatment resistant Parkinsonian patients.

At first glance, it is not clear that panic among Parkinsonian patients contributes to the elucidation of the neural mechanisms associated with panic-like states and/or the putative influence of sensitization. These data merely suggest that panic-like symptoms in Parkinsonian patients follow from some neurochemical cascade elicited by DA denervation. Indeed, the appearance of panic-like symptoms in Parkinsonian patients coincides with the time course of mesolimbic DA denervation (e.g., VTA and prefrontal cortex) (Leenders et al., 1986; Marie et al., 1995; Uhl et al., 1985). In addition to alterations in mesolimbic DA activity, post-mortem analyses of Parkinsonian brain tissue have also provided evidence for altered nigrostriatal CCK activity (Agid and Javoy-Agid, 1985; Bruno et al., 1985; Fernandez et al., 1992; Kontur et al., 1994; Studler et al., 1982). Such changes in nigrostriatal CCK concentrations parallel indices of l-dopa treatment resistance (e.g., l-dopa resistant patients and animal model of Parkinson's disease, Boyce et al., 1990a; 1990b; Brog and Beinfeld, 1992; Carey, 1991; Taylor et al., 1992) and symptom severity (Agid and Javoy-Agid, 1985; Bruno et al., 1985; Fernandez et al., 1992; Kontur et al., 1994). As such, it is conceivable that nigrostriatal DA/CCK and mesolimbic DA alterations contribute to the eventual expression of panic among Parkinsonian patients owing to the gradual denervation of mesocorticolimbic sites from the substantia nigra. In effect, panic associated with nigral denervation and prompted by l-dopa induced psychosis, suggests that a neurochemical depletion threshold may be attained during the latter stages of Parkinson's disease. Available evidence to date has certainly not established a causal role for mesocorticolimbic CCK and panic among Parkinsonian patients. At best, plasma CCK levels and post-mortem CCK-binding provide provisional indices of augmented CCK turnover in specific subject populations experiencing varying levels of anticipatory anxiety (Harro et al., 1992; Phillipp et al., 1992). Nevertheless, anticipatory anxiety among Parkinsonian patients may occur in response to the stressor-like experiences occasioned by the off stages of l-dopa therapy (c.f. stressor induced CCK alterations in nonhuman subjects, Pavlasevic et al., 1993; Pratt and Brett, 1995; Siegel et al., 1987). Indeed, variations of mesocorticolimbic CCK availability between DA-denervated Parkinsonian patients experiencing panic and age, sex and disease matched subjects would be intuitively appealing. While such provisional arguments must be held in abeyance, panic-like symptoms among Parkinsonian patients coincide with (a) changes in nigrostriatal CCK availability during the late stages of the disease and (b) the emergence of presumably enhanced stressor periods among Parkinsonian patients (c.f. DA/CCK interface following stressor imposition in nonhuman subjects, Brodin et al., 1994; Pavlasevic et al., 1993; Rosen et al., 1992; Siegel et al., 1987). However, the appearance of panic among Parkinsonian patients experiencing gradual exacerbation of cognitive function (e.g., impairments in memory and attention and the development of psychoses, White et al., 1992) and motoric debilitation (e.g., during l-dopa off periods and dyskinesias) lends support to a sensitization/conditioning hypothesis in the acquisition and expression of the disorder.

Dopamine and Cholecystokinin in the Mesocorticolimbic System: Anxiety and Panic-like Behavior in Schizophrenia

Paranoid forms of schizophrenia have been associated with elevated anxiety as revealed by the Brief Psychiatric and Hamilton Anxiety Rating Scales (Azorin, 1995; Craig et al., 1985; Donlon et al., 1976; Silverstein et al., 1997; Lysaker et al., 1995; Penn et al., 1994; Shaw et al., 1997). These psychiatric patients routinely report experiencing a high incidence of daily life stressors (e.g., loss of social support, divorce, death of a loved one, impending job and/or residential changes and admission to a psychiatric facility) that exacerbate schizophrenic episodes (Butler et al., 1996; Day, 1981; Docherty, 1996; Dohrenwend and Egri, 1981; Fowles, 1992; Harrow et al., 1994; Hatfield, 1989; Lukoff et al., 1984; Penn et al., 1994; Spring, 1981; Swartz and Myers, 1977). Moreover, repeated exposure to such life stressors increase anticipatory anxiety as revealed by exaggerated startle responsivity among individuals with schizophrenia (Bolino et al., 1994; Patterson et al., 1986). While atypical, severely stressful life events, including active military duty, for example, may precipitate psychotic episodes in vulnerable individuals (Butler et al., 1996), repeated experience with milder, stressful life events (e.g., loss of social support) over a few months has also led to schizophrenic symptom exacerbation, including psychosis (Dohrenwend and Egri, 1981). In effect, elicitation and/or exacerbation of the symptoms of schizophrenia might be occasioned by a broad spectrum of life stressors, varying in severity and chronicity. Interestingly, panic and agoraphobia (e.g., 2.4 ± 1.4 attacks per week) have been reported among individuals with a history of paranoid schizophrenia (e.g., >4 years) by several different laboratories (Argyle et al., 1990; Kahn et al., 1987; Kahn et al., 1988; Kellner et al., 1975; Sandberg and Siris, 1987). The panic symptoms experienced by individuals with schizophrenia appear to represent a moderately severe panic course reminiscent of that experienced by panic patients (Aronson and Logue, 1988). Characteristically, individuals with schizophrenia who experience panic-like symptoms tend to be socially introverted, consistent with pervasive paranoia and/or embarassment associated with psychotic episodes (Argyle et al., 1990; Sandberg and Siris, 1987). The frequency of panic-like symptoms among individuals with schizophrenia coincides with the psychotic episodes that are associated with anxious cognition, including rumination over agoraphobic fears and increased somatic perturbations (Argyle et al., 1990; Lewine et al., 1996; Sandberg and Siris, 1987; Simon et al., 1980).

Indeed, preoccupation with and attention to somatic and cognitive perturbations punctuated with varying degrees of psychosis may contribute to panic symptoms in individuals with schizophrenia. While somatic monitoring in schizophrenia would parallel the physiological vigilance characteristic of panic (Schmidt et al., 1997), cognitive monitoring may be specific to schizophrenia. Individuals with schizophrenia are undoubtedly cognizant of the progression of schizophrenic symptomatology (see Heila et al., 1997 for discussion of suicide prevalence among individuals with schizophrenia). However, schizophrenic illness precludes cognitive intervention strategies with demonstrated efficacy on panic symptomatology in Parkinson's patients (Vazquez et al., 1993) and panic patients (Clum et al., 1993). Nevertheless, panic symptom attenuation in schizophrenia coincides with decreased psychotic episodes (e.g., alprazolam, 2.5 - 5mg/day, Kahn et al., 1988; Sandberg and Siris, 1987) or reduced agoraphobic associated behavior (e.g., imipramine, 50mg/day, Argyle, 1990). At this juncture, it is not readily apparent whether the neural mechanisms underlying schizophrenia are likewise conducive to the expression of panic. For example, psychosis has been demonstrated in panic patients. The appearance of psychosis among panic patients is related to the duration of panic (>10 years), severity (>3 panic attacks/day) of panic symptomatology and the presence of agorophobia (Ciccone and Bellettirie, 1989; Heun and Maier, 1995; Neenan et al., 1986). Moreover, the relative risk for schizophrenia among panic patients appears to be conspicuously increased relative to the general population (Heun and Maier, 1995). Taken together, central neurochemical alterations accompanying psychopathology and/or the gradual emergence of conditioned behavior (e.g., agoraphobia) may influence the course of panic-like symptoms.

Hypersensitivity of mesocorticolimbic DA activity, as measured by DA binding (Mackay et al., 1982; Comings et al., 1991), DA mRNA postmortem (Schmauss et al., 1993), positron emission tomography (PET) (Kapur et al., 1996) and ^{123}I-IBZM SPECT (Busatto et al., 1995; Minabe et al., 1990) among individuals with schizophrenia, appears to coincide closely with the expression of positive schizophrenic symptoms such as delusions and hallucinations (Bench et al., 1990; Cross et al., 1983). Notably, positive symptoms of schizophrenia are associated with social and agoraphobic fear (Penn et al., 1994). It should be underscored that negative symptoms of schizophrenia such as poverty of speech, flatened affect and psychomotor retardation are not associated with hypersensitivity of mesocorticolimbic DA activity (see Maas et al., 1993a for review) or panic. It should be considered that mesocorticolimbic hypersensitivity might follow from the chronic neuroleptic regimens employed to attenuate delusions and hallucinations (see Maas et 1993b). Typically, delusions, hallucinations and phobic avoidance assessed by the Minnesota Multiphasic Personality Inventory (MMPI), Clinical General Impression (CGI) and the Brief Psychiatric Rating Scale (BPRS) (Craig et al., 1985; Maas et al., 1993; Silverstein et al., 1997) are exacerbated over the course of the illness. The gradual exacerbation of schizophrenic symptoms has prompted suggestion that conditioning and/or sensitization of mesocorticolimbic DA (see Cotton and Usher, 1996; Kiyatin, 1995; Simon et al., 1980; White, 1996; and Williams and Goldman-Rakic, 1995, for review of mesocorticolimbic DA and cognition; c.f. amphetamine psychosis, Angrist and Gershon, 1970; Ellison, 1994; Flaum and Schultz, 1996; Leduc and Mittleman, 1995) underlie(s) expression of at least some of the behaviors associated with schizophrenia (Mackay et al., 1982; Pitchot et al., 1990-91; Post et al., 1988; Schatzberg et al., 1995). In addition to alterations of central DA activity, there are some data that outline a putative contribution of central CCK to the etiology and maintenance of schizophrenia (Beinfeld and Garver, 1991; Lotstra et al., 1985; Nair et al., 1985; Wang et al., 1984). Postmortem determinations have revealed increased CCK concentrations in the striatum and mesencephalon (Bourin et al., 1996; Schalling et al., 1990) and reduced CCK availability in the amygdala and hippocampus (Farmery et al., 1985; Ferrier et al., 1983; 1985) as well as concomitant reductions of CCK mRNA in the temporal and frontal cortices in neuroleptic treated individuals with paranoid schizophrenia relative to controls matched for age (65.8 ± 6.8 years), morbidity (e.g., heart disease and cancer) and postmortem delay (16.6 ± 4.2 hours) (Virgo et al., 1995). Available studies to date have clearly not established a relationship between central CCK and panic in individuals with schizophrenia and investigations documenting central CCK variations among individuals with paranoid schizophrenia typically fail to document any symptoms reminiscent of panic. It is interesting, however, that postmortem CCK determinations in brain tissue have verified patterns of CCK activity within specific brain sites associated with positive and negative symptoms of schizophrenia. On the one hand, positive symptoms of schizophrenia, precipitated by increased DA activity (Davis et al., 1985; Davis et al., 1991; Maas et al., 1993), are associated with a greater reduction in frontal cortex CCK mRNA compared to the temporal cortex. On the other hand, negative symptoms of schizophrenia are associated with reduced CCK mRNA in the temporal cortex, amygdala and hippocampus (Virgo et al., 1995). It will be recalled that panic attacks fluctuate with psychosis severity and it would be of interest to determine mesocortical CCK activity (e.g., PET scan) among individuals with schizophrenia during a panic episode. Curiously, neuroleptic strategies for schizophrenia (e.g., haloperidol and clomipramine) increase striatal and mesolimbic CCK concentrations (Brodin et al., 1994; Frey, 1983) and increase CCK binding (e.g., decreasing CCK tissue levels) in several cortical areas in nonhuman subjects that persist for several weeks (Chang et al., 1983; Frey et al., 1983; Suzucki et al., 1993). Panic-like symptoms and exacerbation of schizophrenia following neuroleptic withdrawal (Argyle, 1990; Bachmann and Modestin, 1987; Yergani et al., 1989) has been associated with increased CCK activity and concomitant release of the anxiogenic substances, corticotropin-releasing factor (Forman et al., 1994) and diazepam-binding inhibitor (Payeur et al., 1992; van Kammen et al., 1991).

While the panic properties of CCK-4, a CCK_2 agonist, have been empirically documented among panic patients and healthy volunteers (Bradwejn et al., 1990; Bourin et al., 1993), demonstration of the panic inducing properties of CCK-4 in individuals with schizophrenia is unavailable (c.f. CCK-8S administration in schizophrenia, Albus, 1988; Chase et al., 1985; Hommer et al., 1985; Lostra et al., 1985; Moroji et al., 1985; Nair et al., 1985; Tamminga et al., 1986; van Ree et al., 1984; Verhoeven et al., 1986). Recall that in individuals with schizophrenia, social and agoraphobic fear have been reported to precede panic attacks (Argyle et al., 1990). Interestingly, in rats, social isolation has been associated with an upregulation of CCK_2 receptors in the frontal cortex (Vasar et al., 1993). It is conceivable that some personality variables associated with schizophrenia (e.g., social introversion or social alienation) provide indices of panic susceptibility following CCK-4 challenge. For example, the intensity of somatic, affective and cognitive responsivity to CCK-4 (e.g., Panic Symptom Scale) in panic patients has been related to anxiety sensitivity (e.g., Anxiety Sensitivity Index) and self-alienation scores derived from the MMPI Social Inversion Subscales (Koszycki et al., 1996). It would be of interest to determine the effects of CCK_2 antagonists, which attenuate the panicogenic effects of CCK-4 in panic patients (Bradwejn et al., 1995), on agoraphobic fear and panic symptoms in individuals with schizophrenia (c.f. neuroleptic properties of CCK_2 antagonists in nonhuman preparations, Rasmussen et al., 1991). If CCK_2 antagonists were efficacious in the treatment of panic symptoms among individuals with schizophrenia (e.g., psychosis, agoraphobia and/or social avoidance), it is conceivable that alterations in mesocorticolimbic CCK_2 receptor activity sustain expression of both schizophrenic and panic symptoms. Moreover, it should be considered that current therapeutic interventions (e.g., haloperidol), which promote increases in CCK activity in the frontal cortex of nonhuman subjects, might contribute to panic-like responses among individuals with schizophrenia. Taken together, alienation, introversion, panic and psychotic exacerbation may be associated with variants of enhanced CCK sensitivity and/or overactivity of central DA and contribute to the expression of panic symptoms in individuals with schizophrenia.

Panic-like symptoms among individuals with schizophrenia are reminiscent of those reported by Parkinsonian patients and may be occasioned by (a) the prevalence or perceived prevalence of stressful life events, (b) alterations of central DA/CCK availability associated with chronic illness and/or (c) the chronicity of therapeutic interventions. Interestingly, Parkinsonian panic coincides with reduced l-dopa efficacy and l-dopa induced psychosis. Furthermore, autoradiographic data suggest comparable mesocorticolimbic DA receptor variations (e.g., frontal cortex and nucleus accumbens) in paranoid schizophrenia and Parkinsonian patients experiencing l-dopa psychosis (Bogerts et al., 1983; Holcomb et al., 1996; Klemm et al., 1996; Knable et al., 1996; Pedro et al., 1994; Seeman et al., 1987; Uhl et al., 1985). The saliency of mesocorticolimbic DA/CCK alterations to the promotion of panic in individuals with schizophrenia and Parkinson's disease is obvious. Taken together, the repeated encounters with stressful life events may facilitate panic in Parkinsonian patients, individuals with schizophrenia and panic patients (see Figure 1). The clinical vantage typically asserts that stressful life events do not participate in the precipitation or maintenance of panic. However, panic often emerges in clinical populations with demonstrated vulnerability to stressful life events (e.g., depression, schizophrenia, Parkinson's disease and substance abuse). In order to determine whether stressful life events contribute to the provocation of panic symptomatology in individuals with schizophrenia, Parkinson's disease and panic disorder, the cumulative and proactive influence of stressors must be determined (e.g., sensitization).

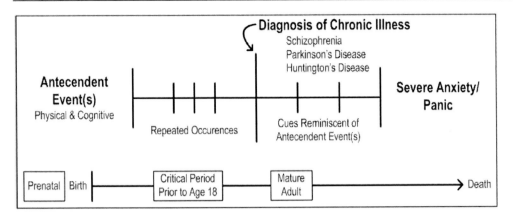

Figure 1. Schematic diagram outlining the progression of events that lead to panic disorder. Initial antecedent events or mild stressful events elicit some physical or cognitive changes following the repeated occurrence of symptoms (subtle physical or cognitive) that culminate in severe anxiety states with disease progression. Interestingly, CCK alterations have been documented in schizophrenia, PD and HD. Events may occur as early as before birth, with a critical period identified as prior to age 18, and span across the lifetime.

Anxiogenic Indices Associated with Stressor Exposure: Nonhuman and Human Experimentation

Anxiety among nonhuman subjects has been defined as the behavioral response to unpredictable, novel or threatening stimuli, including uncontrollable footshock, in anxiety paradigms (Davis, 1989; MacNeil et al., 1997; McBlane and Handley, 1994; Servatius et al., 1995). The induction of anxiety following exposure of rats to an acute session of footshock is supported by the observation that (a) chronic diazepam administration (1.25 - 5.0 mg/kg) following stressor application (e.g., 1 mA every 244 sec with 6 sec duration) prevents disruptions in locomotor activity and rearing to subsequent stressful encounters (e.g., noise, van Dijken et al., 1992), (b) diazepam pretreatment (5 mg/kg) prevents increased DOPAC levels in the frontal cortex following footshock (e.g., 2 mA every 320 msec with 160 msec duration for 20 min) (Fadda et al., 1978; Lavielle et al., 1978; Reinhard et al., 1982) and (c) systemic and central injections of β-CCE, β-CCM and FG-7142, produce neurochemical alterations comparable to those of footshock (see Thiebot et al., 1988 for review of anxiogenic properties of β-CCE, β-CCM and FG-7142). For example, intraperitoneal administration of the benzodiazepine inverse agonists FG-7142 (10.0, 20.0 and 30.0 mg/kg) or β-CCE (1.25 and 2.5 mg/kg) dose dependently elevated DA and DOPAC concentrations in the nucleus accumbens (McCullough and Salamone, 1992). Moreover, subcutaneous administration of β-CCM (4 and 8 mg/kg) or β-CCE (8 mg/kg) increased cortical DOPAC levels among non-stressed rats that were antagonized by the benzodiazepine antagonist RO-151788 (30.0 mg/kg) (Claustre et al., 1986). In addition to provoking changes in DA activity, systemic low dose FG-7142 administration (10 mg/kg cf 20 mg/kg) (Pratt and Brett, 1995 cf Rattray et al., 1993) in rats has been associated with increased CCK mRNA in the amygdala and hippocampus and increased CCK binding in the frontal cortex (Harro et al., 1990, Harro et al., 1993; Vasar et al., 1993). In nonhuman subjects, bolus intravenous injection of FG-7142 (0.001-3 mg/kg) produced a transient (5 min) dose dependent increase in arterial blood pressure that was attenuated by systemic pretreatment with chlordiazepoxide (10 mg/kg) (Webb et al., 1996). Moreover, in rat pups, FG-7142 (50 mg/kg) increased ultrasonic vocalizations and antagonizes the anxiolytic effects of diazepam on ultrasonic vocalizations (Gardner and Budhram, 1987). Clinically, elevated plasma FG-7142 levels following oral ingestion of 400 mg FG-7142 have been associated with panic in 2 healthy volunteers (Dorow et al., 1983). Despite the demonstration that footshock elicits behavioral and neurochemical changes that are mimicked by relatively high doses of the anxiolytic and panicogenic agents FG-7142, β-CCM and β-CCE and are reversed with benzodiazepine administration (c.f. efficacy of benzodiazepines in panic disorder, Hoehn-Saric, 1982), it remains to be determined whether footshock is a suitable stressor in assessing anxiolytic efficacy. Indeed, the influence of anxiolytic interventions on locomotor activity and reactivity to electric shock (e.g., analgesia) may mask the emotive aspects of the noxious stimulation. Moreover, the proconvulsant properties of FG-7142, β-CCE, and β-CCM, may induce behavioral and physiological symptoms that are not pathognomic of anxiety but perhaps indicative of increased discomfort (Thiebot et al., 1988). Taken together, repeated application of relatively mild, uncontrollable stressors in comparison to more severe stressful experiences may provide a more succinct index of the neurochemical and behavioral perturbations associated with anxiogenic states.

Examination of repeated anxiety provoking situations to the provocation of panic necessitates comparison of animal models that parallel the human condition. To date, adequate animal models of panic are lacking. It should be considered that fear conditioning (e.g., startle and freezing) in nonhuman subjects may provide a behavioral analogue of the anticipatory anxiety associated with panic disorder. It has been demonstrated, for example, that rats exposed to apparatus cues previously associated with footshock exhibited increased DA turnover in the prefrontal cortex (Ida et al., 1988) and amygdala (Coco et al., 1992) which was attenuated by low dose diazepam administration (1-5mg/kg). Conditioned fear paradigms employ rather mild stressors relative to paradigms assessing the behavioral repercussions of footshock. In any event, conditioned fear (e.g., freezing) has been reliably associated with elevated plasma ACTH, corticosterone and prolactin concentrations for at least 14 days post-stressor in rats (van Dijken et al., 1992). In humans, conditioned fear or fear-enhanced startle has been linked to psychological disorders in which sustained and exaggerated reactivity to environmental stressors appears fundamental. For example, enhanced startle response has been routinely associated with posttraumatic stress disorder (Morgan et al., 1995), schizophrenia (Shaner and Eth, 1989) and panic (Safadi, 1995; Southwick et al., 1995). In animals, exposure to the cues previously associated with footshock results in exaggerated startle, detectable within minutes following initial stressor exposure. For example, an acute, mild session of footshock (e.g., 1, 5, or 10 shocks, 500 msec duration, 0.2 -1.4 mA, 1 shock/second) increased startle to an acoustically associated cue 20-40 min following initial stressor application in the rat (Davis, 1989). Moreover, brief exposure of animals to contextual cues (e.g., light) previously associated with a more severe stressor (e.g., 1 or 3 days of 40 tailshocks, 2 msec duration, 2 mA over 2 hours) also increased subsequent startle responsivity, albeit with a delayed onset (e.g., 7-10 days, Servatius et al., 1995). It should be considered that delayed startle responsivity (e.g., immediate, 7 days, 10 days) among nonhuman subjects to stressor-associated cues might follow from the nature of the initial stressor encounter (i.e., a mild to severe stressor gradient). Some laboratories have demonstrated differential alterations in DA activity from specific brain regions relative to footshock severity. For example, exposure of rats to 1.5 mA (30 min session, 30 sec intershock interval, and 30 sec shock duration) footshock resulted in selective increases of DOPAC in the medial prefrontal cortex. In contrast, exposure of rats to 2.5 mA (30 min session, 30 sec intershock interval, and 30 sec shock duration) footshock increased DA in the paraventricular nucleus of the hypothalamus and hippocampus and DOPAC and HVA levels within the medial prefrontal cortex, nucleus accumbens, striatum and amygdala. Moreover, rats exposed to the 2.5 mA as opposed to the 1.5 mA footshock regimen displayed more instances of freezing following reexposure to the cues associated with stressor (e.g., shock apparatus, Inoue et al., 1994). Likewise, the appearance of increased startle in response to stressor-associated cues was correlated with the intensity of the initial stressor experience including the frequency of shock imposition and number of stressor sessions employed (Davis et al., 1989; Servatius et al., 1995). Interestingly, clinical investigations have demonstrated an enhanced startle reflex (e.g., eye-blink and heart rate) in response to a startle probe (e.g., binaural burst of 110 dB white noise, 50 msec duration) previously associated with graphic photographic slides (e.g., wounds or mutilated bodies) in normal subjects (Cook et al., 1992). In panic patients, exaggerated fear-potentiated startle response has been detected in response to the threat of electric shock (Grillon et al., 1994). Anticipation of electric shock (e.g., 1.5 mA, 50 msec conducted through the median nerve of the wrist) administered during the final 10 seconds of a 45 second threat but not a 50 second no-threat condition, signaled by differential light cues, increased startle in panic patients relative to healthy controls. This startle response was largest in younger panic patients (e.g., <40 years) who also reported an increased frequency of panic attacks within the week prior to testing relative to older panic patients and age matched control subjects (Grillon et al., 1994). Taken together, the absence of a detailed retrospective clinical characterization of putative stressors and inadequate documentation of salient cue associated variables prevent an accounting of the ensuing panic histories of disparate panic subjects. Ultimately, startle latencies provide a potential measure of the developmental history of anticipatory anxiety and panic emergence. Indeed, Grillon et al. (1994) reported that anticipated cue associated challenges in a simulated startle paradigm among young and older panic subjects elicit variable patterns of experimental compliance which influenced participation and anxiety induction.

Examination of the neurobiological and pharmacological substrates of stressor-induced startle in nonhuman subjects may delineate central neural pathways associated with increased anticipatory anxiety in panic patients. A role for the amygdala in eliciting fear potentiated startle has been empirically demonstrated in nonhuman subjects (Davis et al., 1993) and nonhuman primates (Hoehn-Saric, 1982). For example, bilateral ablation of the central amygdaloid nucleus prevented sensitization of the startle reflex following repeated administration of footshock (i.e., 10, 0.6 mA shocks in rapid succession) (Hitchcock et al., 1989). Anatomical investigations reveal that amygdaloid innervation derived from the VTA and prefrontal cortex may be involved in fear associated conditioning and anxiety. For example, efferent projections from the central and basolateral nuclei of the amygdala to the VTA may mediate conditioned fear associated increases in prefrontal DA turnover and increase vigilance, operationalized by increased cortical EEG activity (Davis, 1992). Moreover, the central and basolateral amygdaloid nuclei (Gelsema et al., 1987; Hopkins and Holstege, 1978; Krettek and Price, 1978; Soltis et al., 1997) and the VTA (Chen et al., 1997) provide prominent parabrachial innervation and accordingly may influence cardiovascular responsivity to environmental challenge. It has been suggested that information concerning putative stressors is conveyed to the amygdala which assigns emotional significance to stimuli and relays stressor-related information to brainstem structures that mediate the behavioral, autonomic and neuroendocrine responsivity to stress (Gray, 1991; Grijalva et al., 1990; Tomaz et al., 1993). More specifically, alterations in amygdaloid CCK and DA activity may promote enhanced behavioral responsivity to stressor-associated cues. For example, administration of the CCK_2 agonist pentagastrin (100 nM, Frankland et al., 1997) and anxiogenic substances colocalized with CCK, including CRF, into the central amygdaloid nucleus increases fear potentiated startle in the rat (Lee and Davis, 1997; Liang et al., 1992). Moreover, systemic administration of the CCK_2 antagonist, L-365,260, dose dependently (0.1, 1.0 and 10.0 mg/kg) reduced fear potentiated startle in rats previously exposed to mild footshock (0.5 mA, 0.5 second duration × 3 days) (Josselyn et al., 1995). Likewise, intra-VTA infusion of quinpirole, a $D_{2/3}$ agonist, attenuated fear potentiated startle in rats, which has suggested a role for DA in the promotion of fear-motivated behavior (Borowski and Kokkinidis, 1996). At this juncture, it is not clear whether attenuation of the enhanced startle response followed from an attenuation of central DA activity (e.g., stimulation of DA autoreceptors in VTA) or concomitant alterations of central CCK activity. Nevertheless, provisional consideration of the argument that exacerbation of fear potentiated startle and conceivably panic follow from alterations of central mesolimbic DA/CCK activity is an appealing one.

Surprisingly, the contribution of mild stressors to anxiety induction in clinical applications has been neglected. It is intriguing that amygdaloid (Gelsema et al., 1987; Hopkins and Holstege, 1978; Krettek and Price, 1978; Soltis et al., 1997) and mesencephalic (Chen et al., 1997) input to the parabrachial nucleus sustains cardiovascular arousal and the VTA participates in the detection of salient and non-salient cues in rats (Oades, 1982). Interestingly, panic patients with frequent panic episodes (e.g., >5.6 ± 2.3 attacks/week) exhibit heightened cardiovascular arousal, increased sympathetic/autonomic alterations and increased anxiety in response to innocuous stimuli relative to panic patients with less frequent panic attacks (1.5 ± 0.5 attacks/week) and normal subjects (Abelson et al., 1996; Kathol et al., 1988). Perhaps, sustained rumination and hypervigilance concerning encounters with situational challenges heighten anxiety. The contribution of such variables to the induction of panic certainly merits consideration. Yet, alterations of central anxiogenic activity accompanying panic and the identification of the parameters of putative stressors or the perceived saliency of environmental stimuli to the evocation of panic attacks have not been established. The demonstration that anticipation of stressful encounters influences CCK activity in humans (Harro et al., 1992; Phillipp et al., 1992) is certainly consistent with such an interpretation. It will be recalled that repeated application of low psychostimulant doses in rats are associated with alterations in CCK concentrations and CCK mRNA expression which can be detected for several weeks following the last injection (Fukamauchi, 1996; Hurd et al., 1992). Likewise, exposure to life stressors prior to age 19 has been documented to precipitate anxiety, depression and/or panic in some individuals (Garnefski et al., 1990; Manfro et al., 1996). Indeed, familial illness and sick role behavior may also be salient to illness onset and the course of the psychological disturbance (Ahmad et al., 1992; Shear, 1996; Whitehead et al., 1994). Moreover, childhood behavioral problems (e.g., social withdrawal, anxiety/depression and aggression/delinquency) and the degree of emotional involvement demonstrated by parents to offspring with schizophrenia have been associated with poor prognosis, including psychotic relapse and comorbid affective disturbances (Baum and Walker, 1995; Bentsen et al., 1996). It should be noted parenthetically that nonhuman primates raised under stressful conditions (e.g., variable foraging demands) reveal aberrant behavior patterns (e.g., hyperactivity, clinging and behavioral inhibition) (Rosenblum and Paully, 1984) and protracted increases in cerebrospinal CRF availability (Coplan et al., 1996) in adulthood compared to age- and sex-matched control subjects. To date, evidence for the enduring influence of site-specific central CCK alterations among human or nonhuman primates exposed to early life stressors are unavailable. In effect, aberrant parental practices, sick-role modeling and excessive rumination may precipitate central CCK alterations that contribute to symptom exacerbation and panic emergence. Moreover, some investigators have suggested that decreased lymphocyte and cerebrospinal CCK-8 concentrations in panic patients may reflect enhanced CCK receptor sensitivity, reduced CCK receptor availability or perhaps compensatory reduction of CCK-8 concentrations secondary to increased CCK-4 activity (Brambilla et al., 1993; Lydiard et al., 1992). It should be considered that neurotransmitters colocalized with CCK, including DA, participate in the production or exacerbation of some of the symptoms associated with panic disorder. It will be recalled that DA alterations may be peculiar to panic patients with considerable anxiety and a relatively severe panic course (Roy-Byrne et al., 1986; Pitchot et al., 1992). Moreover, DA alterations have been linked to the development of social phobia, a severe form of agoraphobia (Johnson et al., 1994; Tiihonen et al., 1997). Taken together, the nature of the panic experience and the frequency of stressful encounters may precipitate CCK release and determine the saliency of environmental conditions to panic induction.

Cholecystokinin, Anxiety and Panic Attacks

Molecular forms of CCK are cleaved from prepro-CCK and include CCK-58, CCK-39, CCK-33, CCK-22, CCK-8 sulfated (S), CCK-8 unsulfated (US), CCK-7S, CCK-7US, pentagastrin (CCK-5) and CCK-4 which are degraded by aminopeptidase (see Crawley et al., 1994 for review). Cholecystokinin-8S is the predominant central form of CCK and CCK or CCK mRNA is found in high concentrations in various nonhuman and human central areas including the cerebral cortex, nucleus accumbens, basal ganglia, thalamus, hypothalamus, periaqueductal grey, olfactory tubercle, olfactory bulb, VTA, some brain stem nuclei and the spinal cord (Beinfeld et al., 1981; Crawley et al., 1985; Emson et al., 1980; Hokfelt et al., 1985; 1987; Lindefors et al., 1993; Zanoveli et al., 2004). Cholecystokinin is colocalized with DA in nonhuman subjects, nonhuman primates and humans in the mesencephalon (Hokfelt et al., 1980), CRF in the paraventricular nucleus of the hypothalamus (Mezey et al., 1985), oxytocin in the supraoptic and paraventricular nucleus of the hypothalamus (Vanderhaeghen et al., 1980), substance P in the central gray projecting to the spinal cord (Skirboll et al., 1982), GABA in the amygdala, frontal cortex and hippocampus (Hendry et al., 1984; Somagyi et al., 1984) and enkephalin in the hippocampus (Gall et al., 1987; see Hebb et al., 2005a and Hebb et al., 2005b for review of antagonistic role of CCK and enkephalin in stress, anxiety, cognition and pain). As such, it is not surprising that CCK has been implicated in nocioception (Baber et al., 1989), learning and memory (Harro and Oreland, 1993) as well as ingestive (Gibbs et al., 1973; Smith and Gibbs, 1992), sexual and reproductive behavior (Ulibarri and Micevych, 1993) and panic (Bradwejn and de Montigny, 1984; Rehfeld et al., 1992; see Crawley and Corwin, 1994 for review).

Central and gastrointestinal CCK receptors have been identified. The CCK_1 receptor distribution predominates in the gastrointestinal tract, area postrema, nucleus tractus solitarius, posterior nucleus accumbens, amygdala, septum, hypothalamus, dorsal raphe, cerebral cortex, ventral tegmental area, substantia nigra and hippocampus in rats and mice (Hill et al., 1987; Honda et al., 1993; Moran and McHugh, 1990). The sedative (Crawley, 1985), ingestive (Dourish et al., 1989), kindling (Burazin and Gundlach, 1996), exploration (Kobayashi et al., 1996), locomotor activity (Hirosue et al., 1992; Wunderlich et al., 1997) and learning and memory (Josselyn et al., 1996) of the CCK_1 receptor have been amply demonstrated. Central CCK_2 receptors are distributed in the brainstem solitary complex, nigrostriatal, mesolimbic and mesocortical sites among nonhuman and human subjects and appear to play an anxiogenic (or pro-panic) role (Branchereau et al., 1992; Durieux et al., 1988). Mice lacking CCK_2 receptors are less anxious, as measured by increased exploratory behavior in the elevated plus maze paradigm, than their wild type littermates (Horinouchi et al., 2004; Raud et al., 2003).

The CCK receptor subtypes have been delineated according to respective affinities for specific CCK fragments. For example, the CCK_1 receptor has conspicuous affinity for CCK-8S and the analogues ceruletide and caerulein but reduced affinity for CCK-8US, CCK-5 (pentagastrin) and CCK-4 while the CCK_2 receptor has a strong affinity for CCK-8S, CCK-8US, CCK-4 and pentagastrin (Durieux et al., 1988; Harhammer et al., 1991). Although the central CCK_1 and CCK_2 receptor distribution is comparable in nonhuman and human subjects, the relative contribution of CCK_1 and CCK_2 receptors to anxiety among nonhuman subjects and clinical populations are ambiguous at best (Rodgers and Johnson, 1995). Indeed, firm conclusions concerning CCK_1 receptors and anxiety are lacking owing to the absence of readily available selective CCK_1 agonists. Consequently, arguments concerning CCK_1 receptors and anxiety are derived from paradigms employing selective CCK_1 antagonists (e.g., devazepide and L364,718) or non-selective CCK_1 agonists. For example, while devazepide possessed marginal anxiolytic properties in the elevated plus maze (Chopin and Briley, 1993), intracerebral administration of CCK-8S (3 fmol) in the CCK_1 receptor dense posteromedial nucleus accumbens significantly reduced open arm entries. This behavioral effect was reversed by the CCK_1 antagonist L364,718 (200 µg/kg, 60 min prior to CCK-8S administration). In contrast, CCK-8US (0.1, 1, 10, 100, 1000 fmol) injected into the posteromedial nucleus accumbens did not modify behavior of rats in the elevated plus maze

(Dauge et al., 1989). Findings such as these are used to support an anxiogenic role for CCK_1 receptor activation. Although, peripheral and central CCK-8S administration in nonhuman subjects has been associated with anxiety in the elevated plus maze (Johnson and Rodgers, 1996; Netto and Guimaraes, 2004) and light-dark paradigms (MacNeil et al., 1997), CCK-8S induces nausea and gastrointestinal malaise in human subjects (de Montigny, 1989; Miaskiewicz et al., 1989). Either "illness behavior" and anxiety are not adequately differentiated in nonhuman subjects following CCK-8S administration or fundamental differences exist between the influence CCK agonists have on peripheral CCK receptors (i.e., those of the alimentary canal) in nonhuman and human subjects. In contrast, the selective CCK_2 agonist, CCK-4, induces anxiety in nonhuman subjects (Harro and Vasar, 1991; Rex et al., 1994) and promotes panic in panic patients and normal subjects (Bradwejn et al., 1990; van Megen et al., 1996). The differential propensity of CCK-8S and CCK-4 to provoke anxiety and/or panic in human subjects as well as rats and mice may be attributable to species variations (Kuwahara et al., 1993), differential brain region sensitivity (e.g., amygdala, prefrontal cortex and nucleus accumbens, Katsuura et al., 1985; Vaccarino et al., 1997), drug route (Adler et al., 1984; Chopin and Briley, 1993) and/or paradigm specificity (Vaccarino et al., 1997). Clearly, discrepancies between clinical and nonhuman studies necessitate examination of methodological variables including drug schedule and experiential factors that influence sensitivity to CCK challenge and anxiety (panic) induction. The ensuing discussion will examine the contributions of CCK-8S, CCK-4 and pentagastrin to the provocation of anxiety in nonhuman and clinical subjects, the evidence supporting the contention that stressful life contribute to CCK-induced panic and the nature of panic symptoms in response to CCK administration. The diverse clinical profiles of panic suggest developmental stages of psychological dysfunction. Sensitization of central DA/CCK activity and cognitive processes (e.g., rumination and anticipatory anxiety) may underlie variability in effective pharmacological management of panic.

Cholecystokinin Induced Anxiety: Nonhuman Models

Chronic diazepam and alprazolam withdrawal has been associated with increased anxiety in human (Fontaine et al., 1984; Otto et al., 1993) and nonhuman subjects (Singh et al., 1992). Interestingly, chronic benzodiazepine treatment in rats decreases neural responsivity to microiontophoretic CCK-8S application in the frontal cortex and hippocampus (Bouthillier and DeMontigny, 1988; Bradwejn and DeMontigny, 1984). In contrast, termination of chronic diazepam treatment increases hippocampal and cortical CCK-8 binding in the rat (Harro et al., 1990). In mice, the CCK_2 receptor antagonist, CI-988, dose dependently (0.001-1.0 mg/kg^{-1}) antagonized the anxiogenic effects associated with diazepam withdrawal (Singh et al., 1992). In rats, flumazenil (4 mg/kg i.p.) significantly antagonized the anxiogenic effects of the CCK_2 agonist, CCK-8US and the anxiolytic-like effects of the CCK_2 antagonist, L-365,260 (Chopin and Briley, 1993). Moreover, rats rated anxious with respect to performance in the elevated plus maze exhibited a reduced benzodiazepine receptor density and increased CCK-8S binding in the frontal cortex relative to non-anxious counterparts (Harro et al., 1990). Although CCK_1 and CCK_2 receptors have been detected in the frontal cortex (Honda et al., 1993; Harro et al., 1990) did not identify the CCK receptor contributing to increased CCK-8S binding in anxious rats. These data only suggest that benzodiazepines suppress CCK-8S activity in the prefrontal cortex of anxious mice (Harro and Vasar, 1991). Moreover, the dose and nature of the CCK fragment employed have suggested site-specific sensitivity to anxiogenic drug administration. Acute administration of caerulein or pentagastrin does not influence mesocortical CCK-8S binding in the rat (Harro et al., 1990). However, site-specific neurochemical alterations to central CCK_1 and CCK_2 receptor activation have been detected among nonhuman subjects. For example, in rats intravenously administered CCK-8S (0.5, 1.0, 2.0 and 4.0 µg/kg) but not CCK-8US (4 and 20 µg/kg) or CCK-4 (70 and 300 µg/kg) dose dependently inhibited DA release from the medial nucleus accumbens. The CCK_1 antagonist, proglumide (0.3 mg/kg i.v.), reduced CCK-8S inhibition of DA availability (Kariya et al., 1994; Kelland et al., 1991; Lane et al., 1986). It is conceivable that CCK fragments, including caerulein and pentagastrin, exert differential influence on central areas and sub-nuclei associated with anxiety emergence. Indeed, the central amygdaloid nucleus is conspicuously more sensitive to CCK-4 than the prefrontal cortex or the nucleus accumbens in the startle paradigm (Vaccarino et al., 1997). Moreover, in exploration paradigms (e.g., light-dark task and elevated plus maze), low doses of ceruletide (100 ng/kg^{-1}) and pentagastrin (500 ng/kg^{-1}) are only anxiogenic among mice previously exposed to the stress of overcrowding. Significantly elevated doses of ceruletide and pentagastrin are required to induce comparable levels of anxiety among rats and mice housed in non-crowded conditions (Harro et al., 1993). Furthermore, investigations in nonhuman primates indicate that intravenously administered CCK-4 dose dependently (0.5- 4 mg/kg^{-1}) increased fear and defensive behaviors according to the baseline anxiety scores of animals and their social hierarchical position (Palmour et al., 1992). Apparently, antecedent environmental experiences interact with the nature of subsequent pharmacological challenges in provoking anxiety.

The demonstration that (a) anxious mice exhibit reduced benzodiazepine receptor density and increased CCK-8S binding in the frontal cortex relative to non-anxious mice (Harro et al., 1990), (b) strain-specific sensitivity in fear-motivated behavior appears among rats (Rex et al., 1996), (c) strain-specific behavioral and neurochemical variations appear among mice exposed to the elevated plus maze (Trullas and Skolnick, 1993) and (d) differential behavioral and neurochemical sensitivity emerges among divergent inbred and outbred mouse strains challenged with anxiogenic agents (e.g., footshock, Shanks et al., 1990) certainly provides evidence for the influence of genetic variables to the expression of anxiety. It is intuitively consistent to suspect that genetic variables and antecedent environmental stressors likewise contribute to the attenuation, exacerbation or maintenance of clinical anxiety. Alterations in CCK_2 receptor sensitivity in panic patients may also accompany increased anxiety following CCK administration. In view of differential post-mortem CCK receptor binding between panic prone Parkinsonian patients and individuals with schizophrenia, panic subjects would likely demonstrate variable central CCK receptor sensitivity to exogenously administered CCK fragments. Current empirical evidence supports altered basal CSF CCK concentrations in panic patients relative to control subjects (Brambilla et al., 1993; Lydiard et al., 1992). The inadequacy of such comparison is apparent and functional indices of CCK turnover and/or CCK receptor sensitivity in discrete central sites among CCK challenged panic subjects are required.

Potential parallels between nonhuman experimentation and clinical data employing CCK-8S is compromised owing to the ineffectiveness of this CCK fragment in provoking anxiety in humans. Accordingly, comparison of nonhuman CCK-induced anxiety with chronic anxiety syndromes, including panic, in human subjects is limited to studies concerned with CCK-4 availability and CCK_2 receptor activation (e.g., van Megen et al., 1994; 1996). However, the functional significance of central CCK_1 receptor sensitivity and density in areas involved in central respiratory and cardiovascular activity (e.g., the nucleus tractus solitarius and parabrachial nucleus) (Chen et al., 1997; Fortin et al., 1992; Jhamandas and Harris, 1992), motivation (e.g., nucleus accumbens) (Derrien et al., 1993), attention (e.g., VTA) (Oades, 1982), and cognition (e.g., prefrontal cortex) (Simon et al., 1980) to anxiety among nonhuman subjects requires consideration. It will be recalled that panic patients engage in considerable somatic monitoring (Schmidt et al., 1997). The neurocircuitry of brainstem sites involved in the modulation of respiratory and cardiovascular function as well as possible neurochemical correlates attending increased vigilance and a possible relation to panic have been discussed previously (Zacharko et al., 1995). Empirical evidence describing CCK_1 receptors and panic is not available. Nevertheless, nonhuman investigations indicate that CCK may exert differential behavioral (e.g., locomotion) (Katsuura et al., 1985) and neurochemical (e.g., DA) effects from the nucleus accumbens (Marshall et al., 1991) mediated by the different types of CCK receptors. It will be recalled that stressors influence central CCK release and conceivably CCK receptor sensitivity. Alterations in CCK_1 receptor sensitivity may temporally exceed or follow from alterations in CCK_2 receptor sensitivity. It is conceivable that hypochondriasis in panic may stem from alterations in CCK_1 receptor sensitivity following protracted vigilance. Such an interpretation may explain the ineffectiveness of CCK_2 receptor antagonists in the management of panic.

Consideration of parallels between behavioral profiles drawn from animal models of anxiety and clinical panic symptoms should focus on behaviors that reflect comparable aspects of anxiety. For example, it appears that conditioned fear (e.g., anticipatory anxiety) and exploratory tendencies in novel environments (e.g., the response of an organism to a potentially threatening stimulus) provide indices of diverse aspects of anxiety (Ravard and Dourish, 1990). Repeated exposure of rats to the elevated plus maze as an analogue of anticipatory anxiety has been criticized owing to the resistance of such behavioral tests to the anxiolytic influence of benzodiazepines (File, 1993; File and Zangrossi, 1993). While questions relating to the validity of the elevated plus maze in evaluating anticipatory anxiety may be relevant, arguments pertaining to the efficacy of benzodiazepine intervention strategies may be misleading. For example, the nature of the anxiety experienced in the plus maze with repeated apparatus exposure undoubtedly varies with successive exposures to the stressor-like influence of the paradigm. It will be recalled that among nonhuman subjects, the pattern of CCK release from specific mesocorticolimbic sites varies according to the nature and severity of the stressor (Brodin et al., 1994; Pavlasevic et al., 1993; Rosen et al., 1992; Siegel et al., 1987). In effect, repeated exposure of animals to the mild, anxiogenic influence of the elevated plus maze may augment CCK release and effect protracted alterations of CCK receptor sensitivity. In effect, the nature of the CCK associated experience has been altered and pharmacological responsivity might likewise be expected to vary. Consistent with this argument, rats exposed to olfactory and auditory cues associated with decapitation of conspecifics exhibited increased CCK concentrations in the hippocampus and ^{3}H-CCK-8 binding in the frontal cortex. Yet, diazepam (5 mg/kg) pretreatment was ineffective in attenuating CCK alterations (Harro et al., 1996). It will be recalled that the pattern of CCK release from specific central sites seems to be correlated with the nature and severity of the stressor. For example, exposure of rats to the smell of a cat (Pavlasevic et al., 1993) but not a 1-minute period of restraint (Rosen et al., 1992) increased CCK-8 concentrations in the nucleus accumbens. Moreover, systemic administration of FG-7142 (10 mg/kg) but not acute elevated plus maze exposure increased CCK mRNA levels in the basolateral nucleus of the amygdala and the hippocampus (Pratt and Brett, 1995). Taken together, reduced propensity of diazepam in alleviating anxiety associated with repeated maze exposure suggests that the neurochemical correlates of the stressor have been altered (e.g., conditioning/sensitization) (Post and Weiss, 1988; 1992).

To date, behavioral sensitization accompanying CCK challenge in conditioned fear paradigms or tasks that assess behavioral change to novel environmental challenge (e.g., light-dark box) has not been attempted. An assessment of behavioral responsivity of animals to previously established non-anxiogenic doses of CCK and a relevant inter-CCK interval is clearly required. It will be recalled that repeated low dose psychostimulant administration in rats is associated with enhanced CCK levels and CCK mRNA expression in the prefrontal cortex, hippocampus (Fukamauchi, 1996), VTA and the medial, caudal aspects of the nucleus accumbens (Hurd et al., 1992) which can be detected for several weeks following the last injection. The temporal parameters of CCK-induced behavioral sensitization have not been ascertained but data derived from nonhuman experimentation suggest that minimal temporal delays are required. For example, data collected in this laboratory suggest that exposure of mice to a mild stressor effects increases in anxiety, initially detected 10 days following initial exposure. Taken together, it is suspected that identification of some of the conditions (e.g., genetic and environmental) contributing to inter-individual sensitivity to CCK challenge paradigms, including efficacious anxiolytic applications, in nonhumans may parallel variable therapeutic efficacy of anti-panic drugs in clinical trials.

Cholecystokinin Challenge, Panic Induction and Clinical Investigations

The selective CCK$_2$ agonists, CCK-4 and pentagastrin, induce panic in healthy volunteers and panic patients (Bradwejn et al., 1990; Lara et al., 2003; van Megen et al., 1994). Acute, oral L365,260 administration (50 mg, 90 minutes prior to CCK-4 challenge) attenuates CCK-4 (50 µg) (Bradwejn et al., 1994) but not lactate (van Megen et al., 1996) induced panic in panic patients. The specificity of L365,260 in attenuating CCK but not lactate-induced panic may suggest that there are different types of panic. Curiously, an acute, oral dose of the CCK$_2$ antagonist CI-988 (50 or 100 mg) 2 hours prior to CCK-4 challenge failed to attenuate CCK-4 (20 µg) induced panic in both normal subjects (Bradwejn et al., 1995) and panic patients (van Megen et al., 1997). At this juncture it is not clear whether the efficacy of L365,260, relative to CI-988, in attenuating CCK-4 panic is attributable to experimental protocol, pharmacological properties or panic profile. Nevertheless, it is likely that CCK-induced panic symptoms including tachycardia, nausea and dyspnea stem from a CCK influence on selective brain stem nuclei. Cognitive variations attending CCK-induced panic, including anticipatory anxiety, are most likely attributable to mesolimbic and cortical sites secondary to brainstem activation (see Benkelfat et al., 1995 and Schunck et al., 2006 for an accounting of such a conclusion with respect to cerebral blood flow and fMRI activity profiles in response to CCK-4 administration, respectively; Bradwejn et al., 1994; van Megen et al., 1994). While clinical responsivity to CCK-4 is well documented, there is considerable behavioral variability in the responsivity of panic patients and healthy volunteers to CCK challenge. For example, the panic inducing properties of relatively large CCK-4 doses (e.g., 25 or 50 μg) or pentagastrin (0.1-0.6 μg/kg) have been reliably demonstrated in several laboratories (Bradwejn et al., 1990, 1992; Lara et al., 2003; de Leeuw et al., 1996; van Megen et al., 1994, 1996). However, elevated anxiogenic drug administration (a) confounds potential central variations describing inter-individual responsivity of clinical patients to CCK challenge and (b) prevents detection of the relative vulnerability of healthy control subjects to panicogenic agents. Indeed, the efficacy of CCK-4 in provoking panic-like symptoms appears to be dose dependent. For example, among panic patients the panic distribution was 17% (10 μg), 64% (15 μg), 75% (20 μg), 75% (25 μg) and 91-100% (50 μg) following the respective CCK challenge doses (Bradwejn et al., 1992). In an accompanying investigation, proportional panic frequencies of 11% (9 μg), 17% (25 μg) and 47% (50 μg) were detected following CCK challenge doses administered in control subjects (Bradwejn et al., 1991). These data suggest varied CCK response thresholds among panic patients that are lower than those of control subjects, which exhibit graded responsivity to CCK challenge. The lower threshold for response found in panic patients relative to controls, with respect to CCK-4 dosage, has been demonstrated directly and recently confirmed (Bradwejn et al., 1991b; Koszycki et al., 2005). Selection of the respective challenge doses of CCK obscures investigation of sensitization and/or conditioning by discounting subject variability and clinical history. Such an approach is unfortunate and counterproductive. In effect, the obvious differential sensitivities of clinical populations to CCK challenge require documentation of threshold CCK doses (e.g., initial challenge). Ensuing responsivity of panic patients to CCK should, at the very least, consider rechallenge with sub-threshold doses of CCK-4. The interval pertaining to CCK re-exposure is not readily available although data derived from nonhuman experimentation suggests that protracted intervals may be required (see MacNeil et al., 1997 for discussion of temporal influences on CCK sensitization). Individuals with panic display variable clinical histories, including age of onset, familial history, frequency and severity of panic as well as comorbid symptoms of depression and/or agoraphobia (see Figure 2). The most appealing of such clinical accounts include instances where panic frequency and the appearance of agoraphobia are temporally exaggerated, suggesting an incremental basis to panic induction (e.g., Keller and Hanks, 1993). Intuitively, it is appealing to consider that sub-threshold doses of CCK-4 in panic patients produce behavioral effects that mirror clinical panic exacerbation. To date, consideration of such factors and the potential contribution of these variables to long-term responsivity to CCK-4 challenge have not been adequately assessed (c.f. Post and Weiss, 1988; 1992). It will be recalled that the anxiogenic efficacy of ceruletide, pentagastrin and CCK-4 in nonhuman animals and nonhuman primates was clearly dependent upon antecedent environmental experiences, including the differential stressor influence of the paradigm considered (Harro et al., 1993; Palmour et al., 1992). Such a comparison to panic patients appears to be a logical one. To be sure, it must be demonstrated that individual stressor and panic histories interact with CCK challenge to influence panic thresholds. Taken together, panic patients and control subjects demonstrate differential sensitivities to the panicogenic properties of CCK-4. Moreover, demonstration of enhanced CCK sensitivity following CCK-4 re-challenge underscores the need to (a) delineate an inter-drug interval conducive to behaviorally enhanced responsivity, (b) establish behavioral sensitivity to previously non-panicogenic doses of CCK-4 and (c) describe patient histories pertaining to effective challenge and rechallenge doses of CCK and the temporal parameters supporting sensitization.

The hypothesis that individuals exhibit differential sensitivities to the panicogenic properties of CCK-4, or to other panicogenic agents, is intriguing. At the very least, these data permit subject characterization according to organismic variables (e.g., baseline anxiety levels) and experiential factors (e.g., age of onset and severity of panic disorder). In effect, age of onset may provide one index of panic severity. For example, panic patients with a history of early life stressors, including childhood separation disorder or a family history of panic disorder with agoraphobia, exhibit an earlier age of onset of panic disorder relative to individuals who fail to report such events (Battaglia et al., 1995). In this respect, severity of panic disorder may be operationally defined according to illness duration. Such an analysis would necessitate assessment of the cognitive repercussions associated with such illness and individual perception of the saliency of such a stressor. In addition to illness duration, the severity of panic may be qualitatively assessed by panic frequency. It will be recalled that Parkinsonian patients and individuals with schizophrenia with panic secondary to chronic illness have a relatively severe panic profile (e.g., 2.4 ± 1.4 panic attacks/week) (Argyle et al., 1990; Vazquez et al., 1993). The appearance of panic attacks, among late-stage Parkinsonian patients is interesting. In the clinical population, it will be recalled that panic attacks rarely occur following age 65. Interestingly, a lower ^{3}H-CCK-8 hippocampal binding density (Harro and Oreland, 1992) as well as decreased CCK mRNA in the hypothalamus and cerebral cortex (Miyasaka et al., 1995) and increased CCK concentrations in the cerebral cortex (Ohta et al., 1995) have been detected among rats 18-29 months of age relative to younger animals (i.e., 2-10 months). It would be of interest to determine if comparable alterations in CCK activity are evident in the amygdala and nucleus accumbens, for example, in animal models of Parkinson's disease. An analysis of mesolimbic sites may provide a CCK associated index of panic susceptibility that addresses the apparent delay of panic onset among Parkinsonian patients. Surely, subjective characteristics including identification of events precipitating panic (e.g., Parkinson's disease, schizophrenia and childhood anxiety separation) would evoke differential sensitivities to the panicogenic properties of CCK-4 among diverse clinical samples.

To date, clinical reports of CCK-4 induced panic, fail to identify subject characteristics or experiential variables that may influence responsivity to CCK in normal subjects and panic patients. It should be noted parenthetically that panic attacks induced by CCK-4 occur within seconds (e.g., 20 ± 3 seconds) following systemic administration and appear to be similar to naturally occurring panic attacks (e.g., mean duration 20.7 ± 7.6 seconds) (Bradwejn et al., 1990). It appears that the assumption of panic spontaneity has been gleaned from the rapid induction of panic following large, bolus injection of CCK-4 (50 μg). Moreover, the onset of "spontaneous" or induced (e.g., CO_2) panic symptoms over a longer period of time (e.g., time to peak intensity >10 minutes) is inconsistent with a panic description afforded by DSM-IV criteria (American Psychological Association, 1994; Scupi et al., 1997). Such clinical definitions are counterintuitive particularly when it is considered that patients exhibiting panic attacks with latencies exceeding 10 minutes achieve peak intensity ratings comparable to those of panic patients with rapid symptom onset (see Bradwejn and Koszycki, 1991; Koszycki et al., 1991 c.f. Scupi et al., 1997). Curiously, immediate panic onset was characterized by increased phobic frequencies and elevated anticipatory anxiety while patients with more protracted latencies prior to panic onset exhibited more generalized anxiety symptoms (Scupi et al., 1997). Persistent fear of anticipated panic episodes has been recently proferred as a diagnostic criterion for panic disorder (American Psychological Association, 1994; Kenardy et al., 1992). While the panic spontaneity is predicated on reduced latencies, it has been well documented that panic patients may experience a paucity of symptoms (e.g., 1-2 symptoms) prior to the emergence of symptom clusters (e.g., >4 symptoms). For example, life-threatening interpretation of vestibular symptoms including fear of fainting, chest pains, breathing difficulty or choking sensations have led to catastrophic interpretations (Kenardy et al., 1992). Not only does the occurrence of limited symptoms prior to the development of panic disorder and the "fear of fear" criterion argue against spontaneity but also is suggestive of a developmental panic course. Recent operational definitions of panic, including limited and situational panic attacks, contradict previous versions of panic spontaneity and inadvertently support the argument that panic attacks evolve from gradual symptom exacerbation. If there were indeed a developmental course of panic, influencing the temporal appearance and severity of symptomatology, panic patients would not only exhibit differential sensitivities to the panicogenic properties of CCK-4 but also exhibit enhanced responsivity to panic-associated cues. Indeed, in some instances the panicogenic properties of placebo have been demonstrated in panic patients (Goetz et al., 1993). Intuitively, panic attacks occurring in response to placebo procedures are suggestive of expectancy and likely reflect augmented basal anxiety levels. At this juncture, available clinical data do not readily identify laboratory setting and procedural details pertaining to blood pressure assessment and/or intravenous protocols as correlates of enhanced behavioral responsivity in clinical samples. Such an interpretation is hardly surprising, despite the accumulation of clinical evidence which argues for the lack of such an effect (c.f. Argyle and Roth, 1989; Bradwejn et al., 1990; Margraf et al., 1987). To be sure, if environmental cues favor panic emergence, illness duration, severity of panic attacks, agoraphobia and associated rumination would likewise be expected to influence behavioral responsivity. Indeed, while a 20 μg oral dose of yohimbine induces panic in panic patients with more than 2.5 panic attacks/week, this identical dose of yohimbine is without effect among panic patients with a panic frequency of less than 2.5 panic attacks/week (Albus et al., 1992; Charney et al., 1984). Likewise, elevated basal indices of anxiety, panic frequency in the week prior to testing and panic associated somatic reporting were reliably associated with yohimbine induced panic attacks relative to panic patients which failed to report such indices

(Albus et al., 1992). Similarly, intravenous lactate elicited panic in 75% of panic patients reporting a panic frequency exceeding 1 panic attack/week while no panic attacks emerged with such challenge among panic patients reporting frequencies of less than 1 panic attack/month (Targum, 1991). It should also be considered that experimental setting and patient expectations including anticipatory reactivity and stressor controllability may influence the course of panicogenic challenge paradigms (Papp et al., 1993; Rapee et al., 1986; Roth et al., 1992, Sanderson et al., 1989). For example, panic patients provided with the expectancy of anxiety in CO_2 challenge investigations have a demonstrable increase in reported distress and elevated panic incidence relative to patients who have been instructed that control over CO_2 inhalation can be achieved (Sanderson et al., 1989). Moreover, experimental protocols that minimize expectancy of panic averted the panicogenic properties of yohimbine (20 μg orally) (Albus et al., 1992). It should be underscored that anxiety rating scales appear to provide inadequate assessment of anticipatory anxiety and are likely influenced by patient compliance and demand characteristics. In contrast, physiological measures (e.g., blood pressure, heart rate and cortisol responses) while providing more objective measures of anxiety (Grillon et al., 1993; Hoehn-Saric et al., 1991; Koszycki et al., 1993; Roth et al., 1992) are not invariably sensitive to expectancy. To be sure, it is rather curious that panic patients fail to report anticipatory anxiety in challenge studies or to provide physiological measures of expectancy yet consistently report a hypervigilant state consisting of somatic monitoring or environmental vigilance which may serve as predictors of panic. It should also be considered that clinical investigation, in some instances, permits patient-assisted low dose benzodiazepine maintenance. In addition, failure to substantiate plasma drug concentrations prior to challenge (e.g., Bradwejn et al., 1992b) may complicate experimental interpretation and mask pre-test anxiety measures. In view of the observation that lactate-, yohimbine- and CO_2-induced panic are influenced by rumination pertaining to panicogenic control and panic expectancy, it is likely that such factors also influence behavioral responsivity to CCK-4 administration. Further to this point, characterization of control subjects responsive to CCK-4 administration may provide salient information regarding panic vulnerability. For example, it has been demonstrated that 6 of 62 normal subjects subsequently reported an unexpected panic attack during the 12 month follow-up period following initial CO_2 challenge (Harrington et al., 1996). Unfortunately, the temporal distribution of life events preceding the panic attack, as well as detailed subjective and familial history were inadequately detailed. Although the proactive influence of CCK-4 on subsequent panic attacks are not available, a parsimonious accounting of this peptide would favor the prediction that CCK-4 experience contributes to the development of panic. Clinical strategies would accordingly employ therapeutic interventions prior to the "second" panic episode that may interrupt, or at best delay, conditioning and/or sensitization of CCK dependent symptoms (Post and Weiss, 1988).

Pharmacological and Cognitive Management of Panic Disorder: Implications for Putative Differential Sensitivities among Panic Patient Samples

Pharmacological management of panic disorder often includes chronic administration of imipramine (150-300 mg/day) with the benzodiazepine alprazolam (2-8 mg) as needed, although amitriptyline (150 mg/day) and clomipramine (150-225 mg/day), the irreversible monoamine oxidase inhibitor phenelzine (45-90 mg/day), the reversible monoamine oxidase inhibitors moclobemide (300-600 mg/day) and brofaromine (150 mg/day) and certain selective 5-HT reuptake inhibitors are also used (Bakish et al., 1993; Bandelow et al., 1995; Buller, 1995; Clum et al., 1993; Curtis et al., 1993; De La Fuente, 1993; Evans et al., 1986; Keck et al., 1993; Nutt and Glue, 1991; Rosenberg et al., 1991; Yonkers et al., 1996). Chronic imipramine administration in nonhuman subjects is associated with reduced cerebrospinal and plasma NE concentrations (Charney and Heninger, 1985; Ko et al., 1983; Sugrue, 1981) and 5-HT (Fuxe et al., 1982; Johanning et al., 1992). In rats, chronic administration of imipramine decreases the electrophysiological activity of the locus coeruleus (Svensson, 1980). Interestingly, imipramine has demonstrable effects on panic frequency with limited effects on phobic and agoraphobic behavior (Zitrin, 1983). In contrast to imipramine, the efficacy of alprazolam in ameliorating panic cannot be attributed to enhanced GABA/benzodiazepine receptor influence (Sethy and Hodges, 1982). Indeed, diazepam and alprazolam augment benzodiazepine receptor density in the frontal cortex, hypothalamus and hippocampus (Miller et al., 1987; c.f. benzodiazepine receptor binding in panic patients, Kaschka et al., 1995) and influence central NE (Charney et al., 1986; Charney and Heninger, 1985) and 5-HT activity (Sevy et al., 1994) to a comparable degree in nonhuman and human subjects. Yet diazepam is therapeutically sterile in the treatment of panic (Jonas and Cohon, 1993) while alprazolam reduces panic frequency, anticipatory anxiety and phobic symptoms (Mellergard et al., 1991). Taken together, these data would suggest that cascading neurochemical alterations associated with benzodiazepine-GABA receptor variations contribute to the therapeutic efficacy of chronic alprazolam treatment. In any event, these data suggest that pharmacological management of panic should be directed toward specific symptoms characterizing the psychological disorder. Nevertheless, the efficacy of pharmacological interventions among panic patients is often confounded by attrition, patient compliance, relapse following progressive drug taper (King et al., 1990; Mavissakalian and Perel, 1992; Pecknold, 1993) and drug side effects (Amrein et al., 1988; Andersch et al., 1991; Fux et al., 1993; Hetem, 1996; Hoehn-Saric et al., 1993; Klein, 1995; Jonas and Cohon, 1993; Taylor et al., 1990). Alprazolam (5%), for example, is associated with a lower attrition than imipramine (20%) or placebo (54%). The enhanced attrition associated with alprazolam is most likely due to its reduced therapeutic latency (e.g., within one week) relative to imipramine (e.g., 4-8 weeks) or placebo on panic frequency, anxiety episodes, anticipatory anxiety and phobic symptoms (Andersch et al., 1991; Rizley et al., 1986; Schweizer et al., 1993; Taylor et al., 1990). In the rat, acute (5 or 10 mg/kg) and chronic (10 mg/kg, 21 days) imipramine administration fails to attenuate fear potentiated startle (Cassella and Davis, 1985). In contrast, acute administration of alprazolam (1.0, 2.0, 3.0 mg/kg) 30 minutes prior to test, dose dependently attenuated startle (Hijzen et al., 1995). The relative efficacies of alprazolam and imipramine in antagonizing fear potentiated startle in rats suggests that alprazolam may be more effective in influencing central sites underlying expression of startle and conditioned behavior, including the central nucleus of the amygdala (c.f. Duncan et al., 1986; Harris and Westbrook, 1995; Pesold and Treit, 1995; Shimazoe et al., 1988; Shirayama et al., 1996). Notably, central and basolateral nuclei amygdaloid neurochemical perturbations associated with benzodiazepine-GABA receptor variations including alterations in GABA and glutamate (Davis et al., 1994; Kunas and Varga, 1995; Soltis et al., 1997; Walker and Davis, 1997) most likely potentiate the anxiolytic and anti-panic properties of alprazolam. The patient characteristics provided by Andersch et al. (1991) as well as Klein (1995) and Taylor et al. (1990), for example, suggest that alprazolam is more effective than imipramine in alleviating anticipatory anxiety preceding panic (e.g., anticipatory intervals associated with panic expectancy, Sheehan Patient-Rated Anxiety Scale). In retrospect, it is curious that clinical reports outlining the panicogenic effects of CCK fail to acknowledge a role for anticipatory anxiety in panic. Such putative differences in anticipatory indices among panic and control subjects participating in CCK challenge paradigms, as well as paradigms that manipulate anticipatory anxiety, pose serious obstacles to detractors of an expectancy hypothesis. In effect, the demonstrable heterogeneity of treatment efficacy associated with chronic imipramine and alprazolam may well follow from the influence of such agents on variable developmental stages of panic disorder.

It is presumed that panic is a heterogeneous disorder comprised of patients who experience uncomplicated panic or, conversely, a complicated panic disorder syndrome consisting of panic with comorbid symptoms of mild or major depression and/or panic with varying degrees of phobic avoidance. While it has been well documented that recurrent anxiety episodes provoke depressive episodes, repeated anxiety episodes together with the affective disturbance of depression may evoke panic (see Keller and Hanks, 1993 for review). In any event, the temporal parameters and the contribution of intra- and inter-individual environmental precipitants have not been clearly established (see Figure 2). Conceptually, the heterogeneity of panic types may coincide with differential stages of panic development. Regardless of psychiatric compartmentalization of panic, panic disorder is invariably progressive with evidence of symptom exacerbation. The adoption of limited panic and situationally provoked panic classifications and arbitrary acceptance of *ad hoc* patient categories provides tacit acceptance of a developmental course in panic. To be sure, it would be reasonable to suggest that premorbid patient characteristics, the duration of the illness, age of onset as well as the frequency and severity of panic episodes influence the expression or exacerbation of depression and phobic avoidance among individuals with panic disorder. Similar comparisons have been provided for depression and schizophrenia and there is no *a priori* reason to suspect a differential developmental course for panic disorder. In fact, uncomplicated panic and panic with comorbid depression and/or extensive phobic avoidance, on the other hand, may operationally define panic severity (see Figure 2). Moreover, while responsivity to CCK challenge may vary with panic history, age of onset, illness duration and panic frequency, the efficacy of panic interventions would also be expected to vary with such variables.

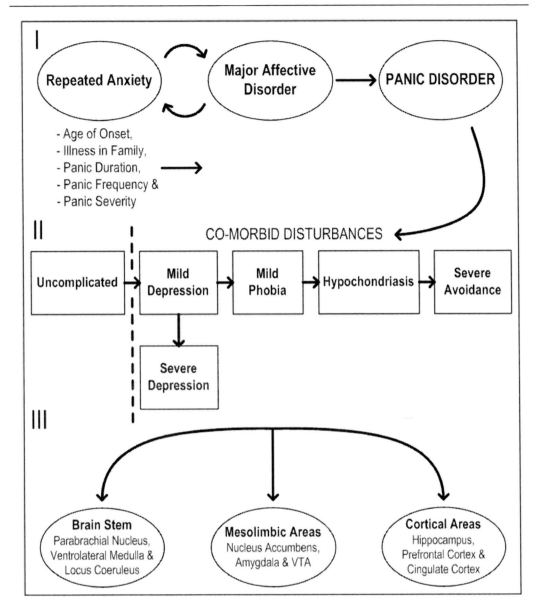

Figure 2. Schematic illustration of the involvement of repeated anxiety episodes in panic (I), the developmental stages, or course, of panic and the precipitating variables that affect its course (II) as well as some of the central sites hypothesized to be involved in panic disorder (III).

Repeated anxiety may precipitate major affective disorder while episodes of depression may lead to further increases in anxiety. Reciprocal influences on individual states of anxiety and depression may be influenced by subjective factors including chronic illness in the family, subject history or other stressors. Panic evolves following some time and the temporal parameters associated with the appearance of panic symptoms among various clinical populations have not been clearly determined. II. Panic symptoms, once present, may consist primarily of autonomic symptoms including cardiovascular perturbations or cognitive symptoms including depersonalization and fear of losing control without accompanying phobic or depressive symptoms (a). More commonly panic disorder is complicated with depression of varying severity (b), mild phobia (c), hypochondriasis (d), and/or severe avoidance behavior (e). The varying types of panic classifications may represent different developmental stages of panic. Moreover, age of onset, illness in the family, panic duration, panic frequency and panic severity may influence the progression of panic from uncomplicated panic episodes to panic with comorbid symptoms of depression and phobia. Moreover, such factors (represented in clouds) may also influence pharmacological management of panic. III. The developmental stages of panic appear to be characterized by prominent symptoms that may involve brain stem structures (a), mesolimbic areas (b) or cortical areas (c). Uncomplicated panic, for example, may be primarily associated with cardiovascular and respiratory perturbations (e.g., brainstem) although anxiety (e.g., amygdala) and rumination (e.g., nucleus accumbens, VTA, prefrontal cortex) are also present. Co-morbidity with depression or phobia would typically involve mesencephalic (e.g., VTA), mesolimbic (e.g., nucleus accumbens, amygdala) and cortical areas (e.g., prefrontal cortex and cingulate gyrus).

Recall that repeated exposure of animals to the elevated plus maze induces anxiogenic behavior that is resistant to previously effective benzodiazepine intervention (File and Zangrossi, 1993). These data suggest that the nature of the anxiety experience has been altered. As such, repeated panic attacks likely alter the neurochemical substrates of the psychological disorder according to the sequence/frequency of panic intrusion or perhaps inter-panic interval. It is intriguing that the effectiveness of imipramine and alprazolam in alleviating panic symptoms varies with the severity of comorbid depressive symptoms or agoraphobia.

Pretreatment measures of uncomplicated panic have revealed diminished panic frequency, anxiety (Hamilton Anxiety Rating scale), depression, phobia, paranoia and help seeking behaviors. Moreover, placebo may be sufficient to attenuate panic symptoms for at least the duration of an eight-week clinical trial (Rosenberg et al., 1991; Woodman et al., 1994). In general, it appears that subjects who respond to placebo have a less severe course of panic and high expectations for pharmacological improvement. Alprazolam and imipramine are equally effective in attenuating panic symptoms associated with uncomplicated panic disorder (Rosenberg et al., 1991; Woodman et al., 1994). It should be noted parenthetically that clinical accounts of panic reveal a depression comorbidity rate of 60-75% (Barlow et al., 1986; Wittchen, 1988). Chronic imipramine intervention (150 mg/day, 4-8 weeks) is relatively effective in ameliorating panic symptoms in panic patients early in the course of the disorder where mild depressive symptoms are also detectable (van Valkenburg et al., 1984; Marks and O'Sullivan, 1989). Conditions favoring imipramine treatment include a relatively short duration of illness (e.g., 1-2 years), younger age of onset (<40 years), comorbid mild depression and panic with no or limited agoraphobia characterized by respiratory distress (Cassano et al., 1994; Keller et al., 1993; Klein, 1988; 1996; Laberge et al., 1992). In contrast, alprazolam is less effective in alleviating panic symptoms among panic patients with comorbid mild depression (Pyke and Kraus, 1988) unless the disorder is accompanied by increased phobic avoidance and increased anticipatory anxiety. In such instances, alprazolam and imipramine are equally effective in alleviating panic symptoms (Rosenberg et al., 1991). Amitriptyline (150 mg/day) and phenelzine (60 mg/day) are also equally effective in alleviating panic symptoms associated with mild depression (Kayser et al., 1988). Patients with panic disorder with comorbid major depression are typically more anxious, fearful of criticism, unassertive and markedly impaired in various social areas compared to non-depressed panic patients (Laberge et al., 1992; Roy-Byrne et al., 1992). Moreover, panic patients with comorbid major depression are more likely to report earlier age of panic onset (<20 years), previous psychiatric hospitalizations, suicidal tendencies and suicide attempts than non-depressed panic patients (Cox et al., 1994; Massion et al., 1993). Typically, the perceived severity (e.g., disability scales) and frequency of panic among such patients is likewise increased (Buffone, 1991; Grunhaus et al., 1994; Kayser et al., 1988) and phenelzine (75 mg/day) is more effective than imipramine and amitriptyline in ameliorating panic symptoms associated with major depression (Davidson et al., 1987; Kayser et al., 1988; Quitkin et al., 1988). Conditions favoring alprazolam treatment include age over 40, lower baseline levels of anxiety (Hamilton Anxiety Rating Scale) and mild phobic symptoms (Phobia Rating Scale) (Woodman et al., 1994). Although the presence of phobic anxiety and avoidance is associated with a longer duration of illness (Scheibe and Albus, 1996) and an increased severity of panic disorder as measured by disability subscales (Klein et al., 1987), panic patients over the age of 40 tend to have a later age of panic onset (e.g., later clinical admission) (Woodman et al., 1994) and evidence suggests that subjects with a later panic onset have a less severe and more treatment responsive illness (Battaglia et al., 1995). Illness severity measures (e.g., disability scale and agoraphobic avoidance) are more pronounced in panic patients who experience a greater frequency of panic attacks (>2 attacks/week) compared to patients who experienced panic attacks at a lesser frequency (<2 attacks/week) and higher doses of alprazolam (5.2 ± 1.5 mg vs. 3.0 ± 1.6 mg) are required to establish panic free periods (Abelson et al., 1995; 1996). At higher doses (150-250 mg/day, 4-8 weeks) imipramine is also effective in attenuating the severity of panic symptoms including measures of fear in nondepressed panic patients with agoraphobia although subjects continued to experience panic attacks (Mavissakalian, 1996). Hypochondriasis may also be a form of sickness behavior that responds favorably to alprazolam. For example, alprazolam (5.8 mg/day 6 weeks) reduced hypochondriasis (e.g. Illness Behaviour Questionnaire, Pilowsky, 1967) including preoccupation with bodily sensations and fear of physical illness yet had no effect on panic frequency (Noyes et al., 1986). Extensive phobic avoidance, hypochondriasis and relatively high levels of anticipatory anxiety have been associated with non-responsiveness of panic symptoms to conventional drug therapies (Albus et al., 1990; Slaap et al., 1995). Data suggests, however, that the reversible MAO inhibitor, brofaromine, may be effective in ameliorating panic attack frequency associated with severe agoraphobia (Bakish, 1994). Typically cognitive and behavioral interventions, in addition to drug therapies, are utilized to reduce panic symptoms in otherwise treatment resistant patients although cognitive interventions may be employed prior to pharmacological therapy early in diagnosis (Barlow et al., 1989; Buffone, 1991; Clark, 1995; Marks and O'Sullivan, 1987; Robins and Hayes, 1993; Yonkers et al., 1996). Moreover, the introduction of cognitive and behavioral or performance-based strategies in the treatment of panic disorder sustains improvement of panic symptoms during drug treatment and following drug taper (Klosko et al., 1990; Nagy et al., 1993; Spiegel et al., 1994). Despite the demonstrated efficacy of most anti-panic medication in the attenuation of panic symptoms early in the disorder, panic progression typically necessitates adoption of protracted cognitive strategies. Such interventions may reduce the saliency of association cues since pharmacotherapy alone does not yield adequate long-term management of panic disorder. In fact, the effectiveness of performance-based treatment in alleviating phobic symptoms relies on subjective perceptions pertaining to performance adequacy or coping ability in specific tasks (Williams et al., 1989). Taken together, baseline symptoms, panic frequency, depression severity, phobic avoidance and anticipatory anxiety are useful predictors of pharmacological efficacy on outcome scales.

It has been well documented that early diagnosis of panic facilitates pharmacological and cognitive intervention strategies (Albus et al., 1990; Jonas and Cohon, 1993; Keller and Hanks, 1993; Mellergard et al., 1991). Indeed, data derived from various laboratories suggest that the duration of panic disorder (Scheibe and Albus, 1996), the severity and frequency of panic attacks and agoraphobic avoidance (Noyes et al., 1989) prior to treatment is negatively correlated with the efficacy of ensuing therapy. In many instances, illness chronicity appears to complicate treatment owing to the induction of agoraphobia and impairments of social interaction (Bakish, 1994; Scheibe and Albus, 1996). Illness severity as measured by patient reports of more severe panic and agoraphobic symptoms, increased psychiatric hospitalizations and longer duration of panic were predictive of poor pharmacological and cognitive management compared to less severe courses of panic disorder (Noyes et al., 1989). Moreover, illness severity may also reflect an earlier age of onset and panic may be precipitated by childhood events. For example, investigators have alluded to a relationship between a history of childhood anxiety, including separation anxiety, school phobia and familial illness and the development of panic in childhood or early adulthood (Bakish, 1994; Buffone, 1991; Free et al., 1993; Klein, 1995; Pollack et al., 1996; Shear, 1996). It will be recalled that nonhuman primates raised under stressful conditions (e.g., variable foraging demands) reveal aberrant behavior (e.g., hyperactivity, clinging and behavioral inhibition among others) (Rosenblum and Paully, 1984). Studies of nonhuman primates also indicate that infant temperament and qualities of the maternal-infant relationship influence the intensity of separation anxiety. For example, peer-raised animals show exaggerated and persistent attachment behaviors (e.g., exhibit more despair on separation) and display alterations in central NE, DA and 5-HT concentrations relative to maternally fostered animals which may impede the infants later ability to cope with life-stressors (Kraemer, 1992). Clinically, increased anxiety in childhood typically follows illness of a primary caregiver, with the imminent perception of possible death (Roth et al., 1996) and appears to be salient to the eventual induction of panic, (Rosenbaum et al., 1988; Roth, 1996; Shear, 1996). Notably, illness and separation can exacerbate the frequency and severity of panic attacks (Buffone, 1991; Roth, 1996). Not surprisingly, familial illness and sick role behavior can also influence the efficacy of anti-panic medications. For example, children who developed panic disorder following a bout of school phobia respond well to the selective 5-HT reuptake inhibitor, citalopram (20 mg/day). Interestingly, however, panic free periods were temporally shorter among children whose mothers also suffered from panic disorder with agoraphobia (Lepola et al., 1996). Presentation of panic symptomatology following a history of childhood anxiety is typically more severe relative to panic symptoms in patients without a history of childhood anxiety (Bakish, 1994; Buffone, 1991; David et al., 1995; Raskin et al., 1982). For example, at the time of initial panic assessment, patients with childhood anxiety are characterized by greater agoraphobic avoidance as measured by agoraphobic avoidance scales (e.g., Fear

Questionnaire), a longer duration of panic (e.g., childhood onset), more frequent panic attacks and more severe anxiety as indicated by clinical global severity scales (e.g., frequency of panic attacks/week, intensity of anticipatory anxiety, degree of avoidance and degree of social role impairment) (Otto et al., 1994). Patients with a childhood history of anxiety disorders also have a significantly higher rate of comorbidity including social phobia, generalized anxiety disorder, obsessive-compulsive disorder, major depression and a family history of anxiety disorders (Pollack et al., 1996). Moreover, panic disorder following a history of childhood anxiety is typically resistant to pharmacological treatment (Bakish, 1994) and requires lengthy cognitive and psychological counseling (Buffone, 1991; Roth et al., 1996). Taken together, clinical accounts of panic and the heterogeneity of individual treatment responses to alprazolam and imipramine, among others, reveal diversity in prominent symptoms associated with panic disorder. The presence of depression and agoraphobia reflect illness severity and influence the responsivity of panic symptoms to treatment. Moreover, untreated or inadequately treated panic symptoms worsen with time and the progression from uncomplicated to complicated instances of panic are predicated on panic frequency, severity of symptoms, age of onset, coping strategies and familial setting.

The clinical manifestation of panic among panic patients, individuals with Parkinson's disease and schizophrenia among others suggests that stressful life events or the perception of uncontrollable or unpredictable aversive events may influence the emergence and exacerbation of anxiety. Repeated panic experiences influence cognitive activity and may enhance vigilance and somatic monitoring. In nonhuman subjects, the intensity, duration, controllability, predictability and chronicity of an aversive encounter as well as experiential factors (Zacharko and Anisman, 1984; 1991) influence the effectiveness of stressors in modifying ensuing behavioral and neurotransmitter activity. Moreover, presentation of the cues associated with the initial stressor experience can influence the expression of pathology. Similarly, among individuals with diverse panic histories, fear motivated behavior including anticipation of subsequent panic attacks and the development of avoidance behavior are modulated by prior stressor experience (e.g., previous panic attacks) and the cues associated with prior panic episodes (e.g., assignment of a weighting scheme to specific environmental events, Cox et al., 1995). The contribution of mild, stressful life events and DA to the emergence and maintenance of panic symptoms requires clarification. It would be difficult to characterize Parkinson's disease, myasthenia gravis, schizophrenia or major affective disorder with comorbid panic symptoms as mild disturbances from either physiological or cognitive vantages. Yet, sensitization of DA mechanisms and putative involvement with panic disorder is predicated on the assumption that pathology may be augmented owing to progressive encounters with mild, unpredictable and/or uncontrollable life events. It is conceivable that cognitive variations immediately preceding onset of Parkinson's disease or schizophrenia, for example, provide rather subtle cues pertaining to alterations in the emotional and/or physical lability of the individual. Nevertheless, repeated or relatively protracted indices of such cues may be sufficient to sensitize central neurochemical substrates. In addition, mild stressors or environmental cues that elicit comparable cognitive variations may sustain the neurochemical correlates of initial experiences. In effect, such a scenario may eventually define the profile of symptoms and determine vulnerability (e.g., latency to the emergence of psychological dysfunction) to anxiety disorders, including panic.

The emergence of panic necessitates the coupling of conditioned/sensitized DA activity, the behavioral manifestation of such neurochemical activity and central CCK. Interestingly, data collected in this laboratory suggest that mild stressors reliably induce anxiety among nonhuman subjects and more importantly that these anxiogenic indices are exaggerated following central CCK administration at protracted intervals. In effect, long-term responsivity to stressful life events, CCK activation or cross-sensitization between CCK and stressors is dependent on the mild nature and the contextual cues associated with anxiogenic challenge. Notably, initial imposition of a severe stressor or re-exposure of animals to an equally severe stressor or a high dose of CCK does not induce a dissociable increase in behavioral responsivity. The duration of panic disorder prior to the emergence of symptom exacerbation would provide (a) an operational index of the time course of neurochemical sensitization and (b) provide evidence for, but not necessarily identification of, the influence of patient-specific stimuli contributing to illness progression. In accordance with such an argument, imipramine and alprazolam would be expected to exert an influence when administered relatively early in the course of the disorder (e.g., soon after sensitization) and likely prior to clinical diagnosis of panic. Moreover, the pharmacological efficacy of imipramine and alprazolam on panic symptoms in CCK-challenge studies would interact with the dose(s) of CCK employed and panic profile. For example, clinical investigations examining the anti-panic influence of imipramine on CCK-4 induced panic among panic patients revealed that a variable dose of imipramine (150-300 mg/day) and a fluctuating duration of imipramine treatment (3-26 months) was necessary to attain an eight week panic free period following a bolus injection of CCK-4 (50 µg) which subsequently attenuated panic attacks to a rechallenge dose of CCK-4 (20 µg). Notably, 18% of panic patients who had previously panicked with CCK-4 (50 µg) reported a panic attack upon rechallenge (20 µg CCK-4) (Bradwejn et al., 1994). Unfortunately, with respect to CCK-induced panic, panic was predicated on large CCK challenge doses and, from a pharmacological vantage, investigators failed to isolate specific patient characteristics and panic profiles that enhance pharmacological responsiveness or at the very least dictate the dose of imipramine required to attenuate panic naturally. At best, imipramine and alprazolam may prevent exacerbation of panic. Indeed, withdrawal of such therapeutic interventions ordinarily results in the re-emergence and in some cases exacerbation of panic symptoms. To date, the role of CCK in the reemergence of panic symptoms following alprazolam withdrawal remains enigmatic (see Abelson et al., 1995; Akiyoshi et al., 1996; Owens et al., 1989; Owens et al., 1993). However, it should be emphasized that the symptoms diagnostic of Parkinson's disease, schizophrenia or other disorders associated with the emergence of panic worsen over time. In parallel, panic symptoms also are temporally exaggerated. In effect, once sensitization has occurred the profile and/or progression of panic symptoms is relatively dependent upon host factors. Notably, the conditioning of both somatic and cognitive panic symptoms over time and the demonstrated long-term resistance of panic symptomatology to therapeutic interventions support an argument for sensitization (Milrod and Busch, 1996; c.f., Post and Weiss, 1988).

Conclusion

There is no evidence that panic attacks are spontaneous. However, available evidence points to a common etiology across disorders associated with panic. Clinically, the gradual exacerbation of anxiety-like behavior and the appearance of panic are reminiscent of the behavioral and neurochemical alterations in nonhuman subjects repeatedly exposed to anxiogenic stimuli. In fact, it is likely that panic disorder represents a constellation of sensitized behavioral responses (e.g., limited symptom attacks to a full blown panic attack with phobic avoidance) and the inter-subject variability may follow from the differential influence of organismic and experiential variables. Such claims are not surprising as sensitization/conditioning models have been offered as explanations for Parkinson's disease (e.g., l-dopa fluctuations), schizophrenia and depression. Moreover, it appears that variations of CCK availability in specific central sites are associated with variable panic profiles. To date, a conditioning/sensitization hypothesis of panic disorder has not been adequately assessed. To be sure, the nature of the challenge stimuli, including dose and drug schedule, as well as possible cross-sensitization of specific anxiogenic challenges with stressful life events and the long-term repercussions associated with challenge-induced panic in both normal and panic patients must be considered in studies. Moreover, adequate measures of anticipatory anxiety are clearly needed. It will be recalled that CCK availability is linked to colocalization of other neurotransmitters in distinct central sites which suggests that CCK may modulate (a) different aspects of anxiety, including anticipatory reactions to anxiogenic stimuli, (b) variations in cognitive arousal and vigilance and (c) sensitization and conditioning of behavior (e.g., phobic associations) and central neurochemical activity (e.g., DA and GABA). Likewise, multiple anxiogenic agents and putative neurotransmitters or neuromodulators in the mesencephalon, the limbic system as well as prefrontal cortex and brain stem sites would appear to participate in the promotion of anxiety. In fact, it may be the failure of clinical investigations to appreciate the complex interaction of CCK with other neurotransmitter systems, the sensitization of such systems and the contributions of subjective factors to the nature and temporal progression of anxiogenic release that prevents adequate treatment of panic disorder. Conversely, it should be considered that elimination of panic might only occur with prophylactic treatment. In any event, identification of specific subject populations at risk for later development of panic disorder, necessitates empirical demonstration of differential thresholds for panic evocation (e.g., challenge studies) and detailed clinical histories which would demonstrate the circumstances under which panic can be reliably induced (e.g., environmental and cognitive). Taken together a comprehensive analysis of panic and panic-like states requires attention to the specific details outlined in this review regarding dose of challenge, inter-challenge intervals, precise subject characteristics and panic history. Undoubtedly, exacerbation and maintenance of panic in chronic conditions, including Parkinson's disease and schizophrenia, and the divergent panic profiles among panic patients involves sensitization and conditioning of neurochemicals (e.g., DA/CCK) and increased rumination that ultimately influence the effectiveness of therapeutic regimens.

References

Abelson, J. L. and Curtis, G. C. (1996). Hypothalamic-pituitary-adrenal axis activity in panic disorder: prediction of long-term outcome by pretreatment cortisol levels. *American Journal of Psychiatry, 153(1),* 69-73.

Abelson, J. L., Curtis, G. C. and Cameron, O. G. (1996). Hypothalamic-pituitary-adrenal axis activity in panic disorder: effects of alprazolam on 24h secretion of adrenocorticotropin and cortisol. *Journal of Psychiatric Research, 30(*2), 79-93.

Abelson, J.L., Curtis, G. C., Nesse, R. M., Fantone, R., Pyke, R. E. and Bammert-Adams, J. (1995). The effects of central cholecystokinin receptor blockade on hypothalamic-pituitary-adrenal and symptomatic responses to overnight withdrawal from alprazolam. *Biological Psychiatry, 37,* 56-59.

Abelson, J. L. and Nesse, R. M. (1994). Pentagastrin infusions in patients with panic disorder. I. Symptoms and cardiovascular responses. *Biological Psychiatry, 36(2),* 73-83.

Abelson, J. L., Nesse, R. M. and Vinik, A. I. (1994). Pentagastrin infusions in patients with panic disorder. II. Neuroendocrinology. *Biological Psychiatry, 36(2),* 84-96.

Adler, M. W., Rowan, C. H. and Geller, E. B. (1984). Intracerebroventricular vs. subcutaneous drug administration: apples and oranges? *Neuropeptides,* 5, 73-76.

Agid, Y. and Javoy-Agid, F. (1985). Peptides and Parkinson's disease. *Trends in Neurosciences,*8(1), 30-35.

Ahmad, T., Wardle, J. and Hayward, P. (1992). Physical symptoms and illness attributions in agoraphobia and panic. *Behavioral Research Therapy, 30(5),* 493-500.

Akiyoshi, J., Moriyama, T., Isogawa, K., Miyamoto, M., Sasaki, I., Kuga, K., Yamamoto, H.,Yamada, K. and Fujii, I. (1996). CCK-4 induced calcium mobilization in T cells is enhanced in panic disorder. *Journal of Neurochemistry, 66(4),* 1610-1616.

Albus, M. (1988). Cholecystokinin. Progress in Neuro-Psychopharmacology and Biological Psychiatry, 12, S5-S21.

Albus, M., Zahn, T. P. and Breier, A. (1992). Anxiogenic properties of yohimbine. I. Behavioral, physiological, and biochemical measures. *European Archives of Psychiatry and Clinical Neuroscience, 241,* 337-344.

Albus, M., Zahn, T. P. and Breier, A. (1992). Anxiogenic properties of yohimbine. II. Influence of experimental set and setting. *European Archives of Psychiatry and Clinical Neuroscience, 241,* 345-351.

Albus, M., Lecrubier, Y., Maier, W., Buller, R., Rosenberg, R. and Hippius, H. (1990). Drug treatment of panic disorder: early response to treatment as a predictor of final outcome. *Acta Psychiatra Scandinavia, 82,* 359-365.

Alho, H., Costa, E., Ferrero, P., Fujimoto, M., Cosenza-Murphy, D. and Guidotti, A. (1985).Diazepam-binding inhibitor: a neuropeptide located in selected neuronal populations of rat brain. *Science, 229(4709),* 179-182.

Altar, C.A. and Boyar, W.C. (1989). Brain CCK-B receptors mediate the suppression of dopamine release by cholecystokinin. *Brain Research, 483,* 321-326.

American Psychiatric Association (1987). *Diagnostic and statistical manual of mental disorders* (DSM-III). Third edition (revised). Washington, D.C.

American Psychiatric Association (1994). *Diagnostic and statistical manual of mental disorders* (DSM-IV). Fourth edition. Washington, D.C.

Amrein, R., Allen, S. R., Vrasanic, D. and Stahl, M. (1988). Antidepressant drug therapy: associated risk. *Journal of Neural Transmission, 26 (suppl)*: 73-86.

Andersch, S., Rosenberg, N. K., Kullingsjo, H., Ottosson, J. O., Bech, P., Bruun-Hansen, J., Hanson, L., Lorentzen, K., Mellergard, M., Rasmussen, S. and Rosenberg, R. (1991). Efficacy and safety of alprazolam and placebo in treating panic disorder. A Scandinavian multicenter study. *Acta Psychiatra Scandinavia, Suppl. 365*, 18-27.

Anderson, S. M., Kant, G. J. and DeSouza, E. B. (1993). Effects of chronic stress on anterior pituitary and brain corticotropin-releasing factor receptors. *Pharmacology, Biochemistry and Behavior, 44*, 755-761.

Andreoli, A., Keller, S. E., Rabaeus, M., Zaugg, L., Garrone, G. and Taban, C. (1992). Immunity, major depression, and panic disorder comorbidity. *Biological Psychiatry, 31*, 896-908.

Angrist, B. M. and Gershon, S. (1970). The phenomenology of experimentally induced amphetamine psychosis-preliminary observations. *Biological Psychiatry, 2(2)*, 95-107.

Antelman, S. M., Eichler, A. J., Black, C. A. and Kocan, D. (1980). Interchangeability of stress and amphetamine in sensitization. *Science, 207 (18)*, 329-331.

Argyle, N. (1990). Panic attacks in chronic schizophrenia. *British Journal of Psychiatry, 157*, 430-433.

Argyle, N. and Roth, M. (1989). The definition of panic attacks, Part I. *Psychiatry Development, 7(3)*, 175-186.

Aronson, T. A. and Logue, C. M. (1988). Phenomenology of panic attacks: a descriptive study of panic disorder patients' self reports. *Journal of Clinical Psychiatry, 49*, 8-13.

Azorin, J. M. (1995). Long-term treatment of mood disorders in schizophrenia. *Acta Psychiatra Scandinavia , 388(Suppl.)*, 20-23.

Baber, N. S., Dourish, C. T. and Hill, D. R. (1989). The role of CCK, caerulein, and CCK antagonists in nocioception. *Pain, 39*, 307-328.

Bachmann, K. M. and Modestin, J. (1987). Neuroleptic-induced panic attacks in a patient with delusional depression. *Journal of Nervous and Mental Disease, 175(6)*, 373-375.

Bakish, D. 1994). The use of the reversible monoamine oxidase-A inhibitor brofaromine in social phobia complicated by panic disorder with or without agoraphobia. *Journal of Clinical Psychopharmacology, 14(1)*, 74-75.

Bakish, D., Saxena, B. M., Bowen, R. and D'Souza, J. (1993). Reversible monoxidase-A inhibitors in panic disorder. *Clinical Neuropharmacology, 16 (Suppl. 2)*, S77-S82.

Bandelow, B., Sievert, K., Rothemeyer, M., Hajak, G. and Ruther, E. (1995). What treatments do patients with panic disorder and agoraphobia get? *European Archives of Psychiatry and Clinical Neuroscience, 245(3)*, 165-171.

Barlow, D. H., Dinardo, P. A., Vermilyea, B. B., Vermilyea, J. and Blanchard, E. B. (1986). Co-morbidity and depression among the anxiety disorders: issues in diagnosis and classification. *Journal of Nervous and Mental Disease, 174*, 63-72.

Barlow, D. H., Craske, M. G., Cerny, J. A. and Klosko, J. S. (1989). Behavioral treatment of panic disorder. *Behavior Therapy, 20*, 261-282.

Battaglia, M., Bertella, S., Politi, E., Bernardeschi, L., Perna, G., Gabriele, A. and Bellodi, L. (1995). Age at onset of panic disorder: influence of familial liability to the disease and of childhood separation anxiety disorder. *American Journal of Psychiatry, 152 (9)*, 1362-1364.

Baum, K. M. and Walker, E. F. (1995). Childhood behavioral precursors of adult symptom dimensions in schizophrenia. *Schizophrenia Research, 16(2)*, 111-120.

Beatty, W. W. and Holzer, G. A. (1978). Sex differences in stereotyped behavior in the rat. *Pharmacology, Biochemistry and Behavior, 9*, 777-783.

Becker, J. B. and Beer, M. E. (1986). The influence of estrogen on nigrostriatal dopamine activity: behavioral and neurochemical evidence for both pre- and postsynaptic components. *Behavioral Brain Research, 19(1)*, 27-33.

Beinfeld, M. C. and Garvey, D. L. (1991). Concentration of cholecystokinin in cerebrospinal fluid is decreased in psychosis: relationship to symptoms and drug response. *Progress in Neuropsychopharmacology and Biological Psychiatry, 15(5)*, 601-609.

Beinfeld, M. C., Meyer, D. K., Eskay, R. L., Jensen, R. T. and Brownstein, M. J. (1981). The distribution of cholecystokinin in the central nervous system of the rat as determined by radioimmunoassay. *Brain Research, 212*, 51-57.

Beitman, B. D., Mukerji, V., Russell, J. L. and Grafing, M. (1993). Panic disorder in cardiology patients: a review of the Missouri panic/cardiology project. *Journal of Psychiatric Research, 27 (Suppl. 1)*, 35-46.

Bench, C. J., Dolan, R. J., Friston, K. J. and Frackowiak, R. S. J. (1990). Positron emission tomography in the study of brain metabolism in psychiatric and neuropsychiatric disorders. *British Journal of Psychiatry, 157*, 82-95.

Benkelfat, C., Bradwejn, J., Meyer, E., Ellenbogen, M., Milot, S., Gjedde, A. and Evans, A. (1995). Functional neuroanatomy of CCK-4-induced anxiety in normal healthy volunteers. *American Journal of Psychiatry, 152 (8)*, 1180-1184.

Bentsen, H., Boye, B., Munkvold, O. G., Notland, T. H., Lersbryggen, A. B., Oskarsson, K. H., Ulstein, I., Uren, G., Bjorge, H., Berg-Larsen, R., Lingjaerde, O. and Malt, U. F. (1996). Emotional overinvolvement in parents of patients with schizophrenia or related psychosis: demographic and clinical predictors. *British Journal of Psychiatry, 169(5)*, 622-630.

Berg, W. K. and Davis, M. (1984). Diazepam blocks fear-enhanced startle elicited electrically from the brain stem. *Physiology and Behavior, 32(2)*, 333-336.

Blanchard, D. C., Griebel, G. and Blanchard, R. J. (1995). Gender bias in the preclinical psychopharmacology of anxiety: male models for (predominantly) female disorders. *Journal of Psychopharmacology, 9(2)*, 79-82.

Blanchard, D. C., Griebel, G. and Blanchard, R. J. (2003). The Mouse Defense Test Battery: pharmacological and behavioral assays for anxiety and panic. *European Journal of Pharmacology, 463*, 97-116.

Bless, E. P., McGinnis, K. A., Mitchell, A.L., Hartwell, A. and Mitchell, J. B. (1997). The effects of gonadal steroids on brain stimulation reward in female rats. *Behavioural Brain Research, 82*, 235-244.

Bogerts, B., Hantsch, J. and Herzer , M. (1983). A morphometric study of the dopamine-containing cell groups in the mesencephalon of normals, Parkinson patients, and schizophrenics. *Biological Psychiatry, 18(9)*, 951-969.

Bolino, F., Di Michele, V., Di Cicco, L., Manna, V., Daneluzzo, E. and Casacchia, M. (1994).Sensorimotor gating and habituation evoked by electro-cutaneous stimulation in schizophrenia. *Biological Psychiatry, 36(10)*, 670-679.

Borowski, T. B. and Kokkinidis, L. (1996). Contribution of ventral tegmental area dopamine neurons to expression of conditional fear: effects of electrical stimulation, excitotoxin lesions, and quinpirole infusion on potentiated startle in rats. *Behavioral Neuroscience, 110(6)*, 1349-1364.

Bourin, M., Bradwejn, J. and Nixon, M. K. (1993). Provacative agents and the biology of anic attacks. In *Anxiety: Neurobiology, Clinic and Therapeutic Perspectives*. M. Hamon, H. Ollat and M. -H. Thiebot, Eds: 257-292. France: John Libby Eurotext Ltd.

Bourin, M., Malinge, M., Vasar, E. and Bradwejn, J. (1996). Two faces of cholecystokinin: anxiety and schizophrenia. *Fundamentals of Clinical Pharmacology, 10*,116-126.

Bouthillier, A. and de Montigny, C. (1988). Long-term benzodiazepine treatment reduces neuronal responsiveness to cholecystokinin: an electrophysiological study in the rat. *European Journal of Pharmacology, 151*, 135-138.

Boyce, S., Rupniak, N. M. J., Steventon, M. and Iversen, S. D. (1990a). CCK-8S inhibits l-dopa-induced dyskinesias in parkinsonian squirrel monkeys. *Neurology, 40*, 717-718.

Boyce, S., Rupniak, N. M. J., Tye, S., Steventon, M. and Iversen, S. D. (1990b). Modulatory role for CCK-B antagonists in Parkinson's disease. *Clinical Neuropharmacology, 13(4)*, 339-347.

Bradwejn, J. and de Montigny, C. (1984). Benzodiazepines antagonize cholecystokinin-induced activation of rat hippocampal neurones. *Nature, 312 (5992)*, 363-364.

Bradwejn, J. and Koszycki, D. (1991). Comparison of the panicogenic effect of cholecystokinin 30-33 and carbon dioxide in panic disorder. *Progress in Neuro-Psychopharmacology and Biological Psychiatry, 15*, 237-239.

Bradwejn, J. and Koszycki, D. (1994). Imipramine antagonism of the panicogenic effects of cholecystokinin tetrapeptide in panic disorder patients. *American Journal of Psychiatry, 151(2)*, 261-263.

Bradwejn, J., Koszycki, D., Annable, L., Couetoux du Tertre, A., Reines, S., Karkanias, C. (1992). A dose-ranging study of the behavioral and cardiovascular effects of CCK-tetrapeptide in PD. *Biological Psychiatry, 32*, 903-912.

Bradwejn, J., Koszycki, D. and Bourin, M. (1991). Dose ranging study of the effect of CCK-4 in healthy volunteers. *Journal of Psychiatry and Neuroscience, 16*, 260-264.

Bradwejn, J., Koszycki, D. and Shriqui, C. (1991b). Enhanced sensitivity to cholcystokinin tetrapeptide in panic disorder. Clinical and behavioral findings. *Archives of General Psychiatry, 48*, 603-610.

Bradwejn, J., Koszycki, D., Couetoux du Tertre, A., van Megen, H. J. G. M., Den Boer, J. A., Westenberg, H. G. M. and Annable, L. (1995). The panicogenic effects of cholecystokinin-tetrapeptide are antagonized by L-365, 260, a central cholecystokinin receptor antagonist, in patients with panic disorder. *Archives of General Psychiatry, 51*, 486-493.

Bradwejn, J., Koszycki, D., Couetoux du Tertre, A., van Megen, H. J. G. M., Westenberg, H. G. M., Den Boer, J.A., Karkanias, C. and Haigh, J. (1994). The panicogenic effects of cholecystonin tetrapeptide are antagonized by L-365, 260, a central cholecystonin receptor antagonist in patients with panic disorder. *Archives of General Psychiatry, 51*, 486-493.

Bradwejn, J., Koszycki, D. and Meterissian, G. (1990). Cholecystonin tetrapeptide induces panic attacks in patients with panic disorder. *Canadian Journal of Psychiatry, 35*, 83-85.

Bradwejn, J., Koszycki, D., Paradis, M., Reece, P., Hinton, J. and Sedman, A. (1995). Effect of CI-988 on cholecystokinin tetrapeptide-induced panic symptoms in healthy volunteers. *Biological Psychiatry, 38*, 742-746.

Bradwejn, J., Koszycki, D., Payeur, R., Bourin, M. and Borthwick, H. (1992b). Replication of action of cholecystokinin tetrapeptide in panic disorder: clinical and behavioral findings. *American Journal of Psychiatry, 149(7)*, 962-964.

Brambilla, F., Bellodi, L., Perna, G., Garberi, A., Panerai, A. and Sacerdote, P. (1993). Lymphocyte cholecystokinin concentrations in panic disorder. *American Journal of Psychiatry, 150*, 1111-1113.

Branchereau, P., Bohme, J., Champagnat, M. P., Morin-Surun, C., Durieux, C., Blanchard, J. C., Roques, R. C. and Denavit-Saubie, M. (1992). Cholecystokinin$_A$ and cholecystokinin$_B$ receptors in neurons of the brainstem solitary complex of the rat: Pharmacological identification. *Journal of Pharmacology and Experimental Therapeutics, 260*, 1433-1440.

Breier, A., Charney, D. and Heninger, G. (1984). Major depression in patients with agoraphobia and panic disorder. *Archives of General Psychiatry, 41*, 1129-1135.

Bremner, J. D., Krystal, J. H., Southwick, S. M. and Charney, D. S. (1996). Noradrenergic mechanisms in stress and anxiety: I. Preclinical studies. *Synapse, 23*, 28-38.

Brodin, E., Rosen, A., Schott, E. and Brodin, K. (1994). Effects of sequential removal of rats from a group cage, and of individual housing of rats, on substance P, cholecystokinin and somatostatin levels in the periaqueductal grey and limbic regions. *Neuropeptides, 26*, 253-260.

Brodin, K., Ogren, S. V. and Brodin, E. (1994). Clomipramine and clonazepam increase cholecystokinin levels in rat ventral tegmental area and limbic regions. *European Journal of Pharmacology, 263*, 175-180.

Brog, J. S. and Beinfeld, M. C. (1992). Cholecystokinin release from the rat caudate-putamen, cortex and hippocampus is increased by activation of the D1 dopamine receptor. *The Journal of Pharmacology and Experimental Therapeutics, 260(1)*, 343-348.

Bruno, G., Ruggieri, S., Chase, T. N., Bakker, K. and Tamminga, C.A. (1985). Caerulein treatment of Parkinson's disease. *Clinical Neuropharmacology, 8 (3)*, 266-270.

Buffone, G. W. (1991). Treatment of panic disorder: an overview. *Medical Psychotherapy, 4*, 131-144.

Buller, R. (1995). Reversible inhibitors of monoamine oxidase A in anxiety disorders. *Clinical Neuropharmacology, 18* (Suppl. 2), S38-S44.

Bunney, B. S. (1987). Central dopamine- peptide interactions: electrophysiological studies.*Neuropharmacology, 26(7B)*, 1003-1009.

Bunney, B. S. and Aghajanian, G. K. (1976). D-Amphetamine-induced inhibition of central dopaminergic neurons: mediation by a striato-nigral feedback pathway. *Science, 192,* 391-393.

Burazin, T. C. and Gundlach, A. L. (1996). Rapid but transient increases in cholecystokinin mRNA levels in cerebral cortex following amygdaloid-kindled seizures in the rat. *Neuroscience Letters, 209(1),* 65-68.

Busatto, G. F., Pilowsky, L. S., Costa, D. C., Ell, P. J., Verhoeff, N. P. L. G. and Kerwin, R. W.(1995). Dopamine D_2 receptor blockade in vivo with the novel antipsychotics risperidone and remoxipride – an ^{123}I-IBZM single photon emission tomography study. *Psychopharmacology, 117,* 55-61.

Butler, R. W., Mueser, K. T., Sprock, J. and Braff, D. L. (1996). Positive symptoms of psychosis in posttraumatic stress disorder. *Biological Psychiatry, 39,* 839-844.

Bystritsky, A. and Shapiro, D. (1992). Continuous physiological changes and subjective reports in panic patients: a preliminary methodological report. *Biological Psychiatry, 32,* 766-777.

Cabib, S., Kempf, E., Schleef, C., Oliverio, A. and Puglisi-Allegra, S. (1988). Effects of immobilization stress on dopamine and its metabolites in different brain areas of the mouse: role of genotype and stress duration. *Brain Research, 441,* 153-160.

Camp, D. M. and Robinson, T. E. (1988). Susceptibility to sensitization. I. Sex differences in the enduring effects of chronic d-amphetamine treatment on locomotion, stereotyped behavior and brain monoamines. *Behavioral Brain Research, 30,* 55-68.

Carey, R. J. (1991). Chronic L-Dopa treatment in the unilateral 6-OHDA rat: evidence for behavioral sensitization. *Brain Research, 568,* 205-214.

Carey, R. J., Dai, H., Huston, J. P., Pinheiro-Carrera, M., Schwarting, R. K. and Tomaz, C. (1995). L-DOPA metabolism in cortical and striatal tissues in an animal model of parkinsonism. *Brain Research Bulletin, 37(3),* 295-299.

Carey, R. J., Pinheiro-Carrera, M., Dai, H., Tomaz, C. and Huston, J. P. (1995). L-DOPA and psychosis: evidence for L-DOPA-induced increases in prefrontal cortex dopamine and in serum corticosterone. *Biological Psychiatry, 38(10),* 669-676.

Cassano, G. B., Toni, C., Musetti, L., Mengali, F. and Perugi, G. (1994). Prophylactic utility and consequences of long-term medication in panic disorder. *Current Therapeutic Approaches to Panic and Other Anxiety Disorders. International Academy of Biomedical Drug Research, 8,* 36-42.

Cassella, J. V. and Davis, M. (1985). Fear-enhanced startle is not attenuated by acute or chronic imipramine treatment in rats. *Psychopharmacology, 87,* 278-282.

Cassens, G., Roffman, M., Kurac, A., Orsulak, A. and Schildkraut, J. J. (1980). Alterations in brain norepinephrine metabolism induced by environmental stimuli previously paired with inescapable shock. *Science, 209 (5),* 1138-1139.

Chang, R. S., Lotti, V. J., Martin, G. E. and Chen, T. B. (1983). Increase in brain 125I-cholecystokinin (CCK) receptor binding following chronic haloperidol treatment, intracisternal 6-hydroxydopamine or ventral tegmental lesions. *Life Sciences, 32(8),* 871-878.

Chappell, P. B., Smith, M. A., Kilts, C. D., Bisette, G., Ritchie, J., Anderson, C. and Nemeroff, C. B. (1986). Alterations in corticotropin-releasing factor-like immunoreactivity in discrete rat brain regions after acute and chronic stress. *Journal of Neuroscience, 6,* 2908-2914.

Charney, D. S. (2003). Neuroanatomical circuits modulating fear and anxiety behaviors. *Acta Psychiatrica Scandinavica. Supplementum, 417,* 38-50.

Charney, D. S., Breier, A., Jatlow, P. I. and Heninger, G. R. (1986). Behavioral, biochemical, and blood pressure responses to alprazolam in healthy subjects: interactions with yohimbine. *Psychopharmacology, 88(2),* 133-140.

Charney, D. S. and Heninger, G. R. (1985). Noradrenergic function and the mechanism of action of antianxiety treatment. The effect of long-term alprazolam treatment. *Archives of General Psychiatry, 42 (5),* 458-467.

Charney, D. S. and Heninger, G. R. (1986). Abnormal regulation of noradrenergic function in panic disorder: Effects of clonidine in healthy subjects and patients with agoraphobia and panic disorder. *Archives of General Psychiatry, 43,* 1042-1054.

Charney, D. S., Heninger, G. R. and Breier, A. (1984). Noradrenergic function in panic anxiety: effects of yohimbine in healthy subjects and patients with agoraphobia and panic disorder. *Archives of General Psychiatry, 41,* 751-763.

Charney, D. S., Heninger, G. R. and Redmond, D. E. (1983). Yohimbine induced anxiety and increased noradrenergic function in humans: effects of diazepam and clonidine. *Life Sciences, 33,* 19-29.

Charney, D. S., Innis, R. B., Duman, R. S., Woods, S. W. and Heninger, G. R. (1989). Platelet alpha-2-receptor binding and adenylate cyclase activity in panic disorder. *Psychopharmacology, 98,* 102-107.

Charney, D. S., Woods, S. W., Nagy, L. M., Southwick, S. M., Krystal, J. H. and Heninger, G. R. (1990). Noradrenergic function in panic disorder. *Journal of Clinical Psychiatry, 51 (12, Suppl A),* 5-11.

Chase, T. N., Barone, P., Bruno, G., Cohen, S. L., Juncos, J., Knight, M., Ruggeri, S., Steardo, L., and Tamminga, C. A. (1985). Cholecystokinin-mediated synaptic function and the treatment of neuropsychiatric disease. *Annals of the New York Academy of Sciences, 448,* 553-561.

Chen, X., Kombian, S. B. and Pittman, Q. J. (1997). Dopamine depresses excitatory synaptic transmission in the rat parabrachial nucleus in vitro. *Society for Neuroscience Abstracts, 23(2),* 1211.

Chignon, J. -M., Lepine, J. -P. and Ades, J. (1993). Panic in cardiac outpatients. *American Journal of Psychiatry, 150(5),* 780-785.

Chopin, P. and Briley, M. (1993). The benzodiazepine antagonist flumazenil blocks the effects of CCK receptor agonists and antagonists in the elevated plus maze. *Psychopharmacology, 110,* 409-414.

Chung, C. K., Remington, N. D. and Suh, B. Y. (1995). Estrogen replacement therapy may reduce panic symptoms. *Journal of Clinical Psychiatry, 56(11),* 533.

Ciccone, P. E. and Bellettirie, G. F. (1989). A patient with panic disorder eventuating in psychosis: nosologic implications. *Psychiatry Journal University of Ottawa, 14(3),* 478-480.

Clark, D. M. (1995). Cognitive therapy in the treatment of anxiety disorders. *Clinical Neuropharmacology, 18 (Suppl. 2),* S27-S37.

Clark, C. R., McFarlane, A. C., Weber, D.L. and Battersby, M. (1996). Enlarged frontal P300 to stimulus change in panic disorder. *Biological Psychiatry, 39*, 845-856.

Clarke, P. B. S., Jakubovic, A. and Fibiger, H. C. (1988). Anatomical analysis of the involvement of mesolimbicocortical dopamine in the locomotor stimulant actions of d-amphetamine and apomorphine. *Psychopharmacology, 96*, 511-520.

Claustre, Y., Rivy, J. P., Dennis, T. and Scatton, B. (1986). Pharmacological studies on stress-induced increase in frontal cortical dopamine metabolism in the rat. *The Journal of Pharmacology and Experimental Therapeutics, 238 (2)*, 693-700.

Clum, G. A., Clum, G. A. and Surls, R. (1993). A meta-analysis of treatments for panic disorder.*Journal of Consulting and Clinical Psychology, 61 (2)*, 317-326.

Coco, M. L., Kuhn, C. M., Ely, T. D. and Kilts, C. D. (1992). Selective activation of mesoamygdaloid dopamine neurons by conditioned stress: attenuation by diazepam. *Brain Research, 590*, 39-47.

Cole, B. J., Hillmann, M., Seidelmann, D., Klewer, M. and Jones, G. H. (1995). Effects of benzodiazepine receptor partial inverse agonists in the elevated plus maze test of anxiety in the rat. *Psychopharmacology, 121*, 118-126.

Comings, D., Comings, B., Muhleman, D., Dietz, G., Shahbahrami, B., Tast, D., Knell, E., Kocsis, P., Baumgarten, R., Kovacs, B. W., Levy, D. L., Smith, M., Borison, R. L., Evans, D. D., Klein, D. N., MacMurray, J., Tosk, J. M., Sverd, J., Gysin, R. and Flanagan, S. D. (1991).The dopamine D_2 receptor locus as a modifying gene in neuropsychiatric disorders. *Journal of the American Medical Association, 266 (13)*, 1793-1800.

Cook, E. W. III, Davis, T. L., Hawk, L. W., Spence, E. L. and Gauthier, C. H. (1992). Fearfulness and startle potentiation during aversive visual stimuli. *Psychophysiology, 29(6)*, 633-645.

Coplan, J. D., Andrews, M. W., Rosenblum, L. A., Owens, M. J., Friedman, S., Gorman, J. M. and Nemeroff, C. B. (1996). Persistant elevations of cerebrospinal fluid concentrations of corticotropin-releasing factor in adult nonhuman primates exposed to early-life stressors: Implications for the pathophysiology of mood and anxiety disorders. *Proceedings of the National Academy of Science, 93*, 1619-1623.

Cotton, J. D. and Usher, M. (1996). A neural network model of stroop interference and facilitation effects in schizophrenia. *Biological Psychology, 39, 568.*

Cox, B. J., Direnfeld, D. M., Swinson, R. P. and Norton, G. R. (1994). Suicidal ideation and suicide attempts in panic disorder and social phobia. *American Journal of Psychiatry, 151 (6)*, 882-887.

Cox, B. J., Endler, N. S. and Swinson, R. P. (1995). An examination of levels of agoraphobic severity in panic disorder. *Behavioral Research Therapy, 33(1)*, 57-62.

Cox, B. J., Swinson, R. P. and Fergus, K. D. (1993). Changes in fear versus avoidance ratings with behavioral treatments for agoraphobia. *Behavior Therapy, 24*, 619-624.

Craig, T. J., Richardson, M. A., Pass, R. and Bregman, Z. (1985). Measurement of mood and affect in schizophrenic inpatients. *American Journal of Psychiatry, 142(11)*, 1272-1277.

Crawley, J. N. (1985). Clarification of the behavioral functions of peripheral and central cholecystokinin: two separate peptide pools. *Peptides, 6 (Suppl. 2)*, 129-136.

Crawley, J. N. (1988). Modulation of mesolimbic dopaminergic behaviors by cholecystokinin. *Annals New York Academy of Sciences, 537*, 380-396.

Crawley, J. N. (1995). Interactions between cholecystokinin and other neurotransmitter systems.In *Cholecystokinin and Anxiety: From Neuron to Behavior.* J. Bradwejn and E. Vasar, Eds: 101-126. Austin: Springer Verlag-R. G. Landes Company.

Crawley, J. N. and Corwin, R.L. (1994). Biological actions of cholecystokinin. *Peptides, 15(4)*, 731-755.

Crawley, J. N., Hommer, D. W. and Skirboll, L. R. (1984). Behavioral and neurophysiological evidence for a facilitatory interaction between co-existing transmitters: cholecystokinin and dopamine. *Neurochemistry International, 6(6)*, 755-760.

Crawley, J. N., Stievers, J. A., Blumstein, L. K. and Paul, S. M. (1985). Cholecystokinin potentiates dopamine-mediated behaviors: evidence for modulation specific to a site of coexistence. *Journal of Neuroscience, 5*, 1972-1983.

Cross, A. J., Crow, T. J., Ferrier, I. N., Johnstone, E. C., McCreadie, R. M., Owen, F., Owens, D. G. and Poulter, M. (1983). Dopamine receptor changes in schizophrenia in relation to the disease process and movement disorder. *Journal of Neural Transmission, Suppl. 18*, 265-272.

Curtis, G. C., Massana, J., Udina, C., Ayuso, J. L., Cassano, G. B. and Perugi, G. (1993).Maintenance drug therapy of panic disorder. *Journal of Psychiatric Research, 27 (Suppl. 1)*, 127-142.

D'Aquila, P. S., Brain, P. and Willner, P. (1994). Effects of chronic mild stress on performance in behavioral tests relevant to anxiety and depression. *Physiology and Behavior, 56(5)*, 861-867.

Dauge, V., Steimes, P., Derrien, M., Beau, N., Roques, B. P. and Feger, J. (1989). CCK8 effects on motivational and emotional states of rats involve CCK_A receptors of the postero-median part of the nucleus accumbens. *Pharmacology, Biochemistry and Behavior, 34*, 157-163.

David, D., Giron, A. and Mellman, T. A. (1995). Panic-phobic patients and developmental trauma. *Journal of Clinical Psychiatry, 56(3)*, 113-117.

Davidson, J., Raft, D. and Pelton, S. (1987). An outpatient evaluation of phenelzine and imipramine. *Journal of Clinical Psychiatry, 48*, 143-146.

Davis, K.L., Davidson, M., Mohs, R. C., Kendler, K. S., Davis, B. M., Johns, C. A., DeNigris, Y. and Horvarth, T. B. (1985). Plasma homovanillic acid concentration and the severity of schizophrenic illness. *Science, 227*, 1601-1602.

Davis, K. L., Kahn, R. S., Ko, G. and Davidson, M. (1991). Dopamine in schizophrenia: review and reconceptualization. *American Journal of Psychiatry, 148(11)*, 1474-1486.

Davis, M. (1989). Sensitization of the acoustic startle reflex by footshock. *Behavioral Neurology, 103*, 495-503.

Davis, M. (1992). The role of the amygdala in fear-potentiated startle: implications for animal models of anxiety. *Trends in Pharmacological Sciences, 13*, 35-41.

Davis, M., Falls, W. A., Campeau, S. and Kim, M. (1993). Fear-potentiated startle: a neural and pharmacological analysis. *Behavioral Brain Research, 58*, 175-198.

Davis, M., Rainnie, D. and Cassell, M. (1994). Neurotransmission in the rat amygdala related to fear and anxiety. *Trends in Neurosciences, 17(5)*, 208-214.

Day, R. (1981). Life events and schizophrenia: the "triggering" hypothesis. *Acta Psychiatra Scandinavia, 64*, 97-122.

De La Fuente, J. R. (1993). Long-term management of panic disorder. *Current Therapeutic Research, 54 (6)*, 838-851.

De Leeuw, A. S., den Boer, J. A., Slaap, B. R. and Westenberg, H. G. (1996). Pentagastrin has panic inducing properties in obsessive-compulsive disorder. *Psychopharmacology, 126(4)*, 339-344.

De Montigny, C. (1989). Cholecystokinin tetrapeptide induces panic-like attacks in healthy volunteers. *Archives of General Psychiatry, 46*, 511-517.

Derrien, M., Durieux, C., Dauge, V. and Roques, B. P. (1993). Involvement of D2 dopaminergic receptors in the emotional and motivational responses induced by injection of CCK-8 in the posterior part of the rat nucleus accumbens. *Brain Research, 617*, 181-188.

Deutch, A. Y., Tam, S. -Y. and Roth, R. H. (1985). Footshock and conditioned stress increase 3, 4-dihydroxyphenylacetic acid (DOPAC) in the ventral tegmental area but not substantia nigra. *Brain Research, 333*, 143-146.

Di Chiara, G. (1993). Searching for the hidden order in chaos. Commentary on Kalivas et al."The pharmacology and neural circuitry of sensitization to psychostimulants. *Behavioral Pharmacology, 4*, 335-337.

Ding, X. Z. and Mochetti, I. (1992). Dopaminergic regulation of cholecystokinin mRNA content in rat striatum. *Molecular Brain Research, 12*, 77-83.

DiPaolo, T., Bedard, P. J., Dupont, A., Poyet, P. and Labrie, F. (1982). Effects of estradiol on intact and denervated striatal dopamine receptors and on dopamine levels: a biochemical and behavioral study. *Canadian Journal of Physiology and Pharmacology, 60(3)*, 350-357.

Docherty, N. M. (1996). Affective reactivity of symptoms as a process discriminator in schizophrenia. *Journal of Nervous and Mental Disease, 184(9)*, 535-541.

Dohrenwend, B. P. and Egri, G. (1981). Recent stressful life events and episodes of schizophrenia. *Schizophrenia Bulletin, 7(1)*, 12-23.

Donlon, P. T., Rada, R. T. and Arora, K. K. (1976). Depression and the reintegration phase of acute schizophrenia. *American Journal of Psychiatry, 133(11)*, 1265-1268.

Dorow, R. (1987). FG 7142 and its anxiety inducing effects in humans. *British Journal of Clinical Pharmacology, 23*, 781-782.

Dourish, C. T., Ruckert, A. S., Tattersall, F. D. and Iversen, S. D. (1989). Evidence that decreased feeding induced by systemic injection of cholecystokinin is mediated by CCK-A receptors. *European Journal of Pharmacology, 173*, 233-234.

Duncan, G. E., Breese, G. R., Criswell, H., Stumpf, W. E., Mueller, R. A. and Covey, J. B. (1986). Effects of antidepressant drugs injected into the amygdala on behavioral responses of rats in the forced swim test. *Journal of Pharmacology and Experimental Therapeutics, 238(2)*, 758-762.

Durieux, C., Pelaprat, D., Charpentier, B., Morgat, J. -L. and Roques, B. P. (1988). Characterization of [^{3}H] CCK$_4$ binding sites in mouse and rat brain. *Neuropeptides, 12,* 141-148.

Eichler, A. J. and Antelman, S. M. (1979). Sensitization to amphetamine and stress may involve nucleus accumbens and medial frontal cortex. *Brain Research, 176,* 412-416.

Ellison, G. (1994). Stimulant-induced psychosis, the dopamine theory of schizophrenia, and the habenula. *Brain Research Reviews, 19,* 223-239.

Emson, P. C., Lee, C. M. and Rehfeld, J. F. (1980). Cholecystokinin octapeptide: vesicular localization and calcium dependent release from rat brain in vitro. *Life Sciences, 26,* 2157-2163.

Eriksson, E., Westberg, P., Alling, C., Thuresson, K. and Modigh, K. (1991). Cerebrospinal fluid levels of monoamine metabolites in panic disorder. *Psychiatry Research, 36,* 243-251.

Evans, L., Kenardy, J., Schneider, P. and Hoey, H. (1986). Effect of a selective serotonin uptake inhibitor in agoraphobia with panic attacks. A double blind comparison of zimeldine, imipramine and placebo. *Acta Psychiatra Scandinavia, 73,* 49-53.

Factor, S. A., Molho, E. S., Podskalny, G. D. and Brown, D. (1995). Parkinson's disease: drug induced psychiatric states. *Advances in Neurology, 65,* 115-138.

Fadda, F., Argiolas, A., Melis, M. R., Tissari, A. H., Onali, P. L. and Gessa, G. L. (1978). Stress induced increase in 3,4-dihydroxyphenylacetic acid (DOPAC) levels in the cerebral cortex and in nucleus accumbens: reversal by diazepam. *Life Sciences, 23,* 2219-2224.

Faravelli, C. (1985). Life events preceding the onset of panic disorder. *Journal of Affective Disorders, 9,* 103-105.

Farmery, S. M., Owen, F., Poulter, M. and Crow, T. J. (1985). Reduced high activity cholecystokinin binding in hippocampus and frontal cortex of schizophrenic patients. *Life Sciences, 36,* 473-477.

Fernandez, A., de Ceballos, M. L., Jenner, P. and Marsden, C. D. (1992). Striatal neuropeptide levels in Parkinson's disease patients. *Neuroscience Letters, 145,* 171-174.

Ferrarese, C., Mennini, T., Pecora, N., Pierpaoli, C., Frigo, M., Marzorati, C., Gobbi, M., Bizzi, A., Codegoni, A., Garattini, S. and Frattola, L. (1991). Diazepam binding inhibitor (DBI) increases after acute stress in rat. *Neuropharmacology, 30(12B),* 1445-1452.

Ferrier, I. N., Crow, T. J., Farmery, S. M., Roberts, G. W., Owen, F., Adrian, T. E. and Bloom, S. R. (1985). Reduced cholecystokinin levels in the limbic lobe in schizophrenia. A marker for pathology underlying the defect state. *Annals of the New York Academy of Sciences, 448,* 495-506.

Ferrier, I. N., Roberts, G. W., Crow, T. J., Johnstone, E. C., Owens, D. G., Lee, Y. C., O'Shaughnessy, D., Adrian, T. E., Polak, J. M. and Bloom, S. R. (1983). Reduced cholecystokinin-like and somatostatin-like immunoreactivity in limbic lobe is associated with negative symptoms in schizophrenia. *Life Sciences, 33(5),* 475-482.

File, S. E. (1993). The interplay of learning and anxiety in the elevated plus maze. *Behavioural Brain Research, 58,* 199-202.

File, S. E. and Zangrossi, H. (1993). "One trial tolerance" to the anxiolytic actions of benzodiazepines in the elevated plus-maze, or the development of a phobic state? *Psychopharmacology, 110,* 240-244.

Flaum, M. and Schultz, S. K. (1996). When does amphetamine-induced psychosis become schizophrenia. *American Journal of Psychiatry, 153(6),* 812-815.

Fontaine, R., Chouinard, G. and Annable, L. (1984). Rebound anxiety in anxious patients after abrupt withdrawal of benzodiazepine treatment. *American Journal of Psychiatry, 141,* 848-852.

Forman, S. D., Bissette, G., Tao, J., Nemeroff, C. B. and van Kammen, D. P. (1994). Cerebrospinal fluid corticotropin-releasing factor increases following haloperidol withdrawal in chronic schizophrenia. *Schizophrenia Research, 12(1),* 43-51.

Fortin, G., Branchereau, P., Araneda, S. and Champagnat, J. (1992). Rhythmic activities in the rat solitary complex in vitro. *Neuroscience Letters, 145,* 23-27.

Fowles, D. C. (1992). Schizophrenia:diathesis-stress revisited. *Annual Reviews in Psychology, 43,* 303-336.

Frankland, P. W., Josselyn, S. A., Bradwejn, J., Vaccarino, F. J. and Yeomans, J. S. (1996). Intracerebroventricular infusion of the CCK_B receptor agonist pentagastrin potentiates acoustic startle. *Brain Research, 733,* 129-132.

Frankland, P. W., Josselyn, S. A., Bradwejn, J., Vaccarino, F. J. and Yeomans, J. S. (1997). Activation of amygdala cholecystokininB receptors potentiates the acoustic startle response in the rat. *The Journal of Neuroscience, 17(5),* 1838-1847.

Free, N. K., Winget, C. N. and Whitman, R. M. (1993). Separation anxiety in panic disorder. *American Journal of Psychiatry, 150 (4),* 595-599.

Frey, P. (1983). Changes in cholecystokinin content in rat brain after subchronic treatment with neuroleptics. *Annals New York Academy of Science, 95(1-2),* 601-603.

Fukamauchi, F. (1996). Changes in cholecystokinin mRNA expression in methamphetamine induced behavioral sensitization. *Neurochemistry International, 28 (4),* 391-394.

Fux, M., Taub, M., Zohar, J. (1993). Emergence of depressive symptoms during treatment for panic disorder with specific 5-hydroxytryptophan reuptake inhibitors. *Acta Psychiatrica Scandinavica, 88,* 235-237.

Fuxe, K., Agnati, L. F., Benefenati, F., Cimmino, M., Algeri, S., Hokfelt, T. and Mutt, V. (1981). Modulation by cholecystokinins of 3H-spiroperidol binding in rat striatum: evidence for increased affinity and reduction in number of binding sites. *Acta Physiologica Scandinavia, 113,* 567-569.

Fuxe, K., Ogren, S. O., Agnati, L. F., Andersson, K. and Eneroth, P. (1982). Effects of subchronic antidepressant drug treatment on central serotonergic mechanisms in the male rat. *Advances in Biochemistry and Psychopharmacology, 31,* 91-107.

Gall, C., Lautervorn, J., Burks, D. and Seroogy, K. (1987). Colocalization of enkephalin and cholecystokinin in discrete areas of rat brain. *Brain Research, 403,* 403-408.

Gardner, C. R. and Budhram, P. (1987). Effects of agents which interact with central benzodiazepine binding sites on stress-induced ultrasounds in rat pups. *European Journal of Pharmacology, 134,* 275-283.

Gardner, W. N. (1996). The pathophysiology of hyperventilation disorders. *Chest, 109,* 516-534.

Garnefski, N., van Egmond, M. and Straatman, A. (1990). The influence of early and recent life stress on severity of depression. *Acta Psychiatra Scandinavia, 81(3)*, 295-301.

Gelsema, A. J., McKitrick, D. J. and Calaresu, F. R. (1987). Cardiovascular responses to chemical and electrical stimulation of amygdala in rats. *American Journal of Physiology,* 253, R712-R718.

Gibbs, J., Young, R. C. and Smith, G. P. (1973). Cholecystokinin decreases food intake in rats. *Journal of Comprehensive Physiological Psychology, 84*, 488-495.

Goetz, R. R., Klein, D. F., Gully, R., Kahn, J., Liebowitz, M. R., Fyer, A. J. and Gorman, J. M. (1993). Panic attacks during placebo procedures in the laboratory. *Archives of General Psychiatry, 50*, 280-285.

Goodwin, R., Lyons, J. S. and McNally, R. J. (2002). Panic attacks in schizophrenia. *Schizophrenia Research, 58*, 213-220.

Gorman, J. M., Liebowitz, M. R., Fyer, A. J. and Stein, J. (1989). A neuroanatomical hypothesis for panic disorder. *American Journal of Psychiatry, 146(2)*, 148-159.

Grant, B. F., Hasin, D. S., Stinson, F. S., Dawson, D. A., Goldstein, R. B., Smith, S., Huang, B. and Saha, T. D. (2006). The epidemiology of DSM-IV panic disorder ad agoraphobia in the United States: results from the national epidemiologic survery on alcohol and related conditions. *The Journal of Clinical Psychiatry, 67*, 363-374.

Gray, T. S. (1991). Limbic pathways and neurotransmitters as mediators of autonomic and neuroendocrine responses to stress. In *Stress: Neurobiology and Neuroendocrinology*. M. R. Brown, G. F. Koob and C. Riviere, Eds. New York: Marcel Dekker Inc.

Griebel, G., Blanchard, D. C. and Blanchard, R. J. (1996). Predator-elicited flight responses in swiss-webster mice: an experimental model of panic attacks. *Progress in Neuro-Psychopharmacology and Biological Psychiatry,* 20, 185-205.

Grijalva, C. V., Levin, E. D., Morgan, M., Roland, B. and Martin, F. C. (1989). Contrasting effects of centromedial and basolateral amygdaloid lesions on stress-related responses in the rat. *Physiology and Behavior, 48*, 495-500.

Grillon, C., Ameli, R., Goddard, A., Woods, S. W. and Davis, M. (1994). Baseline and fear potentiated startle in panic disorder patients. *Biological Psychiatry, 35*, 431-439.

Grillon, C., Ameli, R., Merikangas, K., Woods, S. W. and Davis, M. (1993). Measuring the time course of anticipatory anxiety using the fear-potentiated startle reflex. *Psychophysiology, 30*, 340-346.

Grilo, C. M., Becker, D. F., Fehon, D. C., Walker, M. L., Edell, W. S. and McGlashen, T. H. (1996). Gender differences in personality disorders in psychiatrically hospitalized adolescents. *American Journal of Psychiatry, 153(8)*, 1089-1091.

Grunhaus, L., Harel, Y., Krugler, T., Pande, A. and Haskett, R. F. (1988). Major depressive disorder and panic disorder. *Clinical Neuropharmacology, 11*, 454-461.

Grunhaus, L., Pande, A. C., Brown, M. B. and Greden, J.F. (1994). Clinical characteristics of patients with concurrent major depressive disorder and panic disorder. *American Journal of Psychiatry, 151(4)*, 541-546.

Guidotti, A., Forchetti, C. M., Corda, M. G., Konkel, D., Bennett, C. D. and Costa, E. (1983). Isolation, characterization, and purification to homogeneity of an endogenous polypeptide with agonistic action on benzodiazepine receptors. *Proceeds of the National Academy of Science, 80(11)*, 3531-3535.

Guthrie, S. K., Grunhaus, L., Pande, A. C. and Hariharan, M. (1993). Noradrenergic response to intravenous yohimbine in patients with depression and comorbidity of depression and panic. *Biological Psychiatry, 34,* 558-561.

Hamamura, T. and Fibiger, H. C. (1993). Enhanced stress-induced dopamine release in the prefrontal cortex of amphetamine-sensitized rats. *European Journal of Pharmacology, 237,* 65-71.

Harhammer, R., Schafer, U., Henklein, P., Ott, T. and Repke, H. (1991). CCK-8-related C-terminal tetrapeptides: affinities for central CCK_B and peripheral CCK_A receptors. *European Journal of Pharmacology, 209,* 263-266.

Harrington, P. J., Schmidt, N. B. and Telch, M. J. (1996). Prospective evaluation of panic potentiation following 35% CO_2 challenge in nonclinical subjects. *American Journal of Psychiatry, 153(6),* 823-825.

Harris, J. A. and Westbrook, R. F. (1995). Effects of benzodiazepine microinjection into the amygdala or periaqueductal gray on the expression of conditioned fear and hypoalgesia in rats. *Behavioral Neuroscience, 109(2),* 295-304.

Harro, J., Kiivet, R. A., Lang, A. and Vasar, E. (1990). Rats with anxious or non-anxious type of exploratory behavior differ in their CCK-8 and benzodiazepine receptor characteristics. *Behavioral Brain Research, 39,* 63-71.

Harro, J., Lofberg, C., Rehfeld, J. F. and Oreland, L. (1996). Cholecystokinin peptides and receptors in the rat brain during stress. *Naunyn-Schmiedeberg's Archives of Pharmacology, 354,* 59-66.

Harro, J., Marcussen, J. and Oreland, L. (1992). Alterations in brain cholecystokinin receptors in suicide victims. *European Journal of Pharmacology, 2,* 57-63.

Harro, J. and Oreland, L. (1992). Age-related differences of cholecystokinin receptor binding in the rat brain. *Progress in Neuro-Psychopharmacology and Biological Psychiatry, 16,* 369-375.

Harro, J. and Oreland, L. (1993). Cholecystokinin receptors and memory: a radial maze study. *Pharmacology, Biochemistry and Behavior, 44,* 509-517.

Harro, J. and Vasar, E. (1991). Cholecystokinin-induced anxiety: how is it reflected in studies on exploratory behavior. *Neuroscience and Biobehavioral Reviews, 15,* 473-477.

Harro, J. and Vasar, E. (1991). Evidence that CCK_B receptors mediate the regulation of exploratory behavior in the rat. *European Journal of Pharmacology, 193,* 379-381.

Harro, J., Vasar, E. and Bradwejn, J. (1993). CCK in animal and human research on anxiety. *Trends in Pharmacological Sciences, 14,* 244-249.

Harrow, M., Yonan, C. A., Sands, J. R. and Marengo, J. (1994). Depression in schizophrenia: are neuroleptics, akinesia, or anhedonia involved? *Schizophrenia Bulletin, 20(2),* 327-338.

Hatfield, A. B. (1989). Patients' accounts of stress and coping in schizophrenia. *Hospital Community Psychiatry, 40(11),* 1141-1145.

Hebb, A.L.O., Poulin, J.F., Roach, S.P., Zacharko, R.M., Drolet, G. (2005a). Cholecystokinin and endogenous opioid peptides: interactive influence on pain, cognition, and emotion. *Progress in Neuropsychopharmacology and Biological Psychiatry, 29(8),* 1225-1238.

Hebb, A.L.O., Laforest, S. and G. Drolet. (2005b). Endogenous opioids, stress and psychopathology. In: *Handbook of Stress and the Brain* Vol 15. Part 1 Neurobiology of Stress Edited by T Steckler, N H Kalin, and JMHM Reul , Elsevier, 561-583.

Heila, H., Isometsa, E. T., Henriksson, M. M., Heikkinen, M. E., Marttunen, M. J. and Lonnqvist, J. K. (1997). Suicide and schizophrenia: a nationwide psychological autopsy study on age- and sex-specific clinical characteristics of 92 suicide victims with schizophrenia. *American Journal of Psychiatry, 154(9)*, 1235-1242.

Heinsbroek, R. W., van Haaren, F., Feenstra, M. G. P., Van Galen, H., Boer, G. and Van De Poll, N. E. (1990). Sex differences in the effects of inescapable footshock on central catecholaminergic and serotonergic activity. *Pharmacology, Biochemistry and Behavior, 37*, 539-550.

Hendry, S. H. C., Jones, E. G., DeFelipe, J., Schmechel, D., Brandon, C. and Emson, P. C. (1984). Neuropeptide-containing neurons of the cerebral cortex are also GABAergic. *Proceedings of the National Academy of Science, 81*, 6526-6530.

Hetem, L. A. B. (1996). Addition of d-fenfluramine to benzodiazepines produces a marked improvement in refractory panic disorder- a case report. *Journal of Clinical Psychopharmacology, 16(1),* 77-78.

Heun, R. and Maier, W. (1995). Relation of schizophrenia and panic disorder: evidence from a controlled family study. *American Journal of Medical Genetics (Neuropsychiatric Genetics), 60,* 127-132.

Higgins, G. A., Joharchi, N., Wang, Y., Corrigall, W. A. and Sellars, E. M. (1994). The CCK_A receptor antagonist devazepide does not modify opioid self-administration or drug discrimination: comparison with the dopamine antagonist haloperidol. *Brain Research,* 640, 246-254.

Higgins, G. A., Sills, T. L., Tomkins, D. M., Sellers, E. M. and Vaccarino, F. J. (1994). Evidence for the contribution of CCK_B receptor mechanisms to individual differences in amphetamine-induced locomotion. *Pharmacology, Biochemistry, and Behavior, 48 (4)*, 1019-1024.

Hijzen, T. H., Houtzager, S. W. J., Joordens, R. J. E., Olivier, B. and Slangen, J. L. (1995). Predictive validity of the potentiated startle response as a behavioral model for anxiolytic drugs. *Psychopharmacology, 118*, 150-154.

Hill, D. R., Campbell, N. J., Shaw, T. M. and Soodruff, G. N. (1987). Autoradiographic localization and biochemical characterization of peripheral type CCK receptors in rat CNS using highly selective non-peptide CCK antagonists. *Journal of Neuroscience, 7,* 2967-2977.

Hirosue, Y., Inui, A., Miura, M., Nakajima, M., Okita, M., Himori, N., Baba, S. and Kasuga, M. (1992). Effects of CCK antagonists on CCK-induced suppression of locomotor activity in mice. *Peptides, 13*, 155-157.

Hitchcock, J. M., Sananes, C. B. and Davis, M. (1989). Sensitization of the startle reflex by footshock: blockade by lesions of the central nucleus of the amygdala or its efferent pathway to the brainstem. *Behavioral Neuroscience, 103(3)*, 509-518.

Hoehn-Saric, R. (1982). Neurotransmitters in anxiety. *Archives of General Psychiatry, 39*, 735-742.

Hoehn-Saric, R., McLeod, D. R. and Hipsley, P. A. (1993). Effect of fluvoxamine on panic disorder. *Journal of Clinical Psychopharmacology, 13(5)*, 321-326.

Hoehn-Saric, R., McLeod, D. R. and Zimmerli, W. D. (1991). Psychophysiological response patterns in panic disorder. *Acta Psychiatra Scandinavia, 83(1)*, 4-11.

Hokfelt, T., Johansson, O., Ljungdahl, A., Lundberg, J. M. and Schultzberg, M. (1980). Peptidergic neurones. *Nature, 284*, 165-171.

Hokfelt, T., Morino, P., Verge, V., Castel, M. N., Broberger, C., Zhang, X., Herrera-Marschitz, M., Meana, J. J., Ungerstedt, U., Xu, X. J., Hao, J. X., Puke, M. J. C., Wiesenfeld-Hallin, Z. S., Seigler, A., Hughes, J., Varro, A. and Dockray, G. (1994). CCK in cerebral cortex and at the spinal level. *Annals of the New York Academy of Science, 713*, 157-163.

Hokfelt, T., Rehfeld, J., Skirboll, L., Ivemark, B., Goldstein, M. and Markey, K. (1980). Evidence for coexistence of dopamine and CCK in mesolimbic neurones. *Nature, 285*, 476.

Hokfelt, T., Skirboll, L., Everitt, B., Meister, B., Brownstein, M., Jacobs, T., Faden, A., Kuga, S., Goldstein, M., Markstein, R., Dockray, G. and Rehfeld, J. (1985). Distribution of cholecystokinin-like immunoreactivity in the nervous system. Co-existence with classical neurotransmitters and other neuropeptides. *Annals of the New York Academy of Sciences*, 255-273.

Hokfelt, T., Skirboll, L., Rehfeld, J., Goldstein, M., Markey, K. and Dann, O. (1980). A subpopulation of mesencephalic dopamine neurons projecting to limbic areas contains a cholecystokinin-like peptide: evidence from immunohistochemistry combined with retrograde tracing. *Neuroscience, 5*, 2093.

Hokfelt, T., Tsuruo, Y., Meister, B., Melander, T., Schalling, M. and Everitt, B. (1987). Localization of neuroactive substances in the hypothalamus with special reference to coexistence of messenger molecules. *Advances in Experimental and Medical Biology, 219*, 21-45.

Holcomb, H. H., Cascella, N. G., Thaker, G. K., Medoff, D. R., Dannals, R. F. and Tamminga, C. A. (1996). Functional sites of neuroleptic drug action in the human brain: PET/FDG studies with and without haloperidol. *American Journal of Psychiatry, 153(1)*, 41-49.

Hommer, D. W., Pickar, D., Crawley, J. N., Weingartner, H. and Paul, S. M. (1985). The effects of cholecystokinin-like peptides in schizophrenics and normal human subjects. *Annals of the New York Academy of Sciences, 448*, 542-551.

Hommer, D. W. and Skirboll, L. R. (1983). Cholecystokinin-like peptides potentiate apomorphine induced inhibition of dopamine neurons. *European Journal of Pharmacology, 91*, 151-152.

Honda, T., Wada, E., Battey, J. F. and Wank, S. A. (1993). Differential gene expression of CCK_A and CCK_B receptors in the rat brain. *Molecular Cell Neuroscience, 4*, 143-154.

Horinouchi, Y., Akiyoshi, J., Nagata, A., Matsushita, H., Tsutsumi, T., Isogawa, K., Noda, T. and Nagayama, H. (2004). Reduced anxious behavior in mice lacking the CCK2 receptor gene. *European Neuropsychopharmacology, 14*, 157-161.

Hopkins, D. A. and Holstege, G. (1978). Amygdaloid projections to the mesencephalon, pons and medulla oblongata in the cat. *Experimental Brain Research, 32*, 529-547.

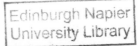

Hruska, R. E. and Silbergeld, E. K. (1980). Estrogen treatment enhances dopamine receptor sensitivity in the rat striatum. *European Journal of Pharmacology, 61(4),* 397-400.

Hurd, Y. L., Lindefors, N., Brodin, E., Brene, S., Persson, H., Ungerstedt, U. and Hokfelt, T. (1992). Amphetamine regulation of mesolimbic dopamine/cholecystokinin neurotransmission. *Brain Research, 578,* 317-326.

Ida, Y., Tsuda, A., Sueyoshi, K., Shirao, I. and Tanaka, M. (1988). Blockade by diazepam of conditioned fear-induced activation of rat mesoprefrontal dopamine neurons. *Pharmacology, Biochemistry and Behavior, 33,* 477-479.

Imperato, A., Puglisi-Allegra, S., Casolini, P., Zocchi, A. and Angelucci, L. (1989). Stress induced enhancement of dopamine and acetylcholine release in limbic structures: role of corticosterone. *European Journal of Pharmacology, 165,* 337-338.

Inoue, T., Tsuchiya, K. and Koyama, T. (1994). Regional changes in dopamine and serotonin activation with various intensity of physical and psychological stress in the rat brain. *Pharmacology, Biochemistry and Behavior, 49(4),* 911-920.

Ivy, A. C. and Oldberg, E. (1928).Hormone mechanism for gallbladder contraction and evacuation. *American Journal of Physiology, 86,* 599-613.

Jackson, D. M. and Westlind-Danielsson, A. (1994). Dopamine receptors: molecular biology, biochemisty and behavioural aspects. *Pharmacological Therapy, 64,* 291-369.

Jackson, H. C. and Nutt, D. J. (1993). A single preexposure produces sensitization to the locomotor effects of cocaine in mice. *Pharmacology, Biochemistry, and Behavior, 45,* 733-735.

Jenck, F., Moreau, J. L. and Martin, J. R. (1995). Dorsal periaqueductal gray-induced aversion as a simulation of panic anxiety:elements of face and predictive validity. *Psychiatry Research, 57(2),* 181-191.

Jhamandas, J. H. and Harris, K. M. (1992). Influence of nucleus tractus solitarius stimulation and baroreceptor activation on rat parabrachial neurons. *Brain Research Bulletin, 28,* 565-571.

Johanning, H., Plenge, P. and Mellerup, E. (1992). Serotonin receptors in the brain of rats treated chronically with imipramine or RU 24969: support for the 5-HTIB receptor being a 5-HT autoreceptor. *Pharmacology and Toxicology, 70(2),* 131-134.

Johnson, M. R., Lydiard, R. B., Zealberg, J. J., Fossey, M. D. and Ballenger, J. C. (1994). Plasma and CSF HVA levels in panic patients with comorbid social phobia. *Biological Psychiatry, 36,* 426-427.

Johnson, N. J. and Rodgers, R. J. (1996). Ethological analysis of cholecystokinin (CCK$_A$ and CCK$_B$) receptor ligands in the elevated plus-maze test of anxiety in mice. *Psychopharmacology, 124(4),* 355-64 1996.

Jonas, J. M. and Cohon, M. S. (1993). A comparison of the safety and efficacy of alprazolam versus other agents in the treatment of anxiety, panic, and depression: a review of the literature. *Journal of Clinical Psychiatry, 54 (10),* 25-45.

Jones, B. C., Campbell, A. D., Radcliffe, R. A. and Erwin, V. G. (1992). Psychomotor stimulant effect of cocaine is affected by genetic makeup and experimental history. In *The Neurobiology of Drug and Alcohol Addiction, 654,* 456-458. New York: Annals of the New York Academy of Sciences.

Jordan, B. K., Schlenger, W. E., Hough, R., Kulka, R. A., Weiss, D., Fairbank, J. A. and Marmar, C. R. (1991). Lifetime and current prevalence of specific psychiatric disorders among vietnam veterans and controls. *Archives of General Psychiatry, 48,* 207-215.

Josselyn, S. A., Franco, V. P. and Vaccarino, F. J. (1996). Devazepide, a CCK$_A$ antagonist, impairs the acquisition of conditioned reward and conditioned activity. *Psychopharmacology, 123(2),* 131-143.

Josselyn, S. A., Frankland, P. W., Petrisano, S., Bush, D. E., Yeomans, J. S. and Vaccarino, F. J. (1995). The CCK$_B$ antagonist, L-365,260, attenuates fear-potentiated startle. *Peptides, 16(7),* 1313-1315.

Kahn, J. P., Krusin, R. E. and Klein, D. F. (1987). Schizophrenia, panic anxiety and alprazolam (letter). *American Journal of Psychiatry, 144,* 527-528.

Kahn, J. P., Puertollano, M. A., Schane, M. D. and Klein, D. F. (1988). Adjunctive alprazolam for schizophrenia with panic anxiety: clinical observation and pathogenetic implications. *American Journal of Psychiatry, 145(6),* 742-744.

Kapur, S., Remington, G., Jones, C., Wilson, A., DaSilva, J., Houle, S. and Zipursky, R. (1996). High levels of dopamine D2 receptor occupancy with low-dose haloperidol treatment: A PET study. *American Journal of Psychiatry, 153 (7),* 948-950.

Kalivas, P. W., Duffy, P., Abhold, R. and Dilts, R. P. (1988). Sensitization of mesolimbic dopamine neurons by neuropeptides and stress. In *Sensitization in the Nervous System.* P. W. Kalivas and C. D. Barnes, Eds: 119-142. New Jersey: Telford Press.

Kalivas, P. W., Sorg, B. A. and Hooks, M. S. (1993). The pharmacology and neural circuitry of sensitization to psychostimulants. *Behavioral Pharmacology, 4,* 315-334.

Kalivas, P. W. and Stewart, J. (1991). Dopamine transmission in the initiation and expression of drug- and stress-induced sensitization of motor activity. *Brain Research Reviews, 16,* 223-244.

Kalivas, P. W., Striplin, C., Steketee, J. D., Klitenick, M. A. and Duffy, P. (1992). Cellular mechanisms of behavioral sensitization to drugs of abuse. *Annals of the New York Academy of Science, 654,* 128-135.

Kariya, K., Tanaka, J. and Nomura, M. (1994). Systemic administration of CCK-8S, but not CCK-4, enhances dopamine turnover in the posterior nucleus accumbens: a microdialysis study in freely moving rats. *Brain Research, 657,* 1-6.

Kasdorf, J. A., Kasdorf, J. L. and Janzen, W. B. (1988). Panic attacks: are they spontaneous? *Phobia Practice and Research Journal, 1 (1),* 32-47.

Kaschka, W., Feistel, H. and Ebert, D. (1995). Reduced benzodiazepine receptor binding in panic disorders measured by iomazenil spect. *Journal of Psychiatric Research, 29 (5),* 427-434.

Kathol, R. G., Noyes, R. and Lopez, A. (1988). Similarities in hypothalamic-pituitary-adrenal axis activity between patients with panic disorder and those experiencing external stress. *Psychiatry Clinical North America, 11(2),* 335-348.

Katsuura, G., Itoh, S. and Hsiao, S. (1985). Specificity of nucleus accumbens to activities related to cholecystokinins in rats. *Peptides, 6,* 91-96.

Kayser, A., Robinson, D. S., Yingling, K., Howard, D. B., Corcella, J. and Laux, D. (1988). The influence of panic attacks on response to phenelzine and amitriptyline in depressed outpatients. *Journal of Clinical Psychopharmacology, 8(4),* 246-253.

Keck, P. E., McElroy, S. L., Tugrul, K. C., Bennett, J. A. and Smith, J. M. R. (1993). Antiepileptic drugs for the treatment of panic disorder. *Neuropsychobiology, 27*, 150-153.

Keefe, K. A., Stricker, E. M., Zigmond, M. J. and Abercrombie, E. D. (1990). Environmental stress increases extracellular dopamine in striatum of 6-hydroxydopamine-treated rats: in vivo microdialysis studies. *Brain Research, 527*, 350-353.

Kelland, M. D., Zhang, J., Chiodo, L. A. and Freeman, A. S. (1991). Receptor selectivity of cholecystokinin effects on mesoaccumbens dopamine neurons. *Synapse, 8*, 137-143.

Keller, M. B. and Hanks, D. L. (1993). Course and outcome in panic disorder. *Progress in Neuro-Psychopharmacology and Biological Psychiatry, 17*, 551-570.

Keller, M. B., Lavori, P. W., Goldenberg, I. M., Baker, L. A., Pollack, M. H., Sachs, G. S., Rosenbaum, J. F., Deltito, J. A., Leon, A., Shear, K. and Klerman, G. L. (1993). Influence of depression on the treatment of panic disorder with imipramine, alprazolam and placebo. *Journal of Affective Disorders, 28*, 27-38.

Kellner, R., Wilson, R. M., Muldawer, M. D. and Pathak, D. (1975). Anxiety in schizophrenia. The responses to chlordiazepoxide in an intensive design study. *Archives of General Psychiatry, 32(10)*, 1246-1254.

Kenardy, J., Evans, L. and Oei, T. P. S. (1992). The latent structure of anxiety symptoms in anxiety disorders. *American Journal of Psychiatry, 149(8)*, 1058-1061.

Kenardy, J., Fried, L., Kraemer, H. C. and Taylor, C. B. (1992). Psychological precursors of panic attacks. *British Journal of Psychiatry, 160*, 668-673.

Kihara, T., Ikeda, M., Matsubara, K. and Matsushita, A. (1993). Differential effects of ceruletide on amphetamine-induced behaviors and regional dopamine release in the rat. *European Journal of Pharmacology, 230*, 271-277.

King, D., Nicolini, H. and De La Fuente, J. R. (1990). Abuse and withdrawal of panic treatment drugs. *Psychiatric Annals, 20(9)*, 525-528.

Kiyatkin, E. A. (1995). Functional significance of mesolimbic dopamine. *Neuroscience and Biobehavioral Reviews, 19(4)*, 573-598.

Klein, D. F. (1988). The cause and treatment of agoraphobia. *Archives of General Psychiatry, 45*, 388-92.

Klein, D. F. (1995). Is panic disorder associated with childhood separation anxiety disorder? *Clinical Neuropharmacology, 18* (Suppl. 2), S7-S14.

Klein, D. F. (1995). Treatment of panic disorder, agoraphobia, and social phobia. *Clinical Neuropharmacology, 18* (Suppl. 2), S45-S51.

Klein, D. F. (1996). Panic attacks: Klein's false suffocation alarm, Taylor and Rachman's data, and Ley's dyspneic-fear theory. *Archives of General Psychiatry, 53*, 83-85.

Klein, D. F., Ross, D. C. and Cohen, P. (1987). Panic and avoidance in agoraphobia. *Archives of General Psychiatry, 44*, 377-389.

Klemm, E., Grunwald, F., Kasper, S., Menzel, C., Broich, K., Danos, P., Reichmann, K., Krappel, C., Rieker, O., Briele, B., Hotze, A. L., Moller, H. J. and Biersack, H. J. (1996). [123I] IBZM SPECT for imaging of striatal D2 dopamine receptors in 56 schizophrenic patients taking various neuroleptics. *American Journal of Psychiatry, 153(2)*, 183-190.

Klosko, J. S., Barlow, D. H., Tassinari, R. and Cerny, J. A. (1990). A comparison of alprazolam and behavior therapy in treatment of panic disorder. *Journal of Consulting and Clinical Psychology, 58(1)*, 77-84.

Knable, M. B., Hyde, T. M., Murray, A. M., Herman, M. M. and Kleinman, J. E. (1996). A postmortem study of frontal cortical dopamine D1 receptors in schizophrenics, psychiatric controls, and normal controls. *Biological Psychiatry, 40(12),* 1191-1199.

Ko, G. N., Elsworth, J. D., Roth, R. H., Rifkin, B. G., Leigh, H. and Redmond, E. (1983). Panic induced elevation of plasma MHPG levels in phobic-anxious patients. Effects of clonidine and imipramine. *Archives of General Psychiatry, 40,* 425-430.

Kobayashi, S., Ohta, M., Miyasaka, K. and Funakoshi, A. (1996). Decrease in exploratory behavior in naturally occurring cholecystokinin (CCK)-A receptor gene knockout rats. *Neuroscience Letters, 214,* 61-64.

Kokkinidis, L. and Anisman, H. (1977). Perseveration and rotational behavior elicited by d-amphetamine in y-maze exploratory task: differential effects of intraperitoneal and unilateral intraventricular administration. *Psychopharmacology, 52(2)*, 123.

Kokkinidis, L. and MacNeill, E. (1982). Stress-induced facilitation of acoustic startle after d-amphetamine administration. *Pharmacology, Biochemistry and Behavior, 17,* 413-417.

Kontur, P. J., Al-Tikriti, M., Innis, R. B. and Roth, R. H. (1994). Postmortem stability of monoamines, their metabolites, and receptor binding in rat brain regions. *Journal of Neurochemistry, 62 (1),* 282-290.

Kopchia, K. L., Altman, H. J. and Commissaris, R. L. (1992). Effects of lesions of the central nucleus of the amygdala on anxiety-related behaviors in the rat. *Pharmacology, Biochemistry and Behavior, 43(2)*, 453-461.

Koszycki, D., Bradwejn, J. and Bourin, M. (1991). Comparison of the effects of cholecystokinin tetrapeptide and carbon dioxide in healthy volunteers. *European Neuropsychopharmacology, 1*, 137-141.

Koszycki, D., Cox, B. J. and Bradwejn, J. (1993). Anxiety sensitivity and response to CCK-4 in healthy volunteers. *American Journal of Psychiatry, 150,* 1881-1883.

Koszycki, D., Torres, S., Swain, J. E. and Bradwejn, J. (2005). Central cholecystokinin activity in irritable bowel syndrome, panic disorder, and health controls. *Advances in Psychosomatic Medicine, 67,* 590-595.

Koszycki, D., Zacharko, R. M. and Bradwejn, J. (1996). Influence of personality on behavioral response to cholecystokinin-tetrapeptide in patients with panic disorder. *Psychiatry Research, 62,* 131-138.

Kraemer, G. W. (1992). A psychobiologic theory of attachment. *Brain and Behavioral Science, 15,* 493-541.

Krettek, J. E. and Price, J. L. (1978). Amygdaloid projections to subcortical structures within the basal forebrain and brainstem of the rat and cat. *Journal of Comprehensive Neurology, 178,* 225-254.

Kulkarni, J., Horne, M., Butler, E., Keks, N. and Copolov, D. (1992). Psychotic symptoms resulting from intraventricular infusion of dopamine in Parkinson's disease. *Biological Psychiatry, 31,* 1225-1227.

Kunas, G. and Varga, K. (1995). The tachycardia associated with the defense reaction involves activation of both GABA$_A$ and GABA$_B$ receptors in the nucleus tractus solitarii. *Clinical and Experimental Hypertension, 17 (1and2)*, 91-100.

Kuribara, H. (1996). Importance of post-drug environmental factors for induction of sensitization to the ambulation-increasing effects of methamphetamine and cocaine in mice. *Psychopharmacology, 126*, 293-300.

Kushner, M. G., MacKenzie, T. B., Fiszdon, J., Valentiner, D. P., Foa, E., Anderson, N. and Wangensteen, D. (1996). The effects of alcohol consumption on laboratory-induced panic and state anxiety. *Archives of General Psychiatry, 53*, 264-270.

Kuwahara, T., Kudoh, T., Nakano, A., Yoshizaki, H., Takamiya, M., Nagase, H. and Arisawa, M. (1993). Species specificity of pharmacological characteristics of CCK-B receptors. *Neuroscience Letters, 158(1)*, 1-4.

Laberge, B., Gauthier, J., Cote, G., Plamondon, J. and Cormier, H. J. (1992). The treatment of coexisting panic and depression: a review of the literature. *Journal of Anxiety Disorders, 6*, 169-180.

Lachuer, J., Gaillet, S., Barbagli, B., Buda, M. and Tappaz, M. (1991). Differential early time course activation of the brainstem catecholaminergic groups in response to various stresses. *Neuroendocrinology, 53*, 589-596.

Lane, R. F., Blaha, C. D. and Phillips, A. G. (1986). In vivo electrochemical analysis of cholecystokinin-induced inhibition of dopamine release in the nucleus accumbens. *Brain Research, 397*, 200-204.

Lane, J. D. (1992). Neurochemical changes associated with the action of acute administration of diazepam in reversing the behavioral paradigm conditioned emotional response (CER). *Neurochemical Research, 17(5)*, 497-507.

Lara, N., Chrapko, W. E., Archer, S. L., Bellavance, F., Mayers, I. and Le Melledo, J. M. (2003). Pulmonary and systemic nitric oxide measurements during CCK-5-induced panic attacks. *Neuropsychopharmacology, 28*, 1840-1845.

Lavielle, S., Tassin, J. -P., Thierry, A. -M., Blanc, G., Herve, D., Barthelemy, C. and Glowinski, J.(1978). Blockade by benzodiazepines of the selective high increase in dopamine turnover induced by stress in mesocortical dopaminergic neurons of the rat. *Brain Research, 168*, 584-594.

La Via, M. F., Munno, I., Lydiard, R. B., Workman, E. W., Hubbard, J. R., Michel, Y. and Paulling, E. (1996). The influence of stress intrusion on immunodepression in generalized anxiety disorder patients and controls. *Psychosomatic Medicine, 58*, 138-142.

Leckman, J. F., Weissman, M. M., Merikangas, K. R., Pauls, D. L. and Prusoff, B. A. (1983). Panic disorder and major depression. *Archives of General Psychiatry, 40*, 1055-1060.

Leduc, P. A. and Mittleman, G. (1995). Schizophrenia and psychostimulant abuse: a review and re-analysis of clinical evidence. *Psychopharmacology, 121*, 407-427.

Lee, Y. and Davis, M. (1997). Role of the hippocampus 'the bed nucleus of the stria terminalis' and the amygdala in the excitatory effect of corticotropin-releasing hormone on the acoustic startle reflex. *Journal of Neuroscience, 17(16)*, 6434-6436.

Leenders, K. L., Palmer, A. J., Quinn, N., Clark, J. C., Firnau, G., Garnett, E. S., Nahmias, C., Jones, T. and Marsden, C. D. (1986). Brain dopamine metabolosim in patients with

Parkinson's disease measured with positron emission tomography. *Journal of Neurology, Neurosurgery, and Psychiatry, 49(8)*, 853-860.

Lepine, J. -P. and Lellouch, J. (1995). Diagnosis and epidemiology of agorophobia and social phobia. *Clinical Neuropharmacology, 18(2)*, S15-S26.

Lepola, U., Jolkkonen, J., Rimon, R. and Riekkinen, P. (1989). Long-term effects of alprazolam and imipramine on cerebral spinal fluid monoamine metabolites and neuropeptides in panic disorder. *Neuropsychobiology, 21*, 182-186.

Lepola, U., Leinonen, E. and Koponen, H. (1996). Citalopram in the treatment of early-onset panic disorder and school phobia. *Pharmacopsychiatry, 29*, 30-32.

Lewine, R. J., Walker, E. F., Shurett, R., Caudle, J. and Haden, C. (1996). Sex differences in neuropsychological functioning among schizophrenic patients. *American Journal of Psychiatry, 153(9)*, 1178-1184.

Ley, R. (1996). Panic attacks: Klein's false suffocation alarm, Taylor and Rachman's data, and Ley's dyspneic-fear theory. *Archives of General Psychiatry, 53*, 83.

Leyton, M., Belanger, C., Martial, J., Beaulieau, S., Corin, E., Pecknold, J., Kin, N.M., Meaney, M., Thavundayil, J., Larue, S. and Nair, N.P. (1996). Cardiovascular, neuroendocrine, and monoaminergic responses to psychological stressors:possible differences between remitted panic disorder patients and healthy controls. *Biological Psychiatry, 40(5)*, 353-360.

Leyton, M. and Stewart, J. (1990). Preexposure to foot-shock sensitizes the locomotor response to to subsequent morphine and intra-nucleus accumbens amphetamine. *Pharmacology, Biochemistry, and Behavior, 37*, 303-310.

Lezak, M. D. (1983). *Neuropsychological Assessment.* New York: Oxford University Press

Liang, K. C., Melia, K. R., Campeau, S., Falls, W. A., Miserendino, M. J. D. and Davis, M. (1992). Lesions of the central nucleus of the amygdala, but not the paraventricular nucleus of the hypothalamus, block the excitatory effects of corticotropin-releasing factor on the acoustic startle reflex. *The Journal of Neuroscience, 12 (6)*, 2313-2320.

Lindefors, N., Linden, A., Brene, S., Sedvall, G. and Persson, H. (1993). CCK peptides and mRNA in the human brain. *Progress in Neurobiology, 40*, 671-690.

Lotstra, F., Verbanck, P. M. P., Gilles, C., Mendlewicz, J. and Vanderhaeghen, J. -J. (1985). Reduced cholecystokinin levels in cerebrospinal fluid of parkinsonian and schizophrenic patients. *Annals of the New York Academy of Sciences, 448*, 507-517.

Ludewig, S., Geyer, M. A., Ramseier, M., Vollenweider, F. X., Rechsteiner, E. and Cattapan-Ludewig, K. (2005). Information-processing deficits and cognitive dysfunction in panic disorder. *Journal of Psychiatry and Neuroscience, 30*, 37-43.

Lukoff, D., Snyder, K., Ventura, J. and Nuechterlein, K. H. (1984). Life events, familial stress, and coping in the developmental course of schizophrenia. *Schizophrenia Bulletin, 10(2)*, 258-292.

Lundberg, J. M. and Hokfelt, T. (1983). Coexistence of peptides and classical neurotransmitters. *Trends in Neurosciences, 6(8)*, 325-333.

Lydiard, R. B., Ballenger, J. C., Laraia, M. T., Fossey, M. D. and Beinfeld, M. C. (1992). CSF cholecystokinin concentrations in patients with panic disorder and in normal comparison subjects. *American Journal of Psychiatry, 149(5)*, 691-693.

Lysaker, P. H., Bell, M. D., Bioty, S. M. and Zito, W. S. (1995). The frequency of associations between positive and negative symptoms and dysphoria in schizophrenia. *Comprehensive Psychiatry, 36(2)*, 113-117.

Maas, J. W., Contreras, S. A., Miller, A. L., Berman, N., Bowden, C. L., Javors, M. A., Seleshi, E. and Weintraub, S. (1993a). Studies of catecholamine metabolism in schizophrenia/psychosis-I. *Neuropsychopharmacology, 8(2)*, 97-109.

Maas, J. W., Contreras, S. A., Miller, A. L., Berman, N., Bowden, C. L., Javors, M. A., Seleshi, E. and Weintraub, S. (1993b). Studies of catecholamine metabolism in schizophrenia/psychosis-II. *Neuropsychopharmacology, 8(2)*, 111-116.

Mackay, A. V. P., Iversen, L. L., Rossor, M., Spokes, E., Bird, E., Arregui, A., Creese, I. and Snyder, S. H. (1982). Increased brain dopamine and dopamine receptors in schizophrenia. *Archives of General Psychiatry, 39*, 991-997.

MacNeil, G., Sela, Y., McIntosh, J. and Zacharko, R. M. (1997). Anxiogenic behavior in the light-dark paradigm following intraventricular administration of cholecystokinin-8S, restraint stress, or uncontrollable footshock in the CD-1 mouse. *Pharmacology, Biochemistry, and Behavior, 58(3)*, 737-746.

Mahurin, R. K., Feher, E. P., Nance, M. L., Levy, J. K. and Pirozzolo, F. J. (1993). Cognition in Parkinson's disease and related disorders. In *Neuropsychology of Alzheimer's Disease and Other Dementias*. R.W. Parks, R. S. Wilson and R. F. Zec, Eds: 308-334. New York: Oxford University Press.

Maier, W. and Lichtermann, D. (1993). The genetic epidemiology of unipolar depression and and panic disorder. *International Clinical Psychopharmacology, 8 (Suppl. 1)*, 27-33.

Maier, W., Minges, J. and Lichtermann, D. (1993). Alcoholism and panic disorder: co-occurrence and co-transmission in families. *European Archives of Psychiatry and Clinical Neurosciences, 243*, 205-211.

Maier, W., Minges, J. and Lichtermann, D. (1995). The familial relationship between panic disorder and unipolar depression. *Journal of Psychiatric Research, 29(5)*, 375-388.

Manfro, G. G., Otto, M. W., McArdle, E. T., Worthington, J. J. III, Rosenbaum, J. F. and Pollack, M. H. (1996). Relationship of antecedent stressful life events to childhood and family history of anxiety and the course of panic disorder. *Journal of Affective Disorders, 41(2)*, 135-139.

Margraf, J., Ehlers, A. and Roth, W. T. (1986). Biological models of panic disorder and agoraphobia - a review. *Behavioral Research and Therapeutics, 24(5)*, 553-567.

Margraf, J., Taylor, B., Ehlers, A., Roth, W. T. and Agras, W. S. (1987). Panic attacks in the natural environment. *Journal of Nervous and Mental Disease, 175(9)*, 558-565.

Maricle, R. A., Nutt, J. G. and Carter, J. H. (1995). Mood and anxiety fluctuation in Parkinson's disease associated with levodopa infusion: preliminary findings. *Movement Disorders, 10(3)*, 329-332.

Maricle, R. A., Nutt, J. G., Valentine, R. J. and Carter, J. H. (1995). Dose-response relationship of levodopa with mood and anxiety in fluctuating Parkinson's disease: a double-blind, placebo-controlled study. *Neurology, 45(9)*, 1757-1760.

Marie, R. M., Barrie, L., Rioux, P., Allain, P., Lechevalier, B. and Baron, J. C. (1995). PET imaging of neocortical monoaminergic terminals in Parkinson's disease. *Journal of Neural Transmission (Parkinson's Disease Dementia Section), 9(1)*, 55-71.

Marks, I. M. and O'Sullivan, G. (1987). Anti-anxiety drug and psychological treatment effects in agoraphobia/panic and obsessive-compulsive disorders. In *Psychopharmacology of Anxiety*. Peter Tyrer, Ed: 197-242. New York: Oxford University Press.

Marshall, F. H., Barnes, S., Hughes, J., Woodruff, G. N. and Hunter, J. C. (1991). Cholecystokinin modulates the release of dopamine from the anterior and posterior nucleus accumbens by two different mechanisms. *Journal of Neurochemistry, 56(3),* 917-922.

Massion, A. O., Warshaw, M. G. and Keller, M. B. (1993). Quality of life and psychiatric morbidity in panic disorder and generalized anxiety disorder. *American Journal of Psychiatry, 150(4),* 600-607.

Mavissakalian, M. R. (1996). Phenomenology of panic attacks: responsiveness of individual symptoms to imipramine. *Journal of Clinical Psychopharmacology, 16(3),* 233-237.

Mavissakalian, M. and Perel, J. M. (1992). Protective effects of imipramine maintenance treatment in panic disorder with agoraphobia. *American Journal of Psychiatry, 149(8),* 1053-1057.

McBlane, J. W. and Handley, S. L. (1994). Effects of two stressors on behavior in the elevated x-maze: preliminary investigation of their interaction with 8-OH-DPAT. *Psychopharmacology, 116,* 173-182.

McCullough, L. D. and Salamone, J. D. (1992). Anxiogenic drugs beta-CCE and FG7142 increase extracellular dopamine levels in nucleus accumbens. *Psychopharmacology, 109,* 379-382.

McDermott, J. L. (1993). Effects of estrogen upon dopamine release from the corpus striatum of young and aged female rats. *Brain Research, 606(1),* 118-125.

McNally, R. J. (1992). Anxiety sensitivity distinguishes panic disorder from generalized anxiety disorder. *Journal of Nervous and Mental Disease, 180,* 737-738.

McNally, R. J. and Lukach, B. M. (1992). Are panic attacks traumatic stressors? *American Journal of Psychiatry, 149(6),* 824-826.

Mellergard, M., Lorentzen, K., Bech, P., Ottosson, J. -O. and Rosenberg, R. (1991). A trend analysis of changes during treatment of panic disorder with alprazolam and imipramine. *Acta Psychiatra Scandinavia, Suppl. 365,* 28-32.

Menza, M., Forman, N., Sage, J. and Cody, R. (1993). Psychiatric symptoms in Parkinson's disease: a comparison between patients with and without "on-off" symptoms. *Biological Psychiatry, 33,* 682-684.

Menza, M., Robertson-Hoffman, D. and Bonapace, A. (1993). Parkinson's disease and anxiety: comorbidity with depression. *Biological Psychiatry, 34,* 465-470.

Mezey, E., Reisine, T. D., Skirboll, L., Beinfeld, M. and Kiss, J. Z. (1985). Cholecystokinin in the medial parvocellular subdivision of the paraventricular nucleus. Coexistence with corticotropin-releasing hormone. *Annals of the New York Academy of Science, 448,* 152-156.

Miaskiewicz, S. L., Stricker, E. M. and Verbalis, J. G. (1989). Neurohypophyseal secretion in response to cholecystokinin but not meal-induced gastric distention in humans. *Journal of Clinical Endocrinology and Metabolism, 68(4),* 837-843.

Miller, L. G., Greenblatt, D. J., Barnhill, J. G., Deutsch, S. I., Shader, R. I. and Paul, S. M. (1987). Benzodiazepine receptor binding of triazolbenzodiazepines in vivo: increased receptor number with low-dose alprazolam. *Journal of Neurochemistry, 49(5),* 1595-1601.

Milrod, B. and Busch, F. (1996). Long-term outcome of panic disorder treatment: a review of the literature. *Journal of Nervous and Mental Disease, 184(12),* 723-730.

Minabe, Y., Kadono, Y. and Kurachi, M. (1990). A schizophrenic syndrome associated with a midbrain tegmental lesion. *Biological Psychiatry, 27,* 661-663.

Miyasaka, K., Kanai, S., Masuda, M., Ohta, M., Kawanami, T., Matsumoto, M. and Funakoshi, A. (1995). Gene expressions of cholecystokinin (CCK) and CCK receptors, and its satiety effect in young and old male rats. *Archives of Gerontology and Geriatrics, 21,* 147-155.

Moran, T. H. and McHugh, P. R. (1990). CCK$_A$ receptors. In: *Handbook of Chemical Neuroanatomy, 9: Neuropeptides in the CNS, Part II.* A. Bjorklund, T. Hokfelt and M. J. Kuher, Eds. Elsevier Science Publishers, New York.

Morgan, C. A. III, Grillon, C., Southwick, S. M., Davis, M. and Charney, D. S. (1995). Fear-potentiated startle in posttraumatic stress disorder. *Biological Psychiatry, 38(6),* 378-385.

Moroji, T., Itoh, K. and Itoh, K. (1985). Antipsychotic effects of ceruletide in chronic schizophrenia: an appraisal of the long-term, intermittent medication of ceruletide in chronic schizophrenia. *Annals of the New York Academy of Sciences, 448,* 518-533.

Nagy, L. M., Krystal, J. H., Charney, D. S., Merikangas, K. R. and Woods, S. W. (1993). Long-term outcome of panic disorder after short-term imipramine and behavioral group treatment: 2.9-year naturalistic follow-up study. *Journal of Clinical Psychopharmacology, 13(1),* 16-24.

Nair, N. P., Bloom, D., Lal, S., Debonnel, G., Schwartz, G. and Mosticyan, S. (1985). Clinical and neuroendocrine studies with cholecystokinin peptides. *Annals of the New York Academy of Sciences, 448,* 535-541.

Nair, N. P., Lal, S. and Bloom, D. M. (1985). Cholecystokinin peptides, dopamine and schizophrenia-a review. *Progress in Neuro-Psychopharmacology and Biological Psychiatry, 9,* 515-524.

Narabayashi, H. (1995). The neural mechanisms and progressive nature of symptoms of Parkinson's disease-based on clinical, neurophysiological and morphological studies. *Journal of Neural Transmission, Parkinson's Disease and Dementia Section, 10(1),* 63-75.

Neenan, P., Felkner, J. and Reich, J. (1986). Schizoid personality traits developing secondary to panic disorder. *The Journal of Nervous and Mental Disease, 174(8),* 483.

Nemeroff, C. B. (1992). New vistas in neuropeptide research in neuropsychiatry: focus on corticotropin-releasing factor. *Neuropsychopharmacology, 6(2),* 69-75.

Netto, C. F. and Guimaraes, F. S. (2004). Anxiogenic effect of cholecystokinin in the dorsal periaqueductal gray. *Neuropsychopharmacology, 29,* 101-107.

Novas, M. L., Wolfman, C., Medina, J. H. and de Robertis, E. (1988). Proconvulsant and 'anxiogenic' effects of n-butyl beta carboline-3-carboxylate, an endogenous benzodiazepine binding inhibitor from brain. *Pharmacology, Biochemistry and Behavior, 30(2),* 331-336.

Noyes, R., Garvey, M. J. and Cook, B. L. (1989). Follow-up study of patients with panic disorder and agoraphobia with panic attacks treated with tricyclic antidepressants. *Journal of Affective Disorders, 16,* 249-257.

Noyes, R., Reich, J., Clancy, J. and O'Gorman, T. W. (1986). Reduction in hypochondriasis with treatment of panic disorder. *British Journal of Psychiatry, 149,* 631-635.

Nutt, D. J. (1989). Altered central α_2-adrenoceptor sensitivity in panic disorder. *Archives of General Psychiatry, 46,* 165-169.

Nutt, D. J. (1990). The pharmacology of human anxiety. *Pharmacology Therapy, 47,* 233-263.

Nutt, D. J. and Glue, P. (1991). Clinical pharmacology of anxiolytics and antidepressants: a psychopharmacological perspective. In *Psychopharmacology of Anxiolytics and Antidepressants.* S. E. File, Ed: 1-28. New York: Pergamon Press.

Oades, R. D. (1982). Search strategies on a hole-board are impaired in rats with ventral tegmental damage: animal models for tests of thought disorder. *Biological Psychiatry, 17,* 243-258.

O'Brien, M. S., Wu, L. T. and Anthony, J. C. (2005). Cocaine use and the occurrence of panic attacks in the community: A case-crossover approach. *Substance Use and Misuse, 40,* 285-297.

Ohta, M., Tanaka, Y., Masuda, M., Miyasaka, K. and Funakoshi, A. (1995). Impaired release of cholecystokinin (CCK) from synaptosomes in old rats. *Neuroscience Letters, 198,* 161-164.

Otto, M. W., Pollack, M. H., Rosenbaum, J. F., Sachs, G. S. and Asher, R. H. (1994). Childhood history of anxiety in adults with panic disorder: association with anxiety sensitivity and avoidance. *Harvard Review of Psychiatry, 1,* 288-293.

Otto, M. W., Pollack, M. H., Sachs, G. S., Reiter, S. R., Meltzer-Brody, S. and Rosenbaum, J. F. (1993). Discontinuation of benzodiazepine treatment: efficacy of cognitive-behavioral therapy for patients with panic disorder. *American Journal of Psychiatry, 150(10),* 1485-1490.

Owens, M. J., Bissette, G. and Nemeroff, C. B. (1989). Acute effects of alprazolam and adinazolam on the concentrations of corticotropin-releasing factor in the rat brain. *Synapse, 4(3),* 196-202.

Owens, M. J., Varfas, M. A. and Nemeroff, C. B. (1993). The effects of alprazolam on corticotropin-releasing factor neurons in the rat brain: implications for a role for CRF in the pathogenesis of anxiety disorders. *Journal of Psychiatric Research, 27, Suppl 1.,* 209-220.

Oyebode, J. R., Barker, W. A., Blessed, G., Dick, D. J. and Britton, P. G. (1986). Cognitive functioning in Parkinson's disease: in relation to prevalence of dementia and psychiatric diagnosis. *British Journal of Psychiatry, 149,* 720-725.

Palermo-Neto, J. and Dorce, V. A. (1990). Influences of estrogen and/or progesterone on some dopamine related behavior in rats. *General Pharmacology, 21(1),* 83-87.

Pallanti, S. and Mazzi, D. (1992). MDMA (Ecstasy) precipitation of panic disorder. *Biological Psychiatry, 32,* 91-95.

Palmour, R., Bradwejn, J. and Ervin, F. (1992). The anxiogenic effects of CCK-4 in monkeys are reduced by CCK_B antagonists, benzodiazepines or adenosine A2 agonists. *European Journal of Neuropsychopharmacology, 2,* 193-195.

Papp, L. A., Klein, D. F. and Gorman, J. M. (1993). Carbon dioxide hypersensitivity, hyperventilation, and panic disorder. *American Journal of Psychiatry, 150(8),* 1149-1157.

Paradis, C. M., Friedman, S., Lazar, R. M. and Kula, R. W. (1993). Anxiety disorders in a neuromuscular clinic. *American Journal of Psychiatry, 150,* 1102-1104.

Patterson, T., Spohn, H. E., Bogia, D. P. and Hayes, K. (1986). Thought disorder in schizophrenia: cognitive and neuroscience approaches. *Schizophrenia Bulletin, 12(3),* 460-472.

Paulson, P. E., Camp, D. M. and Robinson, T. E. (1991). Time course of transient behavioral depression and persistent behavioral sensitization in relation to regional monoamine concentrations during amphetamine withdrawal in rats. *Psychopharmacology, 103,* 480-492.

Pavlasevic, S., Bednar, I., Qureshi, G. A. and Sodersten, P. (1993). Brain cholecystokinin tetrapeptide levels are increased in a rat model of anxiety. *Neuroreport, 5,* 225-228.

Payeur, R., Lydiard, B., Ballenger, J. C., Laraia, M. T., Fossey, M. D. and Zealberg, J. (1992). CSF diazepam-binding inhibitor concentrations in panic disorder. *Biological Psychiatry, 32,* 712-716.

Pecknold, J. C. (1993). Discontinuation reactions to alprazolam in panic disorder. *Journal of Psychiatric Research, 27 (Suppl. 1),* 155-170.

Pedro, B. M., Pilowsky, L. S., Costa, D. C., Hemsley, D. R., Ell, P. J., Verhoeff, N. P. Kerwin, R.W. and Gray, N. S. (1994). Stereotypy, schizophrenia and dopamine D2 receptor binding in the basal ganglia. *Psychological Medicine, 24(2),* 423-429.

Penn, D. L., Hope, D. A., Spaulding, W. and Kucera, J. (1994). Social anxiety in schizophrenia. *Schizophrenia Research, 11(3),* 277-284.

Pesold, C. and Treit, D. (1995). The central and basolateral amygdala differentially mediate the anxiolytic effects of benzodiazepines. *Brain Research, 671(2),* 213-221.

Philipp, E., Wilckens, T., Friess, E., Platte, P. and Pirke, K. -M. (1992). Cholecystokinin, gastrin and stress hormone responses in marathon runners. *Peptides, 13,* 125-128.

Phillips, G. D., Le Noury, J., Wolterink, G., Donselaar-Wolterink, I., Robbins, T. W. and Everitt, B. J. (1993). Cholecystokinin-dopamine interactions within the nucleus accumbens in the control over behavior by conditioned reinforcement. *Behavioral Brain Research, 55,* 223-231.

Pierce, R. C. and Kalivas, P. W. (1995). Amphetamine produces sensitized increases in locomotion and extracellular dopamine preferentially in the nucleus accumbens shell of rats administered repeated cocaine. *The Journal of Pharmacology and Experimental Therapeutics, 275(2),* 1019-1029.

Pilowsky, I. (1967). Dimensions of hypochondriasis. *British Journal of Psychiatry, 113,* 89-93.

Pinel, J. P. J. and Edwards, M. (1998). A colorful introduction to the anatomy of the human brain. *A Brain and Psychology Coloring Book.* Boston: Allyn and Bacon.

Piolti, R., Appollonio, I., Cocco, E., Ferrarese, C., Frattola, L., Rovati, L. and Panerai, A.E. (1991). Treatment of Parkinson's disease with proglumide, a CCK antagonist. *Neurology, 41*, 749-750.

Pirozzolo, F. J., Swihart, A. A., Rey, G., Jankovic, J. and Mortimer, J. A. (1988). Cognitive impairments associated with Parkinson's disease and other movement disorders. In *Parkinson's Disease and Movement Disorders.* J. Jankovic and E. Tolosa , Eds: 425-439. Baltimore-Munich: Urban and Schwarzenberg.

Pitchot, W., Ansseau, M., Moreno, A., Hansenne, M. and von Frenckell, R. (1992). Dopaminergic function in panic disorder: comparison with major and minor depression. *Biological Psychiatry, 32,* 1004-1011.

Pitchot, W., Hansenne, M., Moreno, A., Von Frenckell, R. and Ansseau, M. (1990-91). Psychopathological correlates of dopaminergic disturbances in major depression. *Neuropsychobiology, 24*, 169-172.

Pollack, M. H., Otto, M. W., Sabatino, S., Majcher, D., Worthington, J. J., McArdle, E. T. and Rosenbaum, J. F. (1996). Relationship of childhood anxiety to adult panic disorder: correlates and influence on course. *American Journal of Psychiatry, 153(3),* 376-381.

Post, R. M. (1980). Intermittent versus continuous stimulation: effect of time interval on the development of sensitization or tolerance. *Life Sciences, 26,* 1275-1282.

Post, R. M. and Weiss, S. R (1988). Sensitization and kindling: implications for the evolution of psychiatric symptomatology. In *Sensitization in the Nervous System.* P. W. Kalivas and C. D. Barnes, Eds: 257-292. New Jersey: Telford Press.

Post, R. M. and Weiss, S. R (1992). Sensitization, kindling, and carbamazepine: an update on their implications for the course of affective illness. *Pharmacopsychiatra, 25,* 41-43.

Post, R. M., Weiss, S. R., Fontana, D. and Pert, A. (1992). Conditioned sensitization to the psychomotor stimulant cocaine. In *The Neurobiology of Drug and Alcohol Addiction,* 654, 386-399. New York: Annals of the New York Academy of Sciences.

Post, R., Weiss, S. R. and Pert, A. (1988). Cocaine-induced behavioral sensitization and kindling: implications for the emergence of psychopathology and seizures. In *The Mesolimbic Dopamine System, 537,* 292-307. New York: Annals of the New York Academy of Sciences.

Pratt, J. A. and Brett, R. R. (1995). The benzodiazepine receptor inverse agonist FG 7142 induces cholecystokinin gene expression in rat brain. *Neuroscience Letters, 184*, 197-200.

Price, W. A. and Heil, D. (1988). Estrogen-induced panic attacks. *Psychosomatics, 29(4),* 433-435.

Pyke, R. E. and Kraus, M. (1988). Alprazolam in the treatment of panic attack patients with and without major depression. *Journal of Clinical Psychiatry, 49(2),* 66-68.

Quitkin, F. M., Stewart, J. W., McGrath, P. J., Liebowitz, M. R., Harrison, W. M., Tricamo, E., Klein, D. F., Rabkin, J. G., Markowitz, J. S. and Wager, S. G. (1988). Phenelzine versus imipramine in the treatment of probable atypical depression: defining syndrome boundaries of selective MAOI responders. *American Journal of Psychiatry, 145(3)*, 306-311.

Rafal, R. D., Posner, M. I., Walker, J. A. and Friedrich, F. J. (1984). Cognition and the basal ganglia. *Brain*, 107, 1083-1094.

Raj, A. and Sheehan, D. V. (1990). *Mitral Valve Prolapse and Panic Disorder.* The Menninger Foundation, U.S.A.

Rapee, R., Mattick, R. and Murrell, E. (1986). Cognitive mediation in the affective component of spontaneous panic attacks. *Journal of Behavior Therapy and Experimental Psychiatry, 17(4)*, 245-253.

Raskin, M., Peeke, H., Dickman, W. and Pinsker, H. (1982). Panic and generalized anxiety disorders: developmental antecedents and precipitants. *Archives of General Psychiatry, 39,* 687-689.

Rasmussen, K. (1994). CCK, schizophrenia, and anxiety. CCK-B antagonists inhibit the activity of brain dopamine neurons. *Annals of the New York Academy of Science, 713,* 300-311.

Rasmussen, K., Stockton, M. E., Czachura, J. F. and Howbert, J. J. (1991). Cholecystokinin (CCK) and schizophrenia: the selective CCK_B antagonist LY262691 decreases midbrain dopamine unit activity. *European Journal of Pharmacology, 209,* 135-138.

Rattray, M., Singhvi, S., Wu, P. -Y., Andrews, N. and File, S. E. (1993). Benzodiazepines increaseb preprocholecystokinin messenger RNA in rat brain. *European Journal of Pharmacology (Molecular Pharmacology Section), 245*, 193-196.

Raud, S., Runkorg, K., Veraksits, A., Reimets, A., Nelovkov, A., Abramov, U., Matsui, T., Bourin, M., Volke, V., Koks, S. and Vasar, E. (2003). Targeted mutation of CCK2 receptor gene modifies the behavioural effects of diazepam in female mice. *Psychopharmacology (Berl.), 168,* 417-425.

Ravard, S. and Dourish, C. T. (1990). Cholecystokinin and anxiety. *Trends in Pharmacological Science, 11(7)*, 271-273.

Reich, J., Warshaw, M., Peterson, L. G., White, K., Keller, M., Lavori, P. and Yonkers, K. A. (1993) Comorbidity of panic and major depressive disorder. *Journal of Psychiatric Research, 27 (S1)*, 23-33.

Reinhard Jr., J. F., Bannon, M. J. and Roth, R. H. (1982). Acceleration by stress of dopamine synthesis and metabolism in prefrontal cortex: antagonism by diazepam. *Nauhyn-Schmeideberg's Archives of Pharmacology, 318,* 374-377.

Rex, A., Barth, T., Voigt, J. -P., Domeney, A. M. and Fink, H. (1994). Effects of cholecystokinin tetrapeptide and sulfated cholecystokinin octapeptide in rat models of anxiety. *Neuroscience Letters, 172,* 139-142.

Rex, A., Sondern, U., Voigt, J. P., Franck, S. and Fink, H. (1996). Strain differences in fear-motivated behavior of rats. *Pharmacology, Biochemistry and Behavior, 54(1)*, 107-111.

Rich, S. S., Friedman, J. H. and Ott, B. R. (1995). Risperidone versus clozapine in the treatment of psychosis in six patients with Parkinson's disease and other akinetic-rigid syndromes. *Journal of Clinical Psychiatry, 56(12),* 556-559.

Riley, D. E. and Lang, A. E. (1993). The spectrum of levodopa-related fluctuations in Parkinson's disease. *Neurology, 43,* 1459-1464.

Rizley, R., Kahn, R. J., McNair, D. M.and Frankenthaler, L. M. (1986). A comparison of alprazolam and imipramine in the treatment of agoraphobia and panic disorder. *Psychopharmacology Bulletin, 22,* 167-172.

Rush, A. J., Zimmerman, M., Wisniewski, S. R., Fava, M., Hollon, S. D., Warden, D., Biggs, M. M., Shores-Wilson, K., Shelton, R. C., Luther, J. F., Thomas, B. and Trivedi, M. H.

(2005). Comorbid psychiatric disorders in depressed outpatients: demographic and clinical features. *Journal of Affective Disorders, 87*, 43-55.

Robins, C. J. and Hayes, A. D.(1993). An appraisal of cognitive therapy. *Journal of Consulting and Clinical Psychology, 61(2)*, 205-214.

Robinson, T. E. (1988). Stimulant drugs and stress: factors influencing individual differences in the susceptibility to sensitization. In *Sensitization in the Nervous System*. P. W. Kalivas and C. D. Barnes, Eds: 145-173. New Jersey: Telford Press.

Robinson, T. E., Angus, A. L. and Becker, J. B. (1985). Sensitization to stress: the enduring effects of prior stress on amphetamine-induced rotational behavior. *Life Sciences, 37*, 1039-1042.

Robinson, T. E. and Becker, J. B. (1986). Enduring changes in brain and behavior produced by chronic amphetamine administration: a review and evaluation of animal models of amphetamine psychosis. *Brain Research, 396(2)*, 157-198.

Robinson, T. E., Becker, J. B. and Presty, S. K. (1982). Long-term facilitation of amphetamine induced rotational behavior and striatal dopamine release produced by a single exposure to amphetamine: sex differences. *Brain Research, 253*, 231-241.

Robinson, T. E., Becker, J. B. and Ramirez, V. D. (1980). Sex differences in amphetamine-elicited rotational behavior and the lateralization of striatal dopamine in rats. *Brain Research Bulletin, 5*, 539-545.

Robinson, T. E. and Berridge, K. C. (1993). The neural basis of drug craving: an incentive-sensitization theory of addiction. *Brain Research Reviews, 18*, 247-291.

Rodgers, R. J. and Johnson, N. J. T. (1995). Cholecystokinin and anxiety: promises and pitfalls.*Critical Reviews in Neurobiology, 9 (4)*, 345-369.

Rosen, A., Brodin, K., Eneroth, P. and Brodin, E. (1992). Short-term restraint stress and s.c. saline injection alter the tissue levels of substance P and cholecystokinin in the peri-aqueductal grey and limbic regions of the rat brain. *Acta Physiologica Scandinavia, 146*, 341-348.

Rosenbaum, J. F. (1990).*A psychopharmacologist's perspective on panic disorder*. The Menninger Foundation , U.S.A.

Rosenbaum, J. F., Biederman, J., Gersten, M., Hirschfeld, D. R., Meminger, S. R., Herman, J. B., Kagan, J., Reznick, J. S. and Snidman, N. (1988). Behavioral inhibition in children of parents with panic disorder and agoraphobia; a controlled study. *Archives of General Psychiatry, 45*, 463-470.

Rosenberg, R., Bech, P., Mellegard, M. and Ottosson, J. O. (1991). Alprazolam, imipramine, and placebo treatment of panic disorder: predicting therapeutic response. *Acta Psychiatra Scandinavia, Suppl. 365*, 46-52.

Rosenberg, R., Bech, P., Mellegard, M. and Ottosson, J. O. (1991). Secondary depression in panic disorder: an indicator of severity with a weak effect on outcome in alprazolam and imipramine treatment. *Acta Psychiatra Scandinavia, Suppl. 365*, 39-45.

Rosenberg, N. K., Mellegard, M., Rosenberg, R., Bech, P. and Ottosson, J.O. (1991). Characteristics of panic patients responding to placebo. *Acta Psychiatra Scandinavia, Suppl. 365*, 33-38.

Rosenblum, L. A. and Paully, G. S. (1984). The effects of varying environmental demands on maternal and infant behavior. *Child Development, 55(1)*, 305-314.

Roth, M. (1996). The panic-agoraphobic syndrome: a paradigm of the anxiety group of disorders and its implications for psychiatric practice and theory. *American Journal of Psychiatry, 153(7)*, 111-124.

Roth, R. H., Tam, S. -Y., Ida, Y., Yang, J. -X. and Deutch, A. Y. (1988). Stress and the mesocorticolimbic system. In *The mesocorticolimbic system*. P.W. Kalivas and C.B. Nemeroff, Eds. New York: New York Academy of Sciences.

Roth, W. T., Margraf, J., Ehlers, A., Taylor, C. B., Maddock, R. J., Davies, S. and Agras, W. S.(1992). Stress test reactivity in panic disorder. *Archives of General Psychiatry, 49,* 301-310.

Roy-Byrne, P. P., Geraci, M. and Uhde, T. W. (1986). Life events and the onset of panic disorder disorder. *American Journal of Psychiatry, 143(11)*, 1424-1427.

Roy-Byrne, P. P., Rubinow, D. R. and Linnoila, M. (1986). Relation between plasma prolactin and plasma homovanillic acid in normal subjects. *Neuropsychobiology, 16*, 85-87.

Roy-Byrne, P. P., Uhde, T.W., Post, R.M., Gallucci, W., Chrousos, G.P. and Gold, P.W. (1986). The corticotropin-releasing hormone stimulation test in patients with panic disorder. *American Journal of Psychiatry, 143 (7),* 896-899.

Roy-Byrne, P. P., Uhde, T. W., Sack, D. A., Linnoila, M. and Post, R. M. (1986). Plasma HVA and anxiety in patients with panic disorder. *Biological Psychiatry, 21,* 847-849.

Roy-Byrne, P. P., Vitaliano, P. P., Cowlry, D. S., Luciano, G., Zheng, Y. and Dunner, D. L. (1992). Coping in panic and major depressive disorder. Relative effects of symptom severity and diagnostic comorbidity. *The Journal of Nervous and Mental Disease, 180(3),* 179-183.

Saavedra, J. M. (1982). Changes in dopamine, noradrenaline and adrenaline in specific septal septal and preoptic nuclei after acute immobilization stress. *Neuroendocrinology, 35(5),* 396-401.

Safadi, G. (1995). Relationship of panic disorder to posttraumatic stress disorder. *Archives of General Psychiatry, 52,* 76-77.

Sandberg, L. and Siris, S. G. (1987). Panic disorder in schizophrenia. *The Journal of Nervous and Mental Disease, 175(10)*, 627-628.

Sanderson, W., Rapee, R. and Barlow, D. (1989). The influence of an illusion of control on panic attacks induced via inhalation of 5.5% carbon dioxide enriched air. *Archives of General Psychiatry, 46,* 157-162.

Sandyk, R. (1989). Estrogens and the pathophysiology of Parkinson's disease. *International Journal of Neuroscience, 45(1-2),* 119-122.

Schalling, M., Friberg, K., Seroogy, K., Riederer, P., Bird, E., Schiffman, S. N., Mailleux, P.,Vanderhaeghan, J. J., Kuga, S., Goldstein, M., Kitahama, K., Luppi, P. H., Jouvet, M. and Hokfelt, T. (1990). Analysis of expression of cholecystokinin in dopamine cells in the ventral mesencephalon of several species and in humans with schizophrenia. *Proceedings of the National Academy of Science, 87,* 8427-8431.

Schatzberg, A. F., Posener, J. A. and Rothschild, A. J. (1995). The role of dopamine in psychotic depression. *Clinical Neuropharmacology, 18(Suppl 1),* S66-S73.

Scheibe, G. and Albus, M. (1996). Predictors of outcome in panic disorder: a 5-year prospective follow-up study. *Journal of Affective Disorders, 41,* 111-116.

Schmauss, C., Haroutunian, V., Davis, K. L. and Davidson, M. (1993). Selective loss of dopamine D3-type receptor mRNA expression in parietal and motor cortices of patients with chronic schizophrenia. *Proceedings of the National Academy of Science, 90(19),* 8942-8946.

Schmidt, N. B., Lerew, D. R. and Trakowski, J. H. (1997). Body vigilance in panic disorder: evaluating attention to bodily perturbations. *Journal of Consultive and Clinical Psychology, 65(2),* 214-220.

Schnur, P., Espinoza, M. and Flores, R. (1994). Context-specific sensitization to naloxone-precipitated withdrawal in hamsters: effect of pimozide. *Pharmacology, Biochemistry and Behavior, 48(3),* 791-797.

Schunck, T., Erb, G., Mathis, A., Gilles, C., Namer, I. J., Hode, Y., Demaziere, A., Luthringer, R. and Macher, J. -P. (2006). Functional magnetic resonance imaging characterization of CCK-4-induced panic attack and subsequent anticipatory anxiety. *NeuroImage, 31,* 1197-1208.

Schwartz, C. C. and Myers, J. K. (1977). Life events and schizophrenia. II. Impact of life events and symptom configuration. *Archives of General Psychiatry, 34(10),* 1240-1245.

Schweizer, E., Case, W. G., Garcia-Espana, F., Greenblatt, D. J. and Rickels, K. (1995). Progesterone co-administration in patients discontinuing long-term benzodiazepine therapy: effects on withdrawal severity and taper outcome. *Psychopharmacology, 117,* 424-429.

Schweizer, E., Rickels, K., Weiss, S. and Zavodnick, S. (1993). Maintenance drug treatment of panic disorder. I. Results of a prospective, placebo-controlled comparison of alprazolam and mipramine. *Archives of General Psychiatry, 50,* 51-60.

Scocco, P., Barbieri, I. and Frank, E. (2006). Interpersonal problem areas and onset of panic disorder. *Psychopathology, 40,* 8-13.

Scupi, B. S., Benson, B. E., Brown, L. B. and Uhde, T. W. (1997). Rapid onset: a valid panic disorder disorder criterion? *Depression and Anxiety, 5 (3),* 121-126.

Seeman, P., Bzowej, N. H., Guan, H. C., Bergeron, C., Reynolds, G. P., Bird, E. D., Riederer, P., Jellinger, K. and Tourtellotte, W. W. (1987). Human brain D1 and D2 dopamine receptors in schizophrenia, Alzheimer's, Parkinson's and Huntington's diseases. *Neuropsychopharmacology, 1(1),* 5-15.

Servant, D., Bailly, D., Dewailly, D., Beuscart, R. and Parquet, P. J. (1993). Recent life stress and the corticotropin-releasing factor test in panic disorder. *Anxiety: Neurobiology, Clinic and Therapeutic Perspectives, Colloque Inserm/John Libbey Eurotext Ltd, 232,* 209-210.

Servatius, R., Ottenweller, J. E. and Natelson, B. H. (1995). Delayed startle sensitization distinguishes rats exposed to one or three stress sessions: Further evidence toward an animal model of PTSD. *Biological Psychiatry,38,* 539-546.

Sethy, V. H. and Hodges, D. H. (1982). Alprazolam in a biochemical model of depression. *Biochemical Pharmacology, 31 (19),* 3155-3157.

Sevy, S., Brown, S. -L., Wetzler, S., Kotler, M., Molcho, A., Plutchik, R. and van Praag, H. M.(1994). Effects of alprazolam on increases in hormonal and anxiety levels induced by meta-chlorophenylpiperazine. *Psychiatry Research, 53,* 219-229.

Shaner, A. and Eth, S. (1989). Can schizophrenia cause posttraumatic stress disorder? *American Journal of Psychotherapy, 43(4)*, 588-597.

Shanks, N., Griffiths, J., Zalcman, S., Zacharko, R. M. and Anisman, H. (1990). Mouse strain differences in plasma corticosterone following uncontrollable footshock. *Pharmacology, Biochemistry and Behavior, 36*, 515-519.

Shaw, K., McFarlane, A. and Bookless, C. (1997). The phenomenology of traumatic reactions to psychotic illness. *Journal of Nervous and Mental Disease, 185(7)*, 434-441.

Shear, K. M. (1996). Factors in the etiology and pathogenesis of panic disorder: revisiting the attachment-separation paradigm. *American Journal of Psychiatry, 153(7)*, 125-136.

Sherbourne, C. D., Wells, K. B. and Judd, L. L. (1996). Functioning and well-being of patients with panic disorder. *American Journal of Psychiatry, 153*, 213-218.

Shimazoe, T., Shibata, S., Yatsugi, S. and Ueki, S. (1988). Involvement of the medial amygdaloid nucleus in the action of imipramine in rats subjected to the forced swimming test. *Journal of Pharmacobio-Dynamics, 11*, 137-139.

Shioiri, T., Someya, T., Murashita, J. and Takahashi, S. (1996). The symptom structure of panic disorder: a trial using factor and cluster analysis. *Acta Psychiatrica Scandinavia, 93*, 80-86.

Shirayama, Y., Mitsushio, H., Takashima, M. Ichikawa, H. and Takahashi, K. (1996). Reduction of substance P after chronic antidepressants treatment in the striatum, substantia nigra and amygdala of the rat. *Brain Research, 739(1-2)*, 70-78.

Siegel, R. A., Duker, E. M., Pahnke, U. and Wuttke, W. (1987). Stress-induced changes in cholecystokinin and substance P concentrations in discrete regions of the rat hypothalamus. *Neuroendocrinology, 46*, 75-81.

Siemers, E. R., Shekhar, A., Quaid, K. and Dickson, H. (1993). Anxiety and motor performance in Parkinson's disease. *Movement Disorders, 8(4)*, 501-506.

Silverstein, M. L., Mavrolefteros, G. and Close, D. (1997). BPRS syndrome scales during the course of an episode of psychiatric illness. *Journal of Clinical Psychology, 53(5)*, 455-458.

Simon, H., Scatton, B. and LeMoal, M. (1980). Dopaminergic A10 neurons are involved in cognitive functions. *Nature, 286 (5769)*, 150-151.

Singh, L., Field, M. J., Vass, C. A., Hughes, J. and Woodruff, G. N. (1992). The antagonism of benzodiazepine withdrawal effects by the selective cholecystokinin$_B$ receptor antagonist CI-988. *British Journal of Pharmacology, 105*, 8-10.

Skirboll, L., Hokfelt, T., Rehfeld, J., Cuello, A. C. and Dockray, G. (1982). Coexistence of substance P- and cholecystokinin-like immunoreactivity in neurons of the mesencephalic periaqueductal central gray. *Neuroscience Letters, 28*, 35-39.

Skodol, A. E., Oldham, J. M., Hyler, S. E., Stein, D. J., Hollander, E., Gallagher, P. E. and Lopez, A. E. (1995). Patterns of anxiety and personality disorder comorbidity. *Journal of Psychiatric Research, 29(5)*, 361-374.

Slaap, B. R., van Vliet, I. M. Westenberg, H. G. M. and den Boer, J. A. (1995). Phobic symptoms as predictors of nonresponse to drug therapy in panic disorder patients (a preliminary report). *Journal of Affective Disorders, 33*, 31-38.

Smith, G. P. and Gibbs, J. (1992). The development and proof of the CCK hypothesis of satiety.In *Multiple cholecystokinin receptors in the CNS*. C.T. Dourish, S.J. Cooper, S.D. Iversen and L.L. Iversen, Eds: 166-182. Oxford University Press.

Soltis, R. P., Cook, J. C., Gregg, A. E. and Sanders, B. J. (1997). Interaction of GABA and excitatory amino acids in the basolateral amygdala: role in cardiovascular regulation. *Journal of Neuroscience, 17(23)*, 9367-9374.

Somogyi, P., Hodgson, A. J., Smith, A. D., Nunzi, M. G., Gorio, A. and Wu, J. -Y. (1984). Different populations of GABAergic neurons in the visual cortex and hippocampus of cat contain somatostatin- or cholecystokinin-immunoreactive material. *Journal of Neuroscience*, 4, 2590-2603.

Southwick, S. M., Krystal, J. H. and Charney, D. S. (1995). Reply to "Safadi, G. (1995). Relationship of panic disorder to posttraumatic stress disorder." *Archives of General Psychiatry, 52*, 77-78.

Spiegel, D. A., Bruce, T. J., Gregg, S. F. and Nuzzarello, A. (1994). Does cognitive behavior therapy assist slow-taper alprazolam discontinuation in panic disorder. *American Journal of Psychiatry, 151 (6)*, 876-881.

Spring, B. (1981). Stress and schizophrenia: some definitional issues. *Schizophrenia Bulletin, 7(1)*, 24-33.

Stein, M. B., Heuser, I.J., Juncos, J.L. and Uhde, T.W. (1990). Anxiety disorders in patients with Parkinson's disease. *American Journal of Psychiatry, 147(2)*, 217-220.

Stewart, J. and Vezina, P. (1988). Conditioning and behavioral sensitization. In *Sensitization in the Nervous System*. P.W. Kalivas and C.D. Barnes, Eds: 207-224. New York: Telford Press.

Stewart, S. H. (1992). Chronic use of alcohol and/or benzodiazepines may account for evidence of altered benzodiazepine receptor sensitivity in panic disorder. *Archives of General Psychiatry, 49*, 329-330.

Strakowski, S., Sax, K. W., Setters, K. W. and Keck Jr, P. E. (1996). Enhanced response to repeated d-amphetamine challenge: evidence for behavioral sensitization in humans. *Biological Psychiatry, 40*, 872-880.

Studler, J. M., Javoy-Agid, F., Cesselin, F., Legrand, J. C., Agid, Y. (1982). CCK-8 immuno-reactivity distribution in human brain: selecctive decrease in the substantia nigra from parkinsonian patients. *Brain Research, 243*, 176-179.

Studler, J. M., Reibaud, M., Tramu, G., Blanc, G., Glowinski, J. and Tassin, J. P. (1984). Pharmacological study on the mixed CCK-8/DA meso-nucleus pathway: evidence for the existence of storage sites containing the two neurotransmitters. *Brain Research, 298*, 91.

Sudo, A. and Miki, K. (1993). Dissociation of catecholamine and corticosterone responses to different types of stress in rats. *Industrial Health, 31(3)*, 101-111.

Sugrue, M. F. (1981). Current concepts on the mechanisms of action of antidepressant drugs.*Pharmacological Therapeutics, 13*, 219-247.

Suzuki, T., Moroji, T., Hori, T., Baba, A., Kawai, N. and Koizumi, J. (1993). Autoradiographic localization of CCK-8 binding sites in the rat brain: effects of chronic methamphetamine administration on these sites. *Biological Psychiatry, 34*, 781-790.

Svensson, T. H. (1980). Effect of chronic treatment with tricyclic antidepressant drugs on identified brain noradrenergic and serotonergic neurons. *Acta Psychiatra Scandinavia, 61(Suppl 280)*, 121-131.

Tamminga, C. A., Littman, R. L., Alphs, L. D., Chase, T. N., Thaker, G. K. and Wagman, A. M. (1986). Neuronal cholecystokinin and schizophrenia: pathogenic and therapeutic studies. *Psychopharmacology, 88,* 387-391.

Targum, S. D. (1991). Panic attack frequency and vulnerability to anxiogenic challenge studies.*Psychiatric Research, 36,* 75-83.

Targum, S. D. (1992). Cortisol response during different anxiogenic challenges in panic disorder patients. *Psychoneuroendocrinology, 17 (5)*, 453-458.

Taylor, A. E., Saint-Cyr, J. A. and Lang, A. E. (1986). Frontal lobe dysfunction in Parkinson's disease. *Brain, 109,* 845-883.

Taylor, C. B., Hayward, C., King, R., Ehlers, A., Margraf, J., Maddock, R., Clark, D., Roth, W. T. and Agras, W. S. (1990). Cardiovascular and symptomatic reduction effects of alprazolam and imipramine in patients with panic disorder: results of a double-blind, placebo-controlled trial. *Journal of Clinical Psychopharmacology, 10 (2)*, 112-118.

Taylor, M. D., DeCeballos, M. L., Rose, S., Jenner, P. and Marsden, C. D. (1992). Effects of unilateral 6-hydroxyphenylalanine treatment on peptidergic systems in rat basal ganglia. *European Journal of Pharmacology, 219,* 183-192.

Thiebot, M. -H., Soubrie, P. and Sanger, D. (1988). Anxiogenic properties of beta-CCE and FG 7142: a review of promises and pitfalls. *Psychopharmacology, 94,* 452-463.

Tiihonen, J., Kuikka, J., Bergstrom, K., Lepola, U., Koponen, H. and Leinonen, E. (1997). Dopamine reuptake site densities in patients with social phobia. *American Journal of Psychiatry, 154(2)*, 239-242.

Tomaz, C., Dickinson-Anson, H., McGaugh, J. L., Souza-Silva, M. A., Viana, M. B. and Graeff, F. G. (1993). Localization in the amygdala of the amnestic action of diazepam on emotional memory. *Behavioral Brain Research, 58(1-2)*, 99-105.

Trullas, R. and Skolnick, P. (1993). Differences in fear motivated behaviors among inbred mouse strains. *Psychopharmacology, 111,* 3223-331.

Uhde, T. W., Stein, M. B., Vittone, B. J., Siever, L. J., Boulenger, J. P., Klein, E. and Mellman, T. A. (1989). Behavioral and physiological effects of short-term and long-term administration of clonidine in panic disorder. *Archives of General Psychiatry, 46,* 170-177.

Uhl, G. R., Hedreen, J. C. and Price, D. L. (1985). Parkinson's disease: loss of neurons from the ventral tegmental area contralateral to the therapeutic surgical lesions. *Neurology, 35(8)*, 1215-1218.

Ulibarri, C. and Micevych, P. E. (1993). Role of perinatal estrogens in sexual differentiation of the inhibition of lordosis by exogenous cholecystokinin. *Physiology and Behavior, 54,* 95-100.

Vaccarino, F. J., Arifuzzaman, A. I., Sabijan, S. M., Wunderlich, G. R., DeSousa, N. J., Bush, D. E. A. and Bradwejn, J. (1997). CCK$_B$ receptor activation and anxiogenic behavior: a neuroanatomical analysis. *Society for Neuroscience Abstracts, 23(2)*, 1621.

Vaccarino, F. J. and Rankin, J. (1989). Nucleus accumbens cholecystokinin (CCK) can either attenuate or potentiate amphetamine-induced locomotor activity: evidence for rostral-caudal differences in accumbens CCK function. *Behavioral Neuroscience, 103,* 831-836.

Vanderhaeghen, J. J., Lotstra, F., DeMay, J. and Gilles, C. (1980). Immunohistochemical localization of cholecystokinin- and gastrin-like peptides in the brain and hypophysis of the rat. *Proceedings of the National Academy of Science, 77,* 1190-1194.

van Dijken, H. H., Tilders, F. J. H., Olivier, B. and Mos, J. (1992). Effects of anxiolytic and antidepressant drugs on long-lasting behavioural deficits resulting from one short stress experience in male rats. *Psychopharmacology, 109(4),* 395-402.

van Kammen, D. P., Guidotti, A., Kelley, M. E., Gurklis, J., Guarneri, P., Gilbertson, M. W., Yao, J. K., Peters, J. and Costa, E. (1993). CSF diazepam binding inhibitor and schizophrenia: clinical and biochemical relationships. *Biological Psychiatry, 34,* 515-522.

van Megen, H. J. G. M., Westenberg, H. G. M. and Den Boer, J. A. (1994). Pentagastrin induced panic attacks: enhanced sensitivity in panic disorder patients. *Psychopharmacology, 114,* 449-455.

van Megen, H. J. G. M., Westenberg, H. G. M. and Den Boer, J. A. (1996). Effect of the cholecystokinin-B receptor antagonist L-365, 260 on lactate-induced panic attacks in panic disorder patients. *Biological Psychiatry, 40,* 804-806.

van Megen, H. J. G. M., Westenberg, H. G. M., Den Boer, J. A. and Kahn, R. S. (1996). The panic inducing properties of the cholecystokinin tetrapeptide CCK$_4$ in patients with panic disorder. *European Neuropsychopharmacology, 6,* 187-194.

van Megen, H. J. G. M., Westenberg, H. G. M., Den Boer, J. A., Slaap, B., van Es-Radhakishum, F. and Pande, A. C. (1997). The cholecystokinin-B receptor antagonist CI-988 failed to affect CCK-4 induced symptoms in panic disorder patients. *Psychopharmacology, 129,* 243-248.

van Ree, J. M., Verhoeven, W. M. A., Brouwer, G. and de Wied, D. (1984). Ceruletide resembles antipsychotics in rats and schizophrenic patients. *Neuropsychobiology, 12,* 4-8.

van Valkenburg, C., Winokur, G., Behar, D. and Lowry, M. (1984). Depressed women with panic attacks. *Journal of Clinical Psychiatry, 45(9),* 367-369.

Vasar, E., Peuranen, E., Harro, J., Lang, A., Oreland, L., Mannisto, P. T. (1993). Social isolation of rats increases the density of cholecystokinin receptors in the frontal cortex and abolishes the antiexploratory effect of caerulein. *Naunyn-Schmiedeberg Arch Pharmacology, 348,* 96-101.

Vazquez, A., Jimenez-Jimenez, F. J., Garcia-Ruiz, P. and Garcia-Urra, D. (1993). Panic attacks in Parkinson's disease: a long-term complication of levodopa therapy. *Acta Neurologica Scandinavica, 87(1),* 14-18.

Verhoeven, W. M. A., Westenberg, H. G. M. and van Ree, J. M. (1986). A comparative study on the antipsychotic properties of desenkephalin-γ-endorphin and ceruletide in schizophrenic patients. *Acta Psychiatra Scandinavia, 73,* 372-382.

Vezina, P., Giovino, A. A., Wise, R. A. and Stewart, J. (1989). Environment-specific cross-sensitization between the locomotor activating effects of morphine and amphetamine. *Pharmacology, Biochemistry and Behavior, 32,* 581-584.

Virgo, L., Humphries, C., Mortimer, A., Barnes, T., Hirsch, S. and de Belleroche, J. (1995). Cholecystokinin messenger RNA deficit in frontal and temporal cerebral cortex in schizophrenia. *Biological Psychiatry, 37,* 694-701.

Vogel, H. P. (1982). Symptoms of depression in Parkinson's Disease. *Pharmacopsychiatria, 15* (6), 192-196.

Walker, D. L. and Davis, M. (1997). Double dissociation between the involvement of the bed nucleus of the stria terminalis and the central nucleus of the amygdala in startle increases produced by conditioned versus unconditioned fear. *Journal of Neuroscience, 17(23),* 9375-9383.

Wang, R. Y., White, F. J. and Voigt, M. M. (1984). Cholecystokinin, dopamine and schizophrenia.*Trends in Pharmacological Sciences, 5(9)*, 436-438.

Watanabe, H. (1984). Activation of dopamine synthesis in mesolimbic dopamine neurons by immobilization stress in the rat. *Neuropharmacology, 23 (11)*, 1335-1338.

Wcedzony, K., Mackowiak, M., Fijal, K. and Golembiowska, K. (1996). Evidence that condiotioned conditioned stress enhances outflow of dopamine in rat prefrontal cortex: a search for the influence of diazepam and 5-HTIA agonists. *Synapse, 24(3)*, 240-247.

Webb, J. K., Rupniak, N. M. J. and Boyce, S. (1996). Inhibition of pentagastrin-induced pressor response in conscious rats by the CCK-B receptor antagonist CI-988 and chlordiazepoxide. *Regulatory Peptides, 61*, 71-76.

Weissman, M. M., Canino, G. J., Greenwald, S., Joyce, P. R., Karam, E. G., Lee, C. -K., Rubio-Stipec, M., Wells, J. E., Wickramaratne, P. J. and Wittchen, H. -U. (1995). Current rates and symptom profiles of panic disorder in six cross-national studies. *Clinical Neuropharmacology, 18(S2)*, S1-S6.

Weissman, M. M.,Wickramaratne, P., Adams, P. B., Lish, J. D., Horwath, E., Charney, D., Woods, S. W., Leeman, E. and Frosch, E. (1993). The relationship between panic disorder and major depression: a new family study. *Archives of General Psychiatry, 50,* 767-780.

White, F.J. (1996).Synaptic regulation of mesocorticolimbic dopamine neurons. *Annual Reviews in Neuroscience, 19,* 405-436.

White, R. F., Au, R., Durso, R. and Moss, M. B. (1992). Neuropsychological function in Parkinson's disease. In *Clinical Syndromes in Adult Neuropsychology: The Practitioner's Handbook*. R.F. White, Ed: 253-286. The Netherlands: Elsevier Science.

Whitehead, W. E., Crowell, M. D., Heller, B. R., Robinson, J. C., Schuster, M. M. and Horn, S. (1994). Modeling and reinforcement of the sick role during childhood predicts adult illness behavior. *Psychosomatic Medicine, 56(6),* 541-550.

Williams, G. V. and Goldman-Rakic, P. S. (1995). Modulation of memory fields by dopamine D1 receptors in prefrontal cortex. *Nature, 376,* 572-575.

Williams, S. L., Kinney, P. J. and Falbo, J. (1989). Generalization of therapeutic changes in agoraphobia: the role of perceived self-efficacy. *Journal of Consulting and Clinical Psychology, 57 (3),* 436-442.

Wittchen, H. U. (1988). Natural course and spontaneous remissions of untreated anxiety disorders: results of the Munich follow-up study. In I. Hand and H.U. Wittchen (Eds.), Panic and Phobia 2: *Treatment and Variables Affecting Course and Outcome.* Berlin: Springer-Verlag, 3-17.

Wittchen, H. -U. and Essau, C.A. (1993). Epidemiology of panic disorder: progress and unresolved issues. *Journal of Psychiatric Research, 27(Suppl. 1)*, 47-68.

Wolpe, J. and Rowan, V. C. (1988). Panic disorder: a product of classical conditioning. *Behavioral Research Therapy, 26(6)*, 441-450.

Woodman, C. L., Noyes, R., Ballenger, J. C., Lydiard, R. B., Sievers, G. and Mihalko, D. (1994).Predictors of response to alprazolam and placebo in patients with panic disorder. *Journal of Affective Disorders, 30,* 5-13.

Wunderlich, G. R., DeSousa, N. J. and Vaccarino, F. J. (1997). Microinjection of PD-140,548, a CCK_A antagonist, into the caudal nucleus accumbens attenuates the locomotor response to amphetamine in amphetamine-sensitized animals. *Society for Neuroscience Abstracts, 23(2),* 1621.

Wunderlich, G. R., DeSousa, N. J. and Vaccarino, F. J. (2000). Cholecystokinin modulates both the development and the expression of behavioral sensitization to amphetamine in the rat. *Psychopharmacology (Berl.), 151,* 283-290.

Wunderlich, G. R., Rotzinger, S., Bush, D. E. A., DeSousa, N. J. and Vaccarino, F. J. (2004). Cholecystokinin modulation of locomotor behavior in rats is sensitized by chronic amphetamine and chronic restraint exposure. *Brain Research, 1001(1-2),* 95-107.

Yeragani, V. K., Balon, R. and Pohl, R. (1989). Schizophrenia, panic attacks, and antidepressants.*American Journal of Psychiatry, 146(2),* 279.

Yeragani, V. K., Pohl, R., Balon, R., Ramesh, C., Glitz, D. and Sherwood, P. (1990). Risk factors for cardiovascular illness in panic disorder patients. *Neuropsychobiology, 23,* 134-139.

Yonkers, K. A., Ellison, J. M., Shera, D. M., Pratt, L. A., Cole, J. O., Frierman, E., Keller, M. B.and Lavori, P. W. (1996). Description of antipanic therapy in a prospective longitudinal study. *Journal of Clinical Psychopharmacology, 16(3),* 223-232.

Yoshioka, M., Matsumoto, M., Togashi, H. and Saito, H. (1996). Effect of conditioned fear stress on dopamine release in the rat prefrontal cortex. *Neuroscience Letters, 209(3),* 201-203.

Zacharko, R. M. and Anisman, H. (1984). Motor, motivational and anti-nociceptive consequences of stress: contribution of neurochemical change. In *Stress-Induced Analgesia.* M.D. Tricklebank and G. Curzon, Eds: 33-65. Chichester: Wiley.

Zacharko, R. M. and Anisman, H. (1991). Stressor induced anhedonia in the mesocorticolimbic system. *Neuroscience and Biobehavioral Reviews, 15,* 391-405.

Zacharko, R. M., Koszycki, D., Mendella, P. D. and Bradwejn, J. (1995). Behavioral, neurochemical, anatomical and electrophysiological correlates of panic disorder: multiple transmitter interaction and neuropeptide colocalization. *Progress in Neurobiology, 47,* 371-423.

Zanoveli, J. M., Netto, C. F., Guimaraes, F. S. and Zangrossi, H. (2004). Systemic and intra-dorsal periaqueductal gray injections of cholecystokinin sulfated octapeptide (CCK-8s) induce a panic-like response in rats submitted to the elevated T-maze. *Peptides, 25,* 1935-1941.

Zeigler, S., Lipton, J., Toga, A. and Ellison, G. (1991). Continuous cocaine administration produces persisting changes in brain neurochemistry and behavior. *Brain Research, 552,* 27-35.

Zeitlin, S. B. and McNally, R. J. (1993). Alexithymia and anxiety sensitivity in panic disorder
    and obsessive-compulsive disorder. *American Journal of Psychiatry, 150(4)*, 658-660.m
Zemishlany, Z. and Davidson, M. (1996). Lack of effect of laboratory-provoked anxiety on
    homovanillic acid concentration in normal subjects. *Biological Psychiatry, 40,* 247-252.
Zitrin, C. M. (1983). Differential treatment of phobias: use of imipramine for panic attacks.
    Journal of Behavioral Therapy and Experimental Psychiatry, 14(1), 11-18.

In: Pain Management: New Research
Editors: P. S. Greco, F. M. Conti

ISBN: 978-1-60456-767-0
© 2008 Nova Science Publishers, Inc.

Chapter II

Brain Mechanisms of Placebo Analgesia

Andrea Eugenio Cavanna[1], Stefano Cavanna[2] and Luca Bertero[2]
[1]Institute of Neurology, London, United Kingdom
[2]University of Turin Medical School, Turin, Italy

Abstract

Placebo treatments have proven effective to alleviate pain perception along with a variety of medical conditions. It is currently acknowledged that placebo effects can be induced by expectation of clinical improvement via specific brain mechanisms. Although research in this field has flourished over the last few years, the neurobiological mechanisms underlying placebo-induced clinical responses are not completely understood. This chapter focuses on the current evidence sustaining placebo responses in pain conditions. *In vivo* neurophysiological and functional neuroimaging studies currently shape our understanding of the neural changes associated with placebo effects. Converging evidence suggests that placebo analgesia is linked to the activation of the endogenous opioid network. Within this network, a pivotal role seems to be played by the rostral portion of the anterior cingulate cortex, an area characterized by high density of endogenous opioid receptors. The newborn neuroscience of placebo will likely prove useful in understanding how the context of beliefs and values influences brain processes related to perception and emotion in subjects with both psychological and physical dysfunctions. Further research on the placebo response is needed, both to shed more light on the complexity of mind-body interactions and to improve the efficacy of its applications to clinical practice.

Keywords: *Analgesia; Expectation; Pain; Placebo effect.*

Introduction

The term "placebo" is a Latin word meaning "I shall please". It was first introduced in the English language during the XIII century, but its use in a medical setting has been first reported during the XVIII century. In this context, it acquired a different meaning, i.e. a medicine whose only aim was to please a patient without any real benefit. During the last century, the concept of "placebo effect" was introduced in the scientific literature [1,2]. The placebo effect consists in an actual change in the illness status induced by the medicine's symbolic value rather than by specific therapeutic effects. The placebo effect is currently considered by the medical community as a healing response induced by non-specific verbal or behavioral procedures that operate via the patient's belief in the therapeutic power of placebo itself [3]. It can also be regarded as the effect induced by the psychosocial context in which the therapeutic action takes place [4]. For obvious reasons, sham therapy represents the gold standard to study this effect. The placebo effect has proved effective in a wide range of pathological conditions. It has been pointed out that this phenomenon could represent a privileged window onto the biological bases of mind-brain and brain-body interactions [5]. In other words, a full understanding of these interactions should not leave apart a thorough explanation of the neurobiological mechanisms on which the placebo effect is based. Finally, knowledge of these mechanisms could prove useful in developing new therapies for pain relief with fewer side-effects.

How Does Placebo Analgesia Work?

How does placebo work? According to current theories, placebo-mediated therapeutic efficacy is due mainly to the patient's expectation of a clinical improvement and pavlovian conditioning. Moreover, the term "placebo effect" can refer to several different kinds of placebo effects which are based upon different mechanisms. Placebo analgesia is probably the better understood.

As a matter of fact, placebo analgesia seems to act through the endogenous opioid system. However, it has been shown that the actions of the endogenous opioid system are not limited to pain control. Other physiological functions, including the respiratory, cardiovascular and immune systems, are also influenced by placebo stimulation [6,7]. Research on brain mechanisms underlying the placebo effect is likely to provide us with a better understanding of the complex relationship between mind and body.

Pain relief is one of the most common clinical applications of the placebo effect. Placebo analgesia is the situation in which a substance known to be non-analgesic (usually a biologically inactive substance administered orally, intramuscularly or endovenously) produces an analgesic response in a subject who has been told that it is a painkiller [8]. The existence of an analgesic effect induced by placebo procedures has long been documented in the literature and placebo analgesia is widely used in everyday clinical practice [5]. Moreover, the insights we have into the brain mechanisms underlying the placebo effect come mostly from studies on pain conditions.

The neurobiology of the placebo effect started to be investigated in 1978, when Levine et al. showed that placebo analgesia could be blocked by the opioid antagonist naloxone, thus indicating the involvement of the endogenous opioid system [9]. These findings represent the first suggestion that placebo analgesia is somehow mediated by the release of endogenous opioids, which in turn are responsible for the diminished pain perception. Conversely, ten years ago, Benedetti et al. [10] showed that the opposite phenomenon – called "nocebo effect" - can be reduced through the hidden administration of proglumide, a cholecystokinin antagonist. This was the first evidence showing that cholecystokinin is implicated in the neurobiological mechanisms mediating nocebo-induced hyperalgesia.

The findings of Levine et al.'s experiment showing that the placebo response relies on an endogenous opioid system have been consistently replicated, however further studies indicated that also a non-opioid system could play an important role [11]. This second system does not appear to be influenced by naloxone. Moreover, in an experimental model of pain, the placebo response could be blocked by naloxone if it was induced by strong expectation cues, whereas if the expectation cues were reduced, it was insensitive to naloxone [12]. These findings seem to suggest that the two systems operate in different circumstances. The placebo-activated endogenous opioid systems have been shown to have a somatotopic organization [13].

The Endogenous Opioid System and Placebo Analgesia

The complexity of the endogenous opioid network indicates that it is an important regulatory system for the organism, especially in dangerous or stressful situations. In animal studies, contexts that induce fear and stress have been described as important for the activation of the endogenous opioid system. This response induces a transient analgesic state which prepares the organisms for the flee-or-fight response [14]. This state has also been induced using noxious stimuli. This activation was also induced by conditioned stress-induced analgesia or setting up a context in which fear is thought to be induced in the animal. These triggers will activate an opioid system mediated via the amygdala, which then activates the brainstem opioid system via the periacqueductal gray [14]. It has been hypothesized that several contexts may be important for activating endogenous opioid systems for the induction of analgesia in humans, although a great deal of variability exists in these studies [15,16]. The placebo response is probably the best-described experimental situation in which the endogenous opioid system is naturally activated in humans [17-20] and, thus, research on the placebo response is of general importance also for understanding the endogenous opioid system.

The relationship between placebo analgesia and the endogenous opioid system has also been investigated using functional imaging methods, including positron emission tomography (PET) and magnetic resonance imaging (MRI). Converging evidence suggests that a pivotal role in both exogenous opioid and endogenous opioid-mediated placebo analgesia is played by the rostral portion of the anterior cingulate cortex (rACC), which is strategically positioned to form a loop linking the brainstem with limbic and medial prefrontal regions, and is densely populated with mu-opioid receptors [21]. The ACC, along with the brainstem and the dorsolateral and orbitofrontal cortices, are the most commonly investigated sites in placebo imaging studies [21-27]. Although there is general consensus on the regions involved in placebo analgesia, the exact location of the activation peak in the ACC is debated. However, most authors agree that the rACC, when activated during placebo procedures, enhances descending pain control systems. In fact, the rACC could act as the main interface between the cognitive elaboration of analgesia expectation and endogenous opioid release.

In an initial examination of the neuronal circuitry implicated in these mechanisms, Petrovic et al. (28) described a coincidence of increases in regional cerebral blood flow (CBF) by the systemic administration of a mu-opioid receptor agonist, remifentanil, and placebo with expectation of analgesia in the rACC. Furthermore, individuals who were placebo responders showed more pronounced rACC regional blood flow responses to remifentanil. These data then suggested the presence of variations in the responses of the mu-opioid receptor system as a function of placebo response, localized in the rACC. With regards to the circuitry implicated in placebo analgesia, Wager et al. [29] used functional magnetic resonance imaging (fMRI) to indirectly measure neuronal activity during the administration of a placebo with expectation of analgesia. Placebo administration was associated with reductions in the activity of pain-responsive regions while subjects underwent a painful heat stimulus. The regions involved included the rACC, the insular cortex, and the thalamus. This study used expectancy manipulation to elicit a placebo response, which enhances belief in the placebo itself. This procedure does not involve classical conditioning *per se* (because there is no active unconditioned stimulus), which has been associated with non-opioid-mediated analgesic mechanisms [30]. Although the methodology used does not examine the neurochemical mechanisms inducing the placebo analgesic effect, the regions implicated do present high concentrations of mu-opioid receptors and demonstrate increases in regional blood flow after the exogenous administration of mu-opioid receptor agonists [31-35].

A recent study [36] directly examined whether the introduction of placebo-induced expectation of analgesia activates endogenous opioid neurotransmission, using PET and a mu-opioid receptor-selective radiotracer. Under these conditions, activation of this neurotransmitter system is showed by reductions in the *in vivo* availability of synaptic mu-opioid receptors to bind the radiolabeled tracer [37-40].

The activation of the endogenous opioid system and mu-opioid receptors was compared between sustained pain and sustained pain plus placebo conditions in a sample of 14 healthy males, aged 20–30 years. Significantly higher levels of activation were obtained for the condition in which placebo was administered. After correction for multiple comparisons, statistically significant effects of placebo on mu-opioid system activation were obtained in the left (ipsilateral to pain) dorsolateral prefrontal cortex (DLPFC), pregenual rostral right (contralateral) anterior cingulate, right (contralateral) anterior insular cortex, and left (ipsilateral) nucleus accumbens. A second area within the contralateral insular cortex, in its posterior region, also showed changes in neurotransmission, but it no longer reached statistical significance after correction for multiple comparisons. The psychophysical correlates associated with the placebo-induced activation of the endogenous opioid system were then examined. For these correlates, subjects were selected who showed a substantial placebo effect (i.e. >10% change in the *in vivo* availability of mu-opioid receptors after placebo administration). This threshold was selected as exceeding the typical interexperimental variability in PET mu-opioid receptor measurements [41]. In the pregenual anterior cingulate, placebo-induced mu-opioid system activation above those levels significantly correlated with ratings of visual analog (VAS) pain intensity and pain unpleasantness, McGill Pain Questionnaire (MPQ) sensory subscale scores, and total MPQ scores. Placebo-induced activation of endogenous opioid neurotransmission in this region was also highly and positively correlated with a measure of pain tolerance. In the right anterior insular cortex, significant correlations were obtained with the changes in VAS ratings of pain intensity and MPQ sensory and total MPQ scores. At the level of the left nucleus accumbens, significant correlations were obtained, in the same direction, with the change in VAS pain intensity ratings, MPQ affective subscale, and reductions in negative affect scores experienced during the challenge (Profile of Mood Scale). In the left dorsolateral prefrontal cortex, mu-opioid system activation was negatively correlated with the expected analgesic effect as rated by the subjects before placebo administration.

The regions in which placebo administration increased the endogenous opioid neurotransmission primarily coincided with those observed by Wager et al. [29] as reductions in pain-induced metabolic demands as measured by fMRI during placebo administration (i.e. prefrontal cortex, pregenual anterior cingulate, and insular cortex). The regions implicated in the placebo analgesic effect were part of those in which prominent endogenous opioid neurotransmission and mu-opioid receptor populations are present in humans [42, 43]. The rACC has also been noted to be more prominently activated in high placebo responders after mu-opioid agonist administration [28].

This work takes the investigation of placebo effects directly into the realm of human brain neurotransmission, addressing the effects of cognitive expectations on neural chemical functions. The results presented are consistent with reports implicating the endogenous opioid system in the mediation of placebo analgesic effects, previously examined by their blockade after the systemic administration of naloxone [30, 44-47].

Examination of the individual data also highlighted that changes in neurochemical signaling induced by the introduction of a placebo did not represent an on-off phenomenon but rather a graded effect that was influenced, with relative independence, by a number of brain regions with complex "integrative–motivational" functions. For example, some subjects presented with profound neurochemical responses to the placebo intervention in some but not other regions. Multiple regression analyses were then conducted to examine whether individual differences in the pain experience could be driving some of the variations in the neurochemical response to the placebo (i.e. the analgesic placebo effect serves an adaptive function in the face of increased needs to reduce the individual experience of pain). A multiple regression model that included sensory and affective qualities of pain, a measure of pain sensitivity, and the internal affective state of the volunteers during pain (in the absence of placebo) described 40-65% of the variance in the subsequent regional neurochemical responses to placebo. When the individual items in the model were examined, the internal affective state of the volunteers during pain (as measured with the Positive and Negative Affectivity Scale) and the affective quality of the pain (as measured with the MPQ pain affect subscale) were the only items reaching statistically significant correlations with regional endogenous opioid release after placebo administration. This was the case in the dorsolateral prefrontal cortex, pregenual anterior cingulate, anterior insular cortex, and nucleus accumbens [48].

The Functional Neuroanatomy of the Placebo Effect

The studies and analyses presented above demonstrate that expectation of analgesia is an important factor in the engagement of objective, neurochemical antinociceptive responses to placebo administration. Furthermore, they show that these processes appear to involve the expectations of the perceived analgesic efficacy of the placebo, an effect that is mediated by endogenous opioid neurotransmission within the dorsolateral prefrontal cortex. However, a substantial proportion of the variance in the regional neurochemistry of placebo analgesia can be explained by the experience of pain itself. In this regard, variations in pain sensitivity, in the affective qualities of the pain, as well as the internal affective state of the individual during pain, can explain a substantial proportion of the variance in the formation of the placebo analgesic effect. These findings seem to support the concept that placebo responses form part of adaptive mechanisms engaged as a function of the perceived needs of the organism, with modifiers, such as negative affective states, further regulating those responses. They also suggest that the investigation and understanding of individual variations in placebo responses is further complicated by the individual responses to the process (e.g. clinical pain) for which relief is expected.

These data are consistent with the notion that placebo-responding regions and neurochemical systems (e.g. the endogenous opioid system and mu-opioid receptors) are an intrinsic part of neuronal processes that mediate the interaction between positive environmental conditions (in the present case the suggestion of analgesia) and the corresponding physical and emotional responses of the individual. From a different perspective, disruptions in the function of these normal regulatory processes (e.g. dorsolateral prefrontal atrophy in chronic pain patients [49] may explain the lower rates of placebo responders in the more persistent or severe forms of various illnesses. These may further represent points of vulnerability for the expression or maintenance of various pathological states.

A recent fMRI study investigated the effects of expectations of placebo analgesia in a thermal pain model [29]. It used a single-trial design to separate activity induced by placebo treatment in anticipation of pain from subsequent changes in pain processing. In addition, the investigators defined pain responsive regions of interest in the group of participants and looked for evidence of decreased pain response in these regions following placebo administration. Comparing results across two separate studies in different pain modalities provided convergent evidence for the reliability of findings. Evidence for prefrontal cortex activation during expectation of pain suggests that placebo expectancies are active neurobiological processes that involve the frontal lobes. Evidence for decreases during pain suggests that placebo treatment alters nociceptive sensory and/or affective processing, not just retrospective judgments about pain [50-52].

Placebo treatment decreased both reported pain and pain evoked activity in the brain. There was a 22% reduction in reported pain (p < 0.001), with >70% of participants showing placebo-induced reductions. Although placebo effects were significant in both experiments in this study, these particularly large effects were induced using an expectancy manipulation procedure to enhance belief in the placebo [53]. Placebo also diminished the brain responses in a subset of pain-responsive regions, including the anterior insula and thalamus (contralateral to stimulation) and the anterior cingulate cortex. Furthermore, the greatest placebo effects in pain response were found late in stimulation. These late effects suggest that a substantial portion of the placebo response may reflect a modulation of limbic and paralimbic regions that are involved in the appraisal of pain. Activity in the anterior cingulate and, in particular, the anterior insula is associated with the subjective experience of pain [54] and other aversive emotional states [55-57]. Paradoxically, placebo-induced increases in activity were found in secondary somatosensory cortex. Clearly, future studies will help disentangling the roles of each region of the "pain matrix" in pain processing, and interventions such as the ones described in this chapter can provide leverage points for characterizing the function of the system.

Because placebo-induced expectancies are formed and maintained in anticipation of pain, fMRI signal in the prefrontal cortex during pain anticipation might reflect the generation and maintenance of placebo-related expectancies. It was hypothesized that placebo treatment would induce increases in DLPFC and ventrolateral prefrontal cortex (VLPFC) because of their roles in generating and maintaining cognitive expectancies that guide memory retrieval and attention. Activity in these regions is also thought to play a key role in shaping perceptual processing in posterior brain regions [58-61]. During the anticipation of pain, placebo increased activity in DLPFC, orbitofrontal cortex (OFC), and rACC. Lateral and medial frontal increases with placebo continued through the pain period. These results indicated that placebo treatment engaged active prefrontal processing mechanisms, and their co-localization with activations from studies of working memory and cognitive control suggest that these regions may play a general role in representing expectancies and other elements of situational context across both cognitive and affective domains.

Placebo-Modulated Pain

According to the gate control theory and much subsequent work on central regulation of pain, the periaqueductal gray (PAG) exerts central control over spinal pain pathways [62,63] The PAG receives projections from insula, anterior cingulate, nucleus accumbens, amygdala, and frontal cortex [64-66]. Microstimulation of ventrolateral OFC in rats transiently attenuates nociceptive reflex responses, and this effect is blocked by lesion of the PAG [67, 68]. Consistent with the notion that descending control is a mechanism of placebo analgesia, placebo treatment in the study by Wager et al. [29] induced activity in PAG during anticipation of pain. Surprisingly, the strongest increases were linked in time to the onset of the warning cue signaling upcoming pain. In addition, these increases were positively correlated with increases in OFC and DLPFC, suggesting that opioid systems are engaged by positive expectations of analgesia.

However, this interpretation should be accepted with caution. PAG neurons project upwards to the telencephalon as well as downwards to the spinal cord, and it may well be that PAG modulates the central representation of pain through the activation of opioid release in cortical and limbic regions [36]. Another issue is the timing of PAG activity, which was found during expectation but not during pain. One explanation may be that both placebo and pain itself may increase PAG activity. During pain, placebo-induced increases in PAG may be offset by decreases attributable to reduced pain processing. This issue highlights the potential fruitfulness of separating brain measures of expectation and experience in disentangling the functions of interlocking feedback circuits in the brain.

As reviewed above, there is ample evidence that expectancy-based placebo effects are mediated by endogenous opioids. Future studies may clarify the role of opioids in descending control versus modulation of affective elements of pain. The functions of descending and ascending opioid projections may be closely coupled; indeed, given the recurrent connectivity that is a hallmark of brain circuitry, it would be surprising if they were not. However, they may be functionally separable; the issue at stake is the level of the central nervous system at which nociceptive signals are modulated by placebo.

This chapter focuses on the effects of expectation, which may be directly linked to opioid activity that relieves pain. Positive expectations may also induce changes in several other systems that could impact pain: they could increase positive emotions and activate incentive motivational ("reward") systems, as suggested by the recent results of Zubieta et al.'s study discussed above, or alternatively they could just decrease anxiety. Little is known about the scope of psychological and neural systems that may be affected by placebo. However, the fMRI study by Wager et al. [29] seems to suggest that placebo treatment for pain may act by reducing anxiety: placebo-induced decreases in anticipatory responses were found in the amygdala and temporal poles, both of which have been associated with aversive expectancies [56, 69, 70, 71]. Indeed, a recent study examining placebo-induced anxiolytic effects shares several key activations with regions highlighted by Wager et al. [29], including rACC and OFC [71]. Changes in both anxiety and incentive motivational systems have widespread consequences for the organism, and more research is needed to understand the relationship between brain functions and beliefs and expectations.

Several neurological conditions are associated with pain and have good potential to benefit from placebo treatments. In particular, placebo analgesia in patients suffering from headache is known as a powerful and consistent phenomenon. A recent meta-analysis by de Craen et al. [72] revealed a significant placebo effect in 26-32% of patients with migraine. Overall, results from placebo-controlled clinical trials aimed at the development of new drugs for the abortive treatment of migraine (triptans) have confirmed that placebo effects are highly variable and often substantial in migraine populations [73]. From a clinical perspective, a better knowledge of the neurochemical mechanisms underlying placebo analgesia could be helpful, first in detecting the clinical features of placebo-responder populations and second in refining the use of this additional tool for the treatment of complicated headaches [74].

Conclusions

The usefulness of placebo treatments in alleviating a variety of medical conditions has long been recognized by the scientific community. Generally speaking, the placebo effect can be induced by expectation of clinical improvements and pavlovian conditioning. Although this effect is widely known, the physiological mechanisms underlying this phenomenon are not well understood. Researching these mechanisms could also prove useful in understanding how the context of beliefs and values influences brain processes related to perception and emotion and both mental and physical health. This chapter has focused on the current evidence sustaining placebo responses in pain conditions; however several neurological disorders, including pain, Parkinson's disease, depression, sleep and immune-mediated disorders have been shown to be responsive to placebo. *In vivo* neurophysiological and functional neuroimaging studies conducted over the last decade have considerably deepened our understanding of the neural changes associated with placebo effects. Converging evidence suggests that placebo analgesia is linked to the activation of the endogenous opioid network, the highest density of opioid receptors being located within the brainstem, the DLPFC, the rACC, and limbic structures. Further research on the placebo response is needed, both to shed more light on the complexity of mind-body interactions and to improve the efficacy of its application in clinical practice.

References

[1]   Shapiro AK, Shapiro ED. *The powerful placebo: from ancient priest to modern physician.* Johns Hopkins University Press 1997

[2]   Barsky AJ, Saintfort R, Rogers MP, Borus JF. Nonspecific medication side effects and the nocebo phenomenon. *J. Am. Med. Assoc.* 2002;287:622-627

[3]   Szawarski Z. The concept of placebo. *Sci Eng Ethics* 2004;10:57-64

[4]   Hrobjartsson A. What are the main methodological problems in the estimation of placebo effects? *J. Clin. Epidemiol.* 2002;55:430-435

[5]   Cavanna AE, Monaco F. Placebo treatments: historical overview and current concepts. *Confinia Cephalalgica* 2006;15:3-11

[6]   Benedetti F, Amanzio M, Baldi S, Casadio C, Maggi G. Inducing placebo respiratory depressant responses in humans via opioid receptors. *Eur .J. Neurosci* .1999;11:625–631.

[7]   Pollo A, Vighetti S, Rainero I, Benedetti F. Placebo analgesia and the heart. *Pain* 2003;102:125–133.

[8]   Colloca L, Benedetti F. Placebos and painkillers: is mind as real as matter? *Nat. Rev. Neurosci.* 2004;7:587-588

[9]   Levine JD, Gordon NC, Fields HL. The mechanism of placebo analgesia. *Lancet* 1978;2:654-657

[10]   Benedetti F, Amanzio M, Casadio C, Oliaro A, Maggi G. Blockade of nocebo hyperalgesia by the cholecystokinin antagonist proglumide. *Pain* 1997;71:135-140

[11] Colloca L, Benedetti F Placebos and painkillers: is mind as real as matter? *Nat. Rev. Neurosci.* 2005;6:545–552.

[12] Amanzio M, Benedetti F Neuropharmacological dissection of placebo analgesia: expectation-activated opioid systems versus conditioning-activated specific subsystems. *J. Neurosci.* 1999;19:484–494

[13] Benedetti F, Arduino C, Amanzio M. Somatotopic activation of opioid systems by target-directed expectations of analgesia. *J. Neurosci.* 1999;19:3639 –3648

[14] Fanselow MS. Neural organization of the defensive behavior system responsible for fear. *Psychol. Bull. Rev.* 1994;1:429-438

[15] Fields H, Basbaum A. Central nervous system mechanisms of pain modulation, in Wall P, Melzack R (eds): *Textbook of Pain.* New York, NY, Churchill Livingstone, 1999, pp 309-329

[16] Price D. Placebo analgesia, in Price DD (ed): *Psychological Mechanisms of Pain and Analgesia.* Seattle, WA, IASP Press, 1999, pp 155-181

[17] Levine JD, Gordon NC, Fields HL. The mechanism of placebo analgesia. *Lancet* 1978;2:654-657

[18] Amanzio M, Benedetti F: Neuropharmacological dissection of placebo analgesia: expectation-activated opioid systems versus conditioningactivated specific subsystems. *J. Neurosci.* 1999;19:484-494

[19] Benedetti F, Arduino C, Amanzio M: Somatotopic activation of opioid systems by target-directed expectations of analgesia. *J. Neurosci.* 19: 3639-3648, 1999

[20] Pollo A, Vighetti S, Rainero I, Benedetti F: Placebo analgesia and the heart. *Pain* 2003;102:125-133

[21] Petrovic P. Opioid and placebo analgesia share the same network. *Seminars in Pain Medicine* 2005;3:31-36

[22] Petrovic P, Kalso E, Petersson KM, Ingvar M. Placebo and opioid analgesia: imaging a shared neuronal network. *Science* 2002;295:1737-1740

[23] Wager TD, Rilling JK, Smith EE et al. Placebo-induced changes in fMRI in the anticipation and experience of pain. *Science* 2004;303:1162-1167

[24] Pariente J, White P, Frackowiak RS, Lewith G. Expectancy and belief modulate the neuronal substrate of pain treated by acupuncture. *Neuroimage* 2005;25:1161-1167

[25] Bingel U, Lorentz J, Schoell E, Weiller C. Mechanisms of placebo analgesia: rACC recruitment of a subcortical antinociceptive network. *Pain* 2006;120:8-15

[26] Kong J, Gollub RL, Rosman IS et al. Brain activity associated with expectancy-enhanced placebo analgesia as measured by functional magnetic resonance imaging. *J. Neurosci.* 2006;26:381-388

[27] Zubieta JK, Yau WY, Scott DJ, Stohler CS. Belief or need? Accounting for individual variation in the neurochemistry of the placebo effect. *Brain Behav. Immun.* 2006;20:15-26

[28] Petrovic P, Kalso E, Petersson KM, Ingvar M. Placebo and opioid analgesia—imaging a shared neuronal network. *Science* 2002;295:1737–1740.

[29] Wager TD, Rilling JK, Smith EE, Sokolik A, Casey KL, Davidson RJ, Kosslyn SM, Rose RM, Cohen JD. Placebo-induced changes in FMRI in the anticipation and experience of pain. *Science* 2004;303:1162–1167.

[30] Amanzio M, Benedetti F. Neuropharmacological dissection of placebo analgesia: expectation-activated opioid systems versus conditioning-activated specific subsystems. *J. Neurosc* .1999;19:484–494.

[31] Firestone L, Gyulai F, Mintun M, Adler L, Urso K, Winter P. Human brain activity response to fentanyl imaged by positron emission tomography. *Anesth. Analg.* 1996;82:1247–1251.

[32] Adler LJ, Gyulai FE, Diehl DJ, Mintun MA, Winter PM, Firestone LL. Regional brain activity changes associated with fentanyl analgesia elucidated by positron emission tomography. *Anesth. Analg.* 1997;84:120 –126.

[33] Schlaepfer T, Strain E, Greenberg B, Preston K, Lancaster E, Bigelow G, Barta P, Pearlson G. Site of opioid action in the human brain: mu and kappa agonists' subjective and cerebral blood flow effects. *Am. J. Psychiatry* 1998;155:470–473.

[34] Casey K, Svensson P, Morrow T, Raz J, Jone C, Minoshima S. Selective opiate modulation of nociceptive processing in the human brain. *J. Neurophysiol.* 2000;84:525–533.

[35] Wagner KJ, Willoch F, Kochs EF, Siessmeier T, Tolle TR, Schwaiger M, Bartenstein P. Dose-dependent regional cerebral blood flow changes during remifentanil infusion in humans: a positron emission tomography study. *Anesthesiology* 2001;94:732–739.

[36] Zubieta JK, Bueller JA, Jackson LR, Scott DJ, Xu Y, Koeppe RA, Stohler CS. Placebo effects mediated by endogenous opioid neurotransmission and mu-opioid receptors. *J. Neurosci.* 2005;25:7754 –7762.

[37] Zubieta JK, Smith Y, Bueller J, Xu Y, Kilbourn M, Meyer C, Koeppe R, Stohler C. Regional mu-opioid receptor regulation of sensory and affective dimensions of pain. *Science* 2001;293:311–315.

[38] Zubieta JK, Smith Y, Bueller J, Xu Y, Woike T, Kilbourn M, Meyer C, Koeppe R, Stohler C. Mu-opioid receptor mediated antinociception differs in men and women. *J. Neurosci.* 2002;22:5100–5107.

[39] Zubieta JK, Heitzeg MM, Smith YR, Bueller JA, Xu K, Xu Y, Koeppe RA, Stohler CS, Goldman D. COMT val158met genotype affects mu-opioid neurotransmitter responses to a pain stressor. *Science* 2003;299:1240 –1243.

[40] Bencherif B, Fuchs PN, Sheth R, Dannals RF, Campbell JN, Frost JJ. Pain activation of human supraspinal opioid pathways as demonstrated by [11C]-carfentanil and positron emission tomography (PET). *Pain* 2002;99:589 –598.

[41] Zubieta JK, Bueller JA, Jackson LR, Scott DJ, Xu Y, Koeppe RA, Stohler CS. Placebo effects mediated by endogenous opioid neurotransmission and mu-opioid receptors. *J. Neurosci* .2005;25:7754 –7762.

[42] Gross-Isseroff R, Dillon K, Israeli M, Biegon A. Regionally selective increases in mu opioid receptor density in the brains of suicide victims. *Brain Res.* 1990;530:312–316.

[43] Gabilondo A, Meana J, Garcia-Sevilla J. Increased density of muopioid receptors in the postmortem brain of suicide victims. *Brain Res.* 1995;682:245–250.

[44] Gracely RH, Dubner R, Wolskee PJ, Deeter WR. Placebo and naloxone can alter post-surgical pain by separate mechanisms. *Nature* 1983;306:264 –265.

[45] Grevert P, Albert L, Goldstein A. Partial antagonism of placebo analgesia by naloxone. *Pain* 1983;16:129 –143.

[46] Levine JD, Gordon NC. Influence of the method of drug administration on analgesic response. *Nature* 1984;312:755–756.

[47] Benedetti F. The opposite effects of the opiate antagonist naloxone and the cholecystokinin antagonist proglumide on placebo analgesia. *Pain* 1996;64:535–543.

[48] Zubieta JK, Yau WY, Scott DJ, Stohler CS. Belief or need? Accounting for individual variations in the neurochemistry of the placebo effect. *Brain. Behav. Immun.* 2005

[49] Apkarian AV, Sosa Y, Sonty S, Levy RM, Harden RN, Parrish TB, Gitelman DR. Chronic back pain is associated with decreased prefrontal and thalamic gray matter density. *J. Neurosci.* 2004;24:10410 –10415.

[50] Kienle GS, Kiene H. The powerful placebo effect: fact or fiction? *J. Clin. Epidemiol.* 1997;50:1311–1318.

[51] Hrobjartsson A, Gotzsche PC. Is the placebo powerless? An analysis of clinical trials comparing placebo with no treatment. *N. Engl. J. Med.* 2001;344:1594 –1602.

[52] Hrobjartsson A, Gotzsche PC. Is the placebo powerless? Update of a systematic review with 52 new randomized trials comparing placebo with no treatment. *J. Intern. Med.* 2004;256:91–100.

[53] Price DD, Milling LS, Kirsch I, Duff A, Montgomery GH, Nicholls SS. An analysis of factors that contribute to the magnitude of placebo analgesia in an experimental paradigm. *Pain* 1999;83:147–156.

[54] Craig AD, Chen K, Bandy D, Reiman EM. Thermosensory activation of insular cortex. *Nat. Neurosci* .1999;3:184 –190.

[55] Wager TD, Phan KL, Liberzon I, Taylor SF. Valence, gender, and lateralization of functional brain anatomy in emotion: a meta-analysis of findings from neuroimaging. *NeuroImage* 2003;19:513–531.

[56] Singer T, Seymour B, O'Doherty J, Kaube H, Dolan RJ, Frith CD. Empathy for pain involves the affective but not sensory components of pain. *Science* 2004;303:1157–1162.

[57] Wager TD, Feldman Barrett L. From affect to control: functional specialization of the insula in motivation and regulation. PsycExtra, 2004. Available at http://www.psycinfo.com/psycextra/.

[58] Posner MI. Orienting of attention. *Q. J. Exp. Psychol.* 1980;32:3–25.A

[59] Allport A. Visual attention. In: *Foundations of cognitive science* (Posner MI, ed). Cambridge, MA: MIT 1989.

[60] Desimone R, Duncan J. Neural mechanisms of selective visual attention. *Annu. Rev. Neurosci.* 1995;18:193–222.

[61] Handy TC, Green V, Klein RM, Mangun GR. Combined expectancies: event-related potentials reveal the early benefits of spatial attention that are obscured by reaction time measures. *J. Exp. Psychol. Hum. Percept. Perform.* 2001;27:303–317.

[62] Melzack R, Wall PD. Pain mechanisms: a new theory. *Science* 1965;150:971–979.

[63] Fields H. State-dependent opioid control of pain. *Nat. Rev. Neurosci*. 2004;5:565–575.

[64] Bragin EO, Yeliseeva ZV, Vasilenko GF, Meizerov EE, Chuvin BT, Durinyan RA. Cortical projections to the periaqueductal grey in the cat: a retrograde horseradish peroxidase study. *Neurosci. Lett.* 1984;51:271–275.

[65] Ma QP, Han JS. Neurochemical studies on the mesolimbic circuitry of antinociception. *Brain Res.* 1991;566:95–102.

[66] Rizvi TA, Ennis M, Shipley MT. Reciprocal connections between the medial preoptic area and the midbrain periaqueductal gray in rat: aWGAHRP and PHA-L study. *J. Comp. Neurol.* 1992;315:1–15.

[67] Zhang S, Tang JS, Yuan B, Jia H. Inhibitory effects of electrical stimulation of ventrolateral orbital cortex on the rat jaw-opening reflex. *Brain Res.* 1998;813:359 – 366.

[68] Zhang YQ, Tang JS, Yuan B, Jia H. Inhibitory effects of electrically evoked activation of ventrolateral orbital cortex on the tail-flick reflex are mediated by periaqueductal gray in rats. *Pain* 1997;72:127–135.

[69] Phelps EA, O'Connor KJ, Gatenby JC, Gore JC, Grillon C, Davis M. Activation of the left amygdala to a cognitive representation of fear. *Nat. Neurosci.* 2001;4:437– 441.

[70] Ochsner KN, Ray RD, Cooper JC, Robertson ER, Chopra S, Gabrieli JD, Gross JJ. For better or for worse: neural systems supporting the cognitive down- and up-regulation of negative emotion. *NeuroImage* 2004;23:483– 499.

[71] Petrovic P, Dietrich T, Fransson P, Andersson J, Carlsson K, Ingvar M. Placebo in emotional processing—induced expectations of anxiety relief activate a generalized modulatory network. *Neuron* 2005;46:957–969.

[72] de Craen AJ, Tijssen JG, de Gans J, Kleijnen J. Placebo effect in the acute treatment of migraine: subcutaneous placebos are better than oral placebos. *J. Neurol.* 2000; 247:183-188.

[73] Loder E, Goldstein R, Biondi D. Placebo effects in oral triptan trials: the scientific and ethical rationale for continued use of placebo controls. *Cephalalgia* 2005;25:124-131

[74] Pascual-Lozano AM, Chamarro-Lazaro R, Lainez MJ. Placebo response in a patient with chronic migraine and ergotic overuse. *Cephalalgia* 2005;25:391-394

In: Pain Management: New Research   ISBN: 978-1-60456-767-0
Editors: P. S. Greco, F. M. Conti   © 2008 Nova Science Publishers, Inc.

Chapter III

Treatment for Muscle Pain by Japanese Traditional Medicine (*Acupuncture* and *Kampo*)

Yutaka Takaoka[*]

Laboratory for Applied Genome Science and Bioinformatics,
Clinical Genome Informatics Center, Kobe University Graduate School of Medicine,
Kobe 650-0017, Japan

Abstract

Japanese traditional medicine that consists of *Acupuncture* and *Kampo* (Japanese herbal medicine), is widely used as a complementary and alternative medicine to cure and to care for patients in Japan. The origin of Japanese traditional medicine came from Chinese Medicine over 1500 years ago. However, it has evolved uniquely to develop different method, needles (e.g., smaller diameter), and adaptation of Herb, from those of Chinese Medicine.

We investigate the molecular mechanisms of Japanese traditional medicine especially the efficacy of *Acupuncture* in muscles. At first, the molecular evidence of the acupuncture stimulation in the muscle is explained. Then the clinical manipulation of *Acupuncture* and *Kampo* formulation are introduced.

Introduction

Acupuncture therapy and *Kampo* medicine have long been believed to be a worthy component of routine clinical practice in Japan, and its use for at least 1,500 years can be verified. The usual theory of *Acupuncture* and *Kampo* have been based on a model of energy (*qi*) balance, which involves metaphysical cognition and is quite different from the premise

---

[*] ytakaoka@med.kobe-u.ac.jp.

on which Western medicine is based; for example, acupuncture may correct imbalances of *qi* flow on meridians, which are the routes of *qi*, and it would then lead to disease cures and wound healing [2, 9]. The treated points of *qi* flow are called acupoints, which are placed on meridians. Acupuncture practice is utilized to cure many diseases and to maintain health. Major acupuncture techniques involve penetration of the skin by thin, solid metallic needles, which are manipulated manually or are stimulated electrically (EA, electroacupuncture) [8]. Figure 1A shows routes of acupuncture stimuli between acupoints and organs. Pain and other physical problems such as muscle exhaustion, including stiff shoulders in patients, as well as the conditioning of athletes, have benefited from acupuncture treatment.

1. Molecular Evidence of Acupuncture Treatment in Muscle Pain

In our molecular investigation of acupuncture [12], we show a proliferative effect on muscle satellite cells of long-term EA treatment. Figure 1B shows typical results of electroacupuncture condition in mice and human subjects. We usually use approximately 1 to 10 Hz for clinical practice, sometimes mixed with other frequencies.

EA suppresses the gene expression of the myostatin which function as an endogenous inhibitor of muscle growth and satellite cell-related muscle regeneration [11, 13]. After only one EA treatment at 24 hr—i.e., the study of the short-term EA—expression of the myostatin gene was at most 50% of that of the control group. Indeed, the long-term EA effect in the expression of the myostatin gene is more significantly suppressed by daily EA treatment after 1 day and 1 week, and quite marked suppression of expression was observed after 1 month (Figure 2A). The molecular evidence suggested with some confidence that EA treatment suppresses the myostatin gene expression under the long-term daily EA. Then the myostatin gene suppression is led to a satellite cell-related proliferative reaction and repair in skeletal muscle. Morphological effect in skeletal muscle after EA is shown in Figure 2B to E. It shows the results for EA-treated muscle after 1 month of daily treatment. Nuclei of EA-treated muscle (Figure 2D) had clearly visible nucleoli compared to control muscle that had had no EA treatment. The presence of nucleoli confirmed DNA replication and synthesis of rRNA. Nuclei in cells of muscle treated daily with EA reacted with PCNA (Proliferating Cell Nuclear Antigen) antibody (Figure 2C, E), whereas no reaction occurred in control muscle (Figure 2B). EA-treated muscle showed a proliferative reaction, because PCNA antibody was prominent in nuclei in the S phase [10].

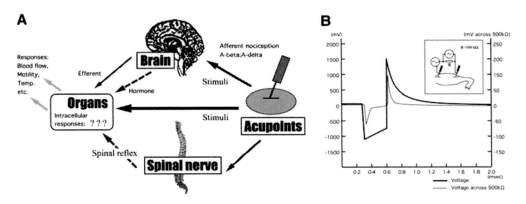

Figure 1. A: Schematic diagram of transmission of acupuncture signals. Solid arrows indicate the nervous system; broken arrows, the extraneural system; gray arrows, organ responses. Modified from Cho et al (1). B: Electrical voltage and current were measured with a digital oscilloscope (LS140, LeCroy Corp., Chestnut Ridge, NY) connected to circuits as shown. Electrical current was calculated (I = E/R) on the basis of voltage across a 500-kΩ resistor in the mouse leg.

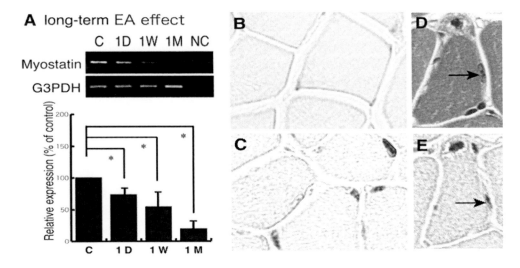

*, $P<0.05$; NS, not significant.

Figure 2. A: RT-PCR analysis of myostatin gene expression after long-term EA. Data were obtained from different individual samples (n=5, except for the 1M group: n=3). G3PDH was used as a loading control. Lanes are as follows: lane C: control; lane 1D: EA stimulation for 1 day; lane 1W: after daily EA stimulation for 1 week; lane 1M: after daily EA stimulation for 1 month. Relative transcript levels of myostatin are shown (means ± SD). B: Immunohistochemical findings indicate the PCNA antibody-negative nuclei were shown in no EA-treated muscle. C: PCNA antibody-positive nuclei were clearly present in EA-treated. D, E: In serial sections, PCNA antibody reacted in satellite cells, and nucleoli were found in the same nuclei by hematoxylin and eosin staining. Original magnifications: ×100.

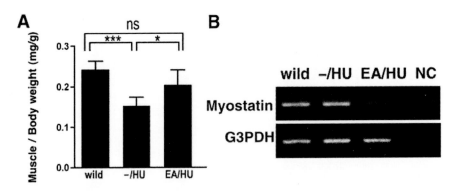

*, *P*<0.05; ***, *P*<0.005; NS, not significant; HU, mouse atrofy model by Hindlimb Unloading method

Figure 3. A: Anti-atrofy analysis in mouse atrofy model (HU) estimated by the relative muscle weight after long-term EA (n=15). Disuse muscle atrophy was suppressed by the EA. B: RT-PCR analysis of myostatin gene expression after long-term EA. Remarkable gene suppression of myostatin was shown in only the muscle of EA-treated mouse atrophy model (EA/HU). NC: negative control.

Indeed, PCNA-positive nuclei (Figure 2D) were found only in satellite cells that had clearly visible nucleoli (Figure 2E) in the nuclei, which confirmed that EA caused a proliferative reaction in skeletal muscle. Tissues collected at the other time points, similar to the control samples, showed no PCNA antibody reactions. In addition, EA-treated disuse muscle atrophy mouse model showed the suppression of muscular atrophy (Figure 3A) with the suppression of myostatin gene expression (Figure 3B). These results indicated with some confidence that long-term EA treatment suppressed the myostatin gene expression and then induced the satellite cell-related proliferative reaction.

From these findings, we can consider simple model of therapeutic effect of EA treatment in skeletal muscle, except neurophysiological pain. The model is as follows: Firstly EA stimulation suppresses the myostatin gene expression and it causes proliferation of skeletal muscle stem cell (satellite cell), and then it facilitates the repair and regeneration of skeletal muscle which leads to the improvement of muscle pain. Thus, our molecular evidence suggested that the EA induce the muscle repair which lead to cure for muscle pain.

2. Clinical Manipulation of Acupuncture: Muscle Pain

We can consider two treatments for muscle pain: (1) EA treatment whose effect is based on molecular evidence, (2) Acupuncture treatment without electrical stimulation. The following sections describe the two practical procedures.

2.1. Electroacupuncture Practice

This section describes the procedure of electroacupuncture practice.

Firstly acupuncture needles are inserted to the subject muscle at the points in the vicinity of its start and stop. The inserted points should not necessarily be acupoints.

Then the needles are stimulated with a low-frequent electrical stimulator for 15 minutes with the repetitions between 1 to 10-Hz. The stimulation repetition should be rather higher unless the patient feels pain.

At the clinical scene, acupuncturist starts with low repetitions, makes it higher gradually, and keeps at slightly lower than the ones that the patient begins to feel pain. If the patient complains pains during 15 minutes stimulation, electrical conditions should be lower.

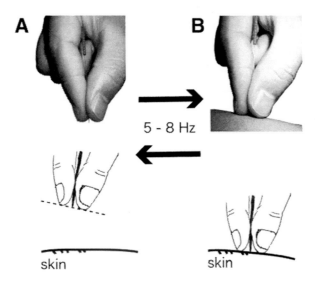

Figure 4. The method of "San-shin". Pick the needle with thumb and forefinger, then touch the surface of the skin without insertion. The dotted line of A designates the end of the thumb and forefinger, and the tip of the needle never comes out of the line. The movement of stimulation (A to B) is repeated at 5-8 Hz frequencies in the pain area.

2.2. Traditional Acupuncture Practice

This section describes the procedure of acupuncture practice without electrical stimulation.

In our previous study, acupuncture with no electrical stimulation did not suppress myostatin gene expression and showed no proliferation of satellite cell. Therefore the effect of acupuncture alone is different from that of EA. Indeed traditional acupuncture practice is known to be effective for suppression of muscle pain after moderating muscle tone based on empirical knowledge. This section introduces two techniques of traditional acupuncture practice for muscle pain: "Tan-shi" and "San-shin".

"Tan-shi" is a technique to simply insert and remove needles without tapping nor twirling.

The practical procedure of this technique is to moderate muscle tone by inserting needles at acupoints, specifically from the ones which patients comparatively feel pain during the examination for muscle tone, and to the ones on the target muscle.

"*San-shin*" is to stimulate by touching the surface of the skin with the end of the needle rhythmically in a wide area including the muscle tone (Figure 4).

We have a variety of "*Tan-shi*" practices which are available when muscle pain is not effectively removed or reduced by "*Tan-shi*" itself: "*Jaku-taku*", tapping a needle (moving slightly up and down) literally meaning sparrows picking their foods; "*Sen-nen*", twirling a needle after inserting it into the skin to a specific degree in depth.

Table 1. Effective *Kampo* for muscle pain

Japanese Name (Chinese Name)	Indications (muscle pain)	Indications (other pain)	Remarks
Shakuyaku-kanzo-to (Shao-Yao-Gan-Cao-Tang)	pain with acute muscle cramp (e.g., muscle cramp in hemodialysis patients, muscle pain or skeletal muscle tremors[3][4][6], nocturnal leg cramps[7], muscle pain from combination chemography with paclitaxel and carboplatin[14])	abdominal pain, thoracic outlet syndrome	
Shakuyaku-kanzo-bushi-to (Shao-Yao-Gan-Cao-Fu-Zi-Tang)	muscle pain from overwork, low back pain, cramp of leg muscles[5]	colic (urinary tract, bile duct, gastrointestinal tract), acute low back pain, gastrocnemial/soleus uscle cramp, sciatic neuralgia, nuchal pain, distortion	Add *bushi* to *Shakuyaku-kanzo-to* when the body being sensitive to cold
Kakkon-to (Ge-Gen-Tang)	shoulder stiffness, muscle tone (mytonia), early symptoms of common cold, coryza, early stage of fabrile disease[5]	neck pain, trigeminal neuralgia, neuralgia for upper body, urticaria, temporomandibular arthritis	Frequently used in daily life in Japan
Keishi-to (Gui-Zhi-Tang)	(the same as *Kakkon-to*)	common cold, influenza	Used at early stage of common cold when physical strength is getting lower
Keishi-ka-bushi-to (Gui-Zhi-Jia-Fu-Zi-Tang)	(the same as *Kakkon-to*)		Add *bushi* to *Keishi-to* when the body being sensitive to cold

3. *Kampo* Treatment: Muscle Pain

Kampo treatment for muscle pain is outlined. Among those herb medicine formulas, *Keishi-to* (*Gui-Zhi-Tang*) is utilized for patients of physical frailty, and the others for patients whose physical strength is relatively high. *Shakuyaku-kanzo-bushi-to* (*Shao-Yao-Gan-Cao-Fu-Zi-Tang*) and *Keishi-ka-bushi-to* (*Gui-Zhi-Jia-Fu-Zi-Tang*) which includes *bushi* (*Fu-Zi*), are utilized when patients feel cold.

In the history of Japanese traditional medicine, pain has been treated by *Acupuncture* while *Kampo* has been utilized for other symptoms. Therefore, there are a few herb medicine for analgesia only. However, there are some options in *Kampo* for muscle pain as shown in Table 1.

In *Kampo*, practitioners should pay attention to the following side effects, although they rarely occur: hypokalemia or syndrome of apparent mineralocorticoid excess for *Shakuyaku-kanzo-to* (*Shao-Yao-Gan-Cao-Tang*), *Kakkon-to* (*Ge-Gen-Tang*), and *Keishi-to* (*Gui-Zhi-Tang*).

Conclusion

Acupuncture therapy is generally thought to be effective only for analgesia. However, our research provided molecular evidence that EA is effective for repair and regeneration of skeletal muscle, whereas *Kampo* efficacy for pain reduction is not noted because acupuncture is mainly utilized for pain treatment.

There are two mechanisms for the treatment of muscle pain by Japanese traditional medicine: muscle repair by EA leading to analgesia, and moderating muscle tone by *Acupuncture* and/or *Kampo*, which facilitates analgesic effect. For a tailor-made treatment, the effective combination of *Acupuncture* and *Kampo* would be needed in the near future.

Acknowledgments

This work was supported by the 20th Grant-in-aid of the Nakatomi Foundation in the fiscal year 2007. I thank Ms. Sachiko Ikemune and Mr. Toshikazu Miyamoto (Tsukuba University Graduate School of Comprehensive Human Sciences) for their experiment of mouse atrophy model, and Dr. Mika Ohta and Ms. Aki Sugano (Kobe University Graduate School of Medicine) for their myostatin gene expression analysis. In addition, I also thank Mr. Hitoshi Nagano (*Ko-jin* Acupuncture Clinic and Kobe University Graduate School of Medicine) for his suggestion of acupuncture practice.

References

[1] Cho, Z.H., Chung, S.C., Jones, J.P., Park, J.B., Park, H.J., Lee, H.J., Wong, E.K. and Min, B.I. (1998). New findings of the correlation between acupoints and corresponding brain cortices using functional MRI. *Proc. Natl. Acad. Sci. USA*, 95, 2670–2673.

[2] Gongwang, L. and Hyodo, A. (1994). Fundamentals of Acupuncture and Moxibustion. Tianjin, China, Tianjin Science and Technology Translation and Publishing.

[3] Hinoshita, F., Ogura Y., Suzuki, Y., Hara, S., Yamada, A., Tanaka, N., Yamashita, A. and Marumo, F. (2003). Effect of orally administered shao-yao-gan-cao-tang (Shakuyaku-kanzo-to) on muscle cramps in maintenance hemodialysis patients: a preliminary study. *Am. J. Chin. Med.*, 31(3), 445-453.

[4] Hyodo, T., Taira, T., Takemura T., Yamamoto, S., Tsuchida, M., Yoshida, K., Uchida, T., Sakai, T., Hidai, H. and Baba, S. (2006). Immediate effect of Shakuyaku-kanzo-to on muscle cramp in hemodialysis patients. *Nephron Clin. Pract.*, 104(1), c28-32.

[5] International Institute of Health and Human Services (Eds.) (2005). Appendix - Composition and Indications of 148 Prescriptions. In: The Journal of Kampo, Acupuncture and Integrative Medicine: Research on Theory, Practice, and Integration Vol. 1. (Special edition, pp.85-101). Berkeley, International Institute of Health and Human Services.

[6] Ito, Y., Murotani, N. Ito, K., Matsuda, Y., Shimada, T., Miyamoto, M., Anzai, K., Ytamashita, K., Yoshida, A. and Ochiai, T. (2003). *J. Jpn. Soc. Dial .The*r., 36(1), 33-39.

[7] Jung, W.S., Moon, S.K., Park, S.U., Ko, C.N. and Cho, K.H. (2004). Clinical assessment of usefulness, effectiveness and safety of jackyakamcho-tang (shaoyaogancao-tang) on muscle spasm and pain: a case series. *Am. J. Chin. Me*d., 32(4), 611-620.

[8] Klein, J.L. and Trachtenberg A.I. (Oct 1997). Acupuncture: Current bibliographies in medicine 97-6 [online]. National Institutes of Health. Available from: http://www.nlm.nih.gov/pubs/cbm/acupuncture.html.

[9] Lock, M.M. (1980) East Asian Medicine in Urban Japan:Varieties of Medical Experience (Comparative Studies of Health Systems and Medical Care). Los Angeles, University of California Press.

[10] Rossi, R., Villa, A., Negri, C., Scovassi, I., Ciarrocchi, G., Biamonti, G. and Montecucco, A. (1999). The replication factory targeting sequence/PCNA-binding site is required in G1 to control the phosphorylation status of DNA ligase I. EMBO J, 18, 5745–5754.

[11] Schuelke, M., Wagner, K.R., Stolz, L.E., Hubner, C., Riebel, T., Komen, W., Braun, T., Tobin, J.F. and Lee, S.J. (2004). Myostatin mutation associated with gross muscle hypertrophy in a child. N. Engl. J. Med., 350, 2682–2688.

[12] Takaoka Y., Ohta M., Ito A., Takamatsu K., Sugano A., Funakoshi K., Takaoka N., Sato N., Yokozaki H., Arizono N., Goto S. and Maeda E. (2007). Electroacupuncture suppresses myostatin gene expression: cell proliferative reaction in mouse skeletal muscle. Physiol. Genomics, 30(2), 102-10.

[13] Wagner, K.R., Liu, X., Chang, X. and Allen, R.E. Muscle regeneration in the prolonged absence of myostatin. (2005). Proc. Natl. Acad. Sci. USA, 102, 2519-2524.

[14] Yamamoto, K., Hoshiai, H. and Noda, K. (2001). Effects of Shakuyaku-kanzo-to on Muscle Pain from Combination Chemotherapy with Paclitaxel and Carboplatin. *Gynecol. Oncol.*, 81(2), 333-334.

Reviewed by Professor Hisahide Nishio (Kobe University Graduate School of Medicine).

In: Pain Management: New Research

Editors: P. S. Greco, F. M. Conti

ISBN: 978-1-60456-767-0

© 2008 Nova Science Publishers, Inc.

Chapter IV

Application of Solution Calorimetry of Nonelectrolytes for the Investigation of Intermolecular Interactions in Solutions

Boris N. Solomonov[*] and Vladimir B. Novikov[+]

Chemical Institute, Kazan State University,
Kremlevskaya 18, Kazan 420008, Russia

Abstract

The solution calorimetry is a valuable instrument for the investigation of intermolecular interactions in condensed media. This chapter is the review of research carried out in this field during the last 50 years. We focused our attention on organic nonelectrolytes as solutes and on individual nonaqueous solvents. The peculiarity of water as a solvent (hydrophobic effect) was also considered.

It is assumed in this chapter that the term 'solution' in distinction from 'mixing' means the transfer of a solute to a solvent at infinite dilution. It allows to exclude the solute-solute interaction in final state. Experimentally obtained enthalpies of solution were recalculated in the majority of cases to solvation enthalpies by subtraction of the vaporization enthalpies of the solutes. It allows to exclude the solute-solute interaction in initial state.

Resulted solvation enthalpies were analyzed using the traditional scheme which assumes that solvation enthalpy can be regarded as the sum of the cavity formation enthalpy and the interaction enthalpy. The former item reflects partial breaking of solvent-solvent interaction during the solvation.

The solute-solvent interaction enthalpy was regarded as the sum of the interaction enthalpies of specific and nonspecific types. Specific interactions are considered as

[*]Boris.Solomonov@ksu.ru

[+]Vladimir.Novikov@ksu.ru

localized donor-acceptor interactions. The examples of specific interactions are hydrogen bonding and charge transfer complex formation.

It was discussed the attempts to correlate the nonspecific solvation enthalpies with the polarity and polarizability parameters of solute and solvent molecules. It was made the attempt to estimate the contribution of polar interactions to the nonspecific solvation enthalpy.

We paid a great attention to the methods of extraction of hydrogen bonding enthalpies from the solvation enthalpy data. The analysis of solvation enthalpies in the solvents associated via hydrogen bonding was performed by taking into consideration the cooperativity of hydrogen bonding formation. Combined use of solution calorimetry and IR spectral methods is especially productive in this case.

1. Introduction

Many chemical and biological processes occur in solutions. The influence of solvent on these processes can be critical. If solvent is not directly engaged in chemical reactions, it influences the dissolved compounds through noncovalent intermolecular interactions. It is obvious that understanding the chemistry of solutions is impossible without studying these interactions.

Many different methods are available to researchers to study the intermolecular interactions. Spectral methods such as NMR-, IR-, UV-VIS spectroscopy are most commonly used. Thermodynamic functions of solution/solvation can also be used to investigate the intermolecular interactions. However, they depend on both solute-solvent and solvent-solvent intermolecular interactions. In order to study the individual types of intermolecular interactions, one needs to have a unified methodology that enables him to extract the contributions of these interactions from the total value of thermodynamic function. Such methodology will allow to develop deeper insights into various physico-chemical processes.

Thermodynamic analysis of the solvation process should be made in terms of enthalpy, Gibbs energy, and entropy of solvation. The Gibbs energy, which is related to the activity coefficients and solubility, often seems to be more interesting magnitude from a practical point of view. For our opinion, to understand the intermolecular interactions, it is equally important to analyze all thermodynamic functions.

The solution enthalpy can be found using direct measurement either from temperature dependence of the solution Gibbs energy. The first way leads, in general, to more accurate results. Modern calorimeters allow to study a very wide range of systems in comparison with the methods used to determine the solution/solvation Gibbs energy.

There exist several approaches to the analysis of the solvation enthalpies. In recent decades multiparameter correlations such as LSER (linear solvation energy relationships) are most commonly used. We have discussed the advantages and disadvantages of these methods in Refs [1; 2]

We think that it is most productive to analyze successively the separate types of intermolecular interactions in solutions. An example of such approach based on the solution enthalpy data is presented in current chapter.

2. Solution, Solvation and Interaction

First of all, we must define some terms used in this chapter. It is necessary because the same terms is used sometimes with diverse meaning and vice versa (e.g. 'partial molar heat of transfer at infinite dilution' in Ref [3] means the same as 'solvation enthalpy' in this chapter).

The properties of any substance in solution differ from ones in gas phase because the molecules in liquids are solvated. *Thermodynamically, the solvation is the of transfer of substance from the state of ideal gas into the solution of definite concentration.* Hence, the solvation enthalpy is the difference between the enthalpic levels of the substance in the solution and in the gas phase. In contrast to solvation, *the solution (as a process) is the of transfer of substance from the standard state into the solution.* For example, the standard state for benzene at 298.15 k is the liquid state. The standard states for methane and anthracene are gaseous and solid (crystalline) states respectively.

The standard molar enthalpies for solvation and solution (as a process) are interrelated by a simple equation:

$$\Delta_{solv}H^{A/S} = \Delta_{soln}H^{A/S} - \Delta_{vap}H^A \qquad (1)$$

where $\Delta_{solv}H^{A/S}$, $\Delta_{soln}H^{A/S}$ and $\Delta_{vap}H^A$ are the standard molar enthalpies for solvation, solution and vaporization respectively.

NB: further as the text goes we will use the term 'enthalpy' having in mind the 'standard molar enthalpy'. Superscripts A and S in Eqn (1) and subsequent equations denote 'any solute' and 'any solvent' respectively.

In view of analysis, solvation enthalpy is essentially more simple than solution enthalpy because the former does not depend on the solute-solute intermolecular interactions in initial state. However, solution enthalpy is simpler for the experimental determination. Therefore, the solvation enthalpy is generally obtained from the data of solution calorimetry using Eqn (1).

In the general case, solvation and solution enthalpies depend on the concentration of resulted solution. It is related with the fact that at sufficiently high concentration of the solute the solute-solute interactions are possible in resulted solution. To simplify the analysis we will consider only the solution (and solvation) enthalpies at infinite dilution. *The infinite dilution conditions imply that the concentration of solute in resulted solution is sufficiently low to neglect the solute-solute interactions.* Experimentally, the infinite dilution conditions is tested by the determination of solution enthalpy at several consecutively growing concentrations.

The driving force of solvation is the solute-solvent intermolecular interactions. Nevertheless, the 'solvation' and 'interaction' are not the identical notions. To penetrate into the solvent the solute molecule must 'pull out' the solvent molecules. That is, the solvation as above defined process implies the partial breaking of the solvent-solvent interactions. Therefore, solvation enthalpy depends not only on solute-solvent interactions but also on solvent-solvent interactions. To segregate these two effects the following model is used. Solvation is considered as it consists of two stages. First, the cavity with size and shape of solute molecule is formed in the solvent. Partial breaking of solvent – solvent interactions take place at this stage. Second, solute molecule is inserted into the cavity formed at previous stage and solute-solvent interactions are turned on. The model is illustrated by the scheme on Figure 1 for the case of equal sizes of solute and solvent molecules.

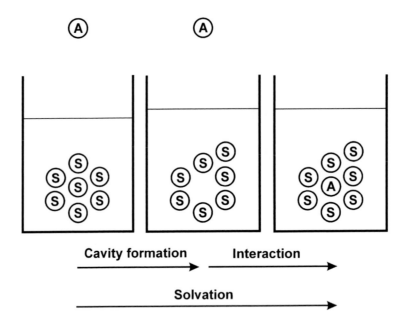

Figure 1. Solvation as it occurs in two stages: cavity formation and interaction.

According to this model, solvation enthalpy is the sum of cavity formation enthalpy ($\Delta_{cav}H^{A/S}$) and interaction enthalpy ($\Delta_{int}H^{A/S}$).

$$\Delta_{solv}H^{A/S} = \Delta_{cav}H^{A/S} + \Delta_{int}H^{A/S} \tag{2}$$

It is easy to show that for the simplest theoretical case (all intermolecular interactions in the solvent are identical and additive) cavity formation enthalpy for solvent itself ($\Delta_{cav}H^{S/S}$) is equal to vaporization enthalpy and interaction enthalpy is equal to doubled vaporization enthalpy with opposite sign. Despite the fact that two stages in above mentioned model are rather speculative the division of solvation enthalpy according to Eqn. (2) is very useful for understanding the influence of solvent nature on solvation enthalpy.

Cavity formation enthalpy can not be measured experimentally, but there are some theoretical approaches which enable to calculate this value [4-7]. Usually such approaches conceive the cavity formation as an inserting to the solvent of hard noninteracting sphere with size and shape of solute molecule. The volume of molecule is commonly considered as the major solute molecule parameter determining the cavity formation enthalpy.

3. Solute-Solvent Intermolecular Interactions

In contrast to solvation enthalpy the solute-solvent interaction enthalpy is closely related to enthalpy of pair intermolecular interactions. Certainly, cooperative nature of solute-solvent interactions must be taken into consideration.

There exist several approaches for division of intermolecular interactions into different types. The most radical point of view is that any division is useless inasmuch as any intermolecular interaction results from interactions of electrons and atomic nucleus and its energy can be calculated by the quantum-chemical methods. We think that quantum-chemical nature of intermolecular interactions is doubtless but such approach to intermolecular interactions at present time is unproductive. Unfortunately, the possibilities of quantum-chemical calculations are far from requirements for real intermolecular interactions in multi-particle condensed systems.

We will consider the enthalpy of solute-solvent interactions first of all as the sum of the enthalpies of specific and nonspecific interactions.

$$\Delta_{int}H^{A/S} = \Delta_{int(nonsp)}H^{A/S} + \Delta_{int(sp)}H^{A/S} \tag{3}$$

Specific interactions enthalpy $\left[\Delta_{int(sp)}H^{A/S}\right]$ is the enthalpy of localized donor-acceptor interactions, including hydrogen bond formation.

According to Eqn (3), solvation enthalpy can be considered as the sum of nonspecific solvation enthalpy $\left[\Delta_{solv(nonsp)}H^{A/S}\right]$ and specific interaction enthalpy:

$$\Delta_{solv}H^{A/S} = \Delta_{solv(nonsp)}H^{A/S} + \Delta_{int(sp)}H^{A/S} \tag{4}$$

where $\Delta_{solv(nonsp)}H^{A/S}$ is the sum of $\Delta_{cav}H^{A/S}$ and $\Delta_{int(nonsp)}H^{A/S}$.

Eqn (4) means that solvation is considered as it consists of two stages: nonspecific solvation and specific interactions. These stages are illustrated by the scheme on figure 2.

In contrast to physical point of view the division of intermolecular interactions into specific and nonspecific ones is quite evident from chemical point of view. The stages on figure 2 are not speculative only. The second stage is well known complexation reaction in the solvent. Solvated but nonbonded specifically molecules in many cases can be detected in the solvent by spectral methods [8-11].

Nonspecific interactions enthalpy is commonly considered as the sum of dispersion, dipolar, and inductive contributions:

$$\Delta_{int(nonsp)}H^{A/S} = \Delta_{int(disp)}H^{A/S} + \Delta_{int(dip)}H^{A/S} + \Delta_{int(ind)}H^{A/S} \tag{5}$$

The second term $\left[\Delta_{int(dip)}H^{A/S}\right]$ on the right-hand side of Eqn (5) reflects the electrostatic solute-solvent interaction arising from dissymmetry of charge distribution in the molecules. This type of interaction is often named the orientational or dipolar interaction. The parameters of such dissymmetry are first of all the dipole moments of the molecules and secondly the multipole moments of higher order. The third term $\left[\Delta_{int(ind)}H^{A/S} \right]$ is also of electrostatic nature, but one of two interacting dipoles (or multipoles) arises from the polarization of initially nonpolar molecule in the electrostatic field of another molecule. In addition to the parameters of charge dissymmetry of second molecules the polarizability of first molecule play decisive role.

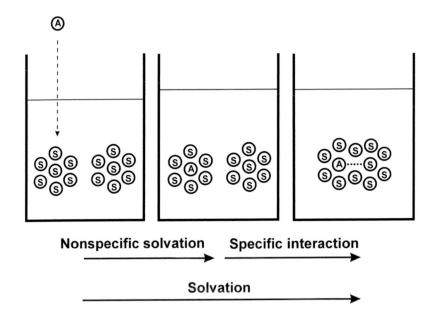

Figure 2. Solvation as it occurs in two stages: nonspecific solvation and specific interaction.

Sometimes the sum of electrostatic contributions is named the enthalpy of polar interactions:

$$\Delta_{int(polar)}H^{A/S} = \Delta_{int(dip)}H^{A/S} + \Delta_{int(ind)}H^{A/S} \tag{6}$$

The first term on the right-hand side of Eqn (5) $\left[\Delta_{int(disp)}H^{A/S} \right]$ is the enthalpy of dispersion interaction which is of quantum-chemical nature. The particular feature of dispersion interaction is that it is attributed to all molecules without any exceptions. For simplest pair molecular systems the value of this term is strongly computable and depends on polarizability and ionization potential of both partners. Sometimes the term 'van der Waals interactions' is used as the synonym of 'dispersion interactions' [12-20]. But in other papers [21-25] the term 'van der Waals interactions' is used as the synonym of 'nonspecific interactions'.

The separation of polar and specific interaction contributions to various physico-chemical parameters including the solvation enthalpy is very often performed by using the homomorph concept [26-33].The latter can be expressed mathematically by the equation:

$$\Delta_{solv}H^{A/S} - \Delta_{solv}H^{h/S} = \Delta_{int(polar)}H^{A/S} + \Delta_{int(sp)}H^{A/S} \tag{7}$$

where $\Delta_{solv}H^{h/S}$ is the solvation enthalpy of homomorph.

Homomorph is the compound with similar dispersion forces but incapable of polar and specific interactions [26]. Assuming this definition of homomorph, the Eqn (7) can be considered as rigorous. Unfortunately, the enthalpy of dispersion interaction can not be measured directly and this definition is partially useless for choice of definite compound as homomorph. Another definition formulated in papers [33-35] states that *homomorphs are the molecules which have the same or closely similar molecular geometry*. For example, alkanes with similar molar volume or ethers with the same number of carbon atoms were often used as homomorphs for aliphatic alcohols. It must be understood that the second definition of homomorph being applied to Eqn (7) means that dispersion interaction enthalpy depends only on the size (volume) and shape (branching) of solute molecule. Despite high allure of such supposition it is not proven and we consider it as erroneous.

Before extracting the polar and specific contributions from solvation enthalpies we will consider the systems for which the dispersion interactions play the decisive role.

4. Systems with Predominance of Dispersion Solute-Solvent Interactions

Solute-solvent dispersion interaction is of quantum-chemical nature. The energy of this interaction should be calculated by quantum-chemical methods. Unfortunately, the rigorous calculations are limited by rather the simplest pairs of molecules such as two atoms of hydrogen. Calculations for real multi-electron and multi-nuclear molecules is possible only by using of several approximations whose validity is often the subject of discussion. It must be noted that quantum-chemical calculation of pair intermolecular interaction is the higher-order problem than calculation of the energy of unique molecule owing to plurality of mutual orientations. The obstacles increase dramatically for the solutions because of nonadditivity of pair intermolecular interactions. There exist some methods for estimating the energy of dispersion interactions. It is reputed that energy of dispersion interactions depends on electronic polarizability, ionization potential [36] and magnetic susceptibility of interacting molecules [6]; and can be calculated by using of certain pair intermolecular potentials such as Lennard-Jones potential [6] or solubility parameter [12]. The essential difficulty is that verification of any estimation according to Eqn (2) depends on the correctness of cavity formation term determination. In other words, the problems of dispersion interactions and cavity formation are closely interrelated.

If there exist among a great many of organic nonelectrolytes the substances capable of dispersion solute-solvent interaction only (or predominantly), then these substances are first of all the alkanes. Indeed, it is generally accepted that alkanes do not interact specifically with common organic compounds. Molecular dipole moments of alkanes are practically equal to zero. The polarity of C-H and C-C bonds is low, so the multipole moments of alkanes must be minimal. Besides, alkanes have the minimal polarizability among all organic substances. This allows us to suppose the minor contribution of inductive interaction. Moreover, inductive interactions must depend not only on the polarizability of first interacting molecule but also on the dipole moment of second molecule and, as it will be shown below, such contribution to solvation enthalpy is negligible.

We will consider both cases: (i) alkane is a solute and (ii) alkane is a solvent.

4.1. Solvation Enthalpies of Alkanes in Various Solvents

Solution and solvation enthalpies of alkanes in various media were studied thermochemically in a series of works [37-41]. It was ascertained that solvation enthalpy of alkyl derivatives of various substances is the additive function of the number of methylene groups in solute molecule [37;40]. Besides, it was shown in Refs. [38;42] that solution enthalpy for alkanes of various structure is proportional to the volume of alkane molecule. Molar volume(V_M), molar refraction (MR, Lorentz–Lorenz equation) or characteristic volume (V_X)[43] can be used as the measure of alkane molecule volume. Example of such proportional dependence is shown in figure 3, where the solution enthalpy values were obtained from Ref. [38].

In contrast to the solution enthalpies, the solvation enthalpies of alkanes depend significantly on the degree of branching of the carbon skeleton, groups of alkanes with the same degree of branching giving rise to several almost parallel lines on the plot of $\Delta_{solv}H^{Alk/S}$ against V_M, MR or V_X. The influence of the branching on the solvation enthalpy of alkane has been investigated in Ref. [38] and it has been shown that the solvation enthalpy of normal alkanes is greater in absolute magnitude than that of branched alkanes with the same number of carbon atoms in the molecule. This phenomenon was explained by the steric hindrances in the interaction of tertiary or quaternary carbon atoms with solvent molecules. The influence of carbon skeleton branching on solvation enthalpy was described in Ref. [47] using the topological index $^A\chi^S$.

Fuchs and Stephenson [40] founded an empirical relation between the solvation enthalpies of the alkane methylene group in various solvents and solvent parameters such as Kamlet–Abboud–Taft π^* constant and function of refractive index $\left[(n^2-1)/(2n^2+1)\right]$:

$$\Delta_{solv}H^{-CH_2-/S} = -3.68 + 1.61 \cdot \pi^* - 5.99 \cdot (n^2-1)/(2n^2+1) \qquad (8)$$

Solvation enthalpies of alkanes in various solvents are very important for the investigation of intermolecular interactions in solutions of organic nonelectrolytes. Several examples are considered below.

Fuchs et al. [38] concluded that an n-alkane and a branched isomer having one or more quaternary carbon atoms have similar molar volumes, and should, therefore, as solutes, cause the expenditure of about the same amount of cavity formation energy in a given solvent. On the other hand, the molecular surface area, and opportunities for effective short range dispersion interactions with solvents, are considerably greater for the n-alkane. The observation that the quantity $\left[\Delta_{solv} H^{Alk(normal)/S} - \Delta_{solv} H^{Alk(branched)/S} \right]$ has nearly the same value for methanol, DMF, benzene, and cyclohexane would be likely only if the dispersion interactions between the n-alkane and each of four solvents were also similar [38]. It means that interaction enthalpy of an alkane as a solute is approximately the same in the solvents of various polarity and the differences in solvation or solution enthalpies in these cases arise primarily from the differences in cavity formation energy. This result was used as a basis of the method for determining the relative cavity formation enthalpy of a solvent [48;49].

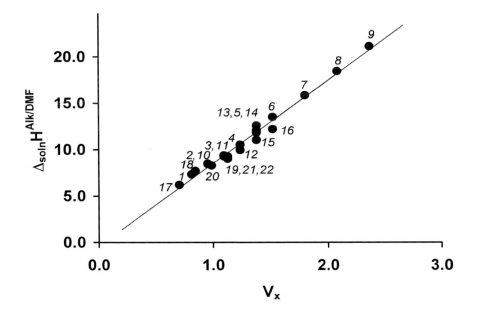

Figure 3. Correlation of solution enthalpies in DMF ($\Delta_{soln} H^{Alk/DMF}$, kJ mol-1) for some alkane solutes with their characteristic volumes (V_x , cm3 mol-1 102). Solutes: 1 - n-pentane, 2 - n-hexane, 3 - n-heptane, 4 - n-octane, 5 - n-nonane, 6 - n-decane, 7 - n-dodecane, 8 - n-tetradecane, 9 - n-hexadecane, 10 - 2,2-dimethylbutane, 11 - 2,2-dimethylpentane, 12 - 2,2,4-trimethylpentane, 13 - 2-methyloctane, 14 - 3,3-diethylpentane, 15 - 2,2,4,4-tetramethylpentane, 16 - 2,2,5,5-tetramethylhexane, 17 - cyclopentane, 18 - cyclohexane, 19 - cyclooctane, 20 - methylcyclohexane, 21 - 1,1-dimethylcyclohexane, 22 - cis-1,2-dimethylcyclohexane. $\Delta_{soln} H^{Alk/DMF}$ values taken from Ref. [38]. V_x values calculated according Ref. [43] and divided by 100 as it is accepted in further papers [44-46].

If the solute is alkane (Alk) Eqns **(1)** and **(2)** gives:

$$\Delta_{soln}H^{Alk/S} = \Delta_{vap}H^{Alk} + \Delta_{cav}H^{Alk/S} + \Delta_{int}H^{Alk/S} \qquad (9)$$

In a series of solvents, vaporization enthalpy is a constant. Any solvent of the series can be defined as the standard solvent (S_0) for the comparison with other solvents. Assuming the constancy of interaction enthalpy of alkane with various solvents it can be written:

$$\Delta_{soln}H^{Alk/S} - \Delta_{soln}H^{Alk/S_0} = \Delta_{cav}H^{Alk/S} - \Delta_{cav}H^{Alk/S_0} = \left\{\delta_{cav}H^{Alk}\right\}_{S_0}^{S} \qquad (10)$$

where $\left\{\delta_{cav}H^{Alk}\right\}_{S_0}^{S}$ is the relative cavity formation enthalpy. It is convenient to define the standard solvent as the hypothetical solvent (n-hexane is good approximation) for which the solution enthalpies of any n-alkane are equal to zero. In this case the relative cavity formation enthalpy is equal to solution enthalpy of n-alkane with the same volume [49].

$$\left\{\delta_{cav}H^{Alk}\right\}_{S_0}^{S} = \Delta_{soln}H^{Alk/S} \qquad (11)$$

The specific relative cavity formation enthalpy ($\delta_{cav}h^S$)[49] was defined owing to proportionality between the solution enthalpy of alkanes and volume of their molecules.

In addition to molar refraction the characteristic volume was used as a measure of solute molecule volume. We consider that validities of both functions are approximately the same. But characteristic volume being strongly additive from atomic and bond contributions is simpler for calculation. So, the specific relative cavity formation enthalpy can be calculated:

$$\delta_{cav}h^S = \frac{\Delta_{soln}H^{Alk/S}}{V_x^{Alk}} \qquad (12)$$

It should be emphasized that the value calculated using Eqns (11) and (12) is not absolute but relative cavity formation enthalpy; nevertheless, it can be used for calculation of the solute-solvent interaction enthalpy relatively to any standard solvent.

The values of specific relative cavity formation enthalpy for some solvents [50] are shown in table 1.

Parameter $\delta_{cav}h^S$ reflects the solvent-solvent intermolecular interactions. In this respect, it is somewhat similar to the Hildebrand solubility parameter calculated by Eqn (13).

$$\delta_H = \sqrt{\frac{\Delta_{vap}H - RT}{V_M}} \qquad (13)$$

where V_M is molar volume of solute or solvent.

**Table 1. Relative cavity formation enthalpies
per unit of McGowan characteristic volume**

Solvent (S)	$\delta_{cav}h^S$ kJ cm^{-3} 10^2
Acetone	7.65
Acetonitrile	10.66
Acetophenone	5.31
Anisole	5.69
Benzene	5.02
Benzonitrile	4.01
Benzylamine	7.85
Chlorobenzene	2.56
1-Chlorobutane	2.07
Cyclohexane	1.42
Cyclohexanone	4.66
Dibutyl Ether	0.53
1,2-Dichlorobenzene	3.47
N,N-Dimethylacetamide	7.66
1,4-Dioxane	7.57
Dipropyl Ether	0.70
DMF	8.62
DMSO	13.87
Ethyl Acetate	5.98
Mesitylene	1.10
Nitrobenzene	4.99
Nitromethane	13.74
Pyridine	6.66
Tetrachloromethane	1.91
Toluene	2.65
1,1,1-Trichloroethane	2.57
Triethylamine	0.43
Trifluoromethylbenzene	3.50
p-Xylene	1.31

However, the Hildebrand parameter for real solvents reflects both nonspecific and specific solvent-solvent interactions being obtained from vaporization enthalpy, while $\delta_{cav}h^S$ seems to reflect only the nonspecific interactions.

The using of relative cavity formation enthalpy allows sometimes the alternative point of view for understanding of some aspects of solvent effect on various physico-chemical processes. For example, it was found [51] the linear correlations between $\delta_{cav}h^S$ and the differences in energies of gauche- and trans- conformers of 1,2-dichloroetane, 1,1,3-

trichloroethane and 1,1,2,2-tetrachloroethane in a series of solvents. Supposing that gauche-conformer occupies the smaller volume in the solvent than trans-conformer, we can conclude that the ratio of conformers in various solvents is controlled by not only the differences in its conformer dipole moment but also the cavity formation term. Both explanations are alternative because of rough correlation of Kirkwood function of the solvent and $\delta_{cav}h^{S}$, nevertheless, the later seems as preferable owing to the absence of anomalous falling out of some points for nonpolar solvents such as 1,4-dioxane and benzene. This conclusion is especially interesting taking into consideration the contribution of electrostatic interactions into the solvation enthalpy which will be considered below.

Very old Berthelot rule [52] states that the interaction potential between two different molecules 1 and 2, U_{12}, is in many cases proportional to the square root of potential between two equal components 1...1 or 2...2: U_{11} or U_{22}:

$$U_{12} = \sqrt{(U_{11}U_{22})} \tag{14}$$

Assuming this approximation we can suppose that square root from relative cavity formation enthalpy is the parameter which describes the possibility of the nonspecific interaction with various solutes. We denote this parameter as S_{vdW} stressing that it related to solvent and van der Waals interactions (as synonym of nonspecific interactions).

$$S_{vdW} = \sqrt{\delta_{cav}h^{S}} \tag{15}$$

This parameter was used to describe the solvent effect on IR stretching vibration frequencies [53;54]. The correlation of OH-frequency shift for pyridine- methanol complex with S_{vdW} is shown on figure 4.

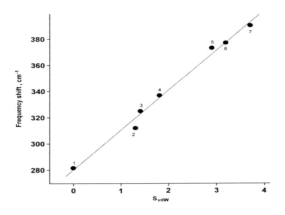

Figure 4. Correlation of OH-frequency shifts for pyridine- methanol complex in several solvents with the values of solvent parameter S_{vdW}. Solvents: 1 - n-hexane; 2 – diethyl ether; 3 – tetrachloromethane; 4 – THF; 5 – 1,2-dichloroethane; 6 – acetonitrile; 7 – nitromethane.

The using of the new thermochemical parameter S_{vdW} allows to extract the frequency shift induced by van der Waals interaction from the total solvent effect. This provides a series of new opportunities for experimental IR spectroscopy [53;54].

4.2. Solvation Enthalpies of Various Nonelectrolytes in Alkanes

The thermochemistry of solvation of various non-electrolytes in alkanes has been studied in a number of works [22;41;55-61]. The most remarkable result [57;60] is the linear correlation of the solvation enthalpies in cyclohexane for solutes of various classes with their molar refraction:

$$-\Delta_{solv}H^{A/C_6H_{12}}\left[kJ/mol\right]=5.09+1.03\cdot MR^A\left[cm^3/mol\right]$$

$$N=102,\quad r=0.994,\quad s=1.6$$

(16)

where N, r and s are number of points, correlation coefficient and standard deviation respectively; molar refraction was calculated by the Lorentz–Lorenz equation:

$$MR=V_M\cdot\frac{n^2-1}{n^2+2}$$

(17)

The analysis of experimental calorimetric data shows that solution and solvation enthalpy of any organic nonelectrolyte in a range of saturated hydrocarbons depends only slightly on the nature of hydrocarbon. Therefore, Eqn (16) can be considered also as a good approximation for the calculation of solvation enthalpies in other saturated hydrocarbons such as normal and branched hexanes, heptanes etc.

The existence of linear correlation (16) is the indirect confirmation of the thesis about the constancy of interaction energy of alkane with various organic nonelectrolytes which was discussed in previous section. Indeed, solvation enthalpy of any solute in alkane can be considered as the sum of cavity formation term and interaction enthalpy:

$$\Delta_{solv}H^{A/Alk}=\Delta_{cav}H^{A/Alk}+\Delta_{int}H^{A/Alk}$$

(18)

Cavity formation term ($\Delta_{cav}H^{A/Alk}$) must be proportional to the volume of solute molecule. If interaction enthalpy of alkane does not depend on the nature of second molecule but only on its size then $\Delta_{int}H^{A/Alk}$ must also be proportional to the volume of solute molecule. Therefore, solvation enthalpy of any solute in alkane must be proportional to the volume of solute molecule. In reality, Eqn (16) shows not the proportional but the linear dependence. The fact that intercept differs from zero can not discredit the constancy of interaction energy. We consider that there are at least two apparent reasons of nonzero intercept. First, the volume of solute molecule is the thing in itself. Molar refraction is only a measure of solute molecule volume. We think that it is more adequate measure than molar volume, since solvation enthalpy in cyclohexane correlates with the latter substantially worse. Nevertheless, it is probably nonideal measure. Second, it is very probable that $\Delta_{int}H^{Al/Alk}$ must be proportional not to volume of molecule but its surface. It is confirmed by the differences in solvation enthalpies for normal and branched alkanes in various solvents. Moreover, the enthalpies of solvation in cyclohexane for substances with branched alkyl groups fall out from the correlation (16). The branching of carbon skeleton of solute molecule can be taken into account using the increments to intercept in Eqn (16) for corresponding solutes [60]. Unfortunately, the surface of molecule is the thing in itself in even a greater degree than volume of molecule.

The solutes involved in correlation (16) widely vary in dipole moment of molecule (from 0 to 3.8 D). Therefore, it can be concluded that contribution of dipolar interactions to solvation enthalpies in alkane as a solvent is absent or not exceeds 1.6 kJ mol[-1] (standard deviation of regression). The same reason allows to exclude the contribution of inductive interactions. Despite the fact that molar refraction can be interpreted as the electronic polarizability of the molecule, it seems as very improbable that product of solute polarizability by small dipole moment of alkane is greater than product of alkane polarizability (comparable with one of solute) by dipole moment of solute. Any allusion to collective character of interaction with a great number of solvent molecules in solvation sphere must be rejected in this as contradicting the results discussed in previous section (solvation of alkanes in a various solvents).

Thus the existence of linear correlation (16) shows that solvation enthalpies of various organic nonelectrolytes in saturated hydrocarbons are controlled by dispersion solute-solvent interactions.

Eqn (16) was the first quantitative correlation between the thermodynamic parameter of solvation and the solute structural parameter for a wide range of organic nonelectrolytes.

It were made several attempts to describe the solvation enthalpies in cyclohexane using another solute parameters which can be associated with dispersion interactions [62]. These parameters are molar volume (V_M^A), molar magnetic susceptibility (χ_M^A) and molecule surface area calculated by Bondi method (A_W). Resulted equations and regression parameters are shown below.

$$-\Delta_{solv}H^{Al/C_6H_{12}}\left[kJ/mol\right]=13.3+0.207\cdot V_M^A\left[cm^3/mol\right]$$
$$N=72,\ r=0.92,\ s=26.6 \tag{19}$$

$$-\Delta_{solv}H^{Al/C_6H_{12}}\left[kJ/mol\right]=15.21+1.995\cdot\chi_M^A\left[cm^3/mol\right]$$
$$N=41,\ r=0.95,\ s=16.4 \tag{20}$$

$$-\Delta_{solv}H^{Al/C_6H_{12}}\left[kJ/mol\right]=6.4+3.51\cdot A_W\left[cm^2/mol\right]$$
$$N=74,\ r=0.80,\ s=8.0 \tag{21}$$

These correlations shows that molar refraction is yet the preferable empiric parameter for describing the dispersion interactions in solutions.

The regular solution theory [63;64] is the most widely used among the semiempirical approaches to analyze the thermodynamic parameters of solvation. It establishes the cohesive energy density (Hildebrand solubility parameter, δ_H) as the parameter characterizing the ability of solute (δ_H^A) and solvent (δ_H^S) to intermolecular interaction.

$$\delta_H = \sqrt{\frac{\Delta_{vap}H - RT}{V_M}} \tag{22}$$

where V_M is molar volume of solute or solvent.

This approach gives us the Eqn (23) for calculation of solvation enthalpy [37;65].

$$\Delta_{solv}H = V_M^A \cdot \left(\delta_H^S\right)^2 - 2 \cdot V_M^A \cdot \delta_H^S \cdot \delta_H^A - RT \tag{23}$$

where $\left[V_M^A \cdot \left(\delta_H^S\right)^2\right]$ and $\left(2 \cdot V_M^A \cdot \delta_H^S \cdot \delta_H^A\right)$ are the internal energies of cavity formation and interaction respectively.

It was found [60] that Eqn (23) describes satisfactorily the solvation enthalpies of n-hexane in a wide range of solvents. On the other hand, it describes rather poorly the solvation enthalpies of wide range of solutes (especially of polar and associated solutes) in cyclohexane. The cause of this discrepancy is that Eqn (23) describes the energy of solute-solvent interaction as proportional to the product of δ_H^S by δ_H^A. It is of course contradicting the above discussed thesis about the constancy of interaction energy of alkane with various organic nonelectrolytes. This contradiction is of little significance for nonpolar substances. But for the polar and associated liquids, Hildebrand solubility parameter being calculated from vaporization enthalpy overestimates the possibility of substance to dispersion interaction. If solute is n-hexane and solvent is polar or associated liquid than Eqn (23) overestimates also the cavity formation term. So it take place some compensation if alkane is a solute. Such compensation is apparently absent if alkane is a solvent.

The method for estimation of vaporization enthalpies from solution enthalpies in cyclohexane was obtained using the Eqns (16) and (1) [57;60]:

$$\Delta_{vap}H^A = \Delta_{soln}H^{A/C_6H_{12}} + 5.09 + 1.03 \cdot MR^A \tag{24}$$

where $\Delta_{vap}H^A$ and $\Delta_{soln}H^{A/C_6H_{12}}$ are the enthalpies (kJ mol^{-1}) of vaporization and of solution in cyclohexane respectively; MR^A is Lorentz–Lorenz molar refraction (cm^3 mol^{-1}) that can be easily calculated using Eqn (17) or some additive schemes [66].

Comparison of vaporization enthalpies calculated by Eqn (24) with experimental values obtained from literature is shown in figure 5.

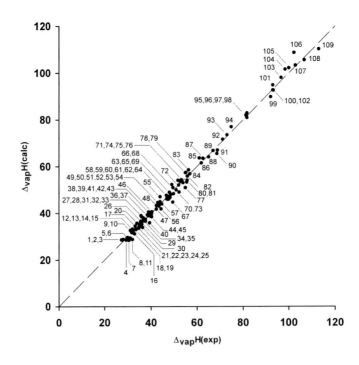

Figure 5. Comparison of vaporization enthalpies (kJ mol^{-1}, 289.15 K) calculated by Eqn (24) with experimental values obtained from literature. Dashed line on the plot corresponds to equality of calculated $\left[\Delta_{vap}H^A(calc) \right]$ and experimental $\left[\Delta_{vap}H^A(exp) \right]$ values. Numerical data are obtained from Refs [60;62]. Substances: 1 — dichloromethane; 2 — carbon disulfide; 3 — iodomethane; 4 — trans-1,2-dichloroethylene; 5 — propanal; 6 — propionaldehyde; 7 — chloroform; 8 — cis-1,2-dicloroethylene; 9 — acetone; 10 — methyl acetate; 11 — THF; 12 — thiophene; 13 — propanethiol-1; 14 — allyl amine; 15 — tetrachloromethane; 16 — acetonitrile; 17 — 1-chlorobutane; 18 — cyclohexene; 19 — acrylonitrile; 20 — benzene; 21 — trichloroethylene; 22 — butanone; 23 — ethyl acetate; 24 — fluorobenzene; 25 — 1-aminobutane; 26 — 1,4-difluorobenzene; 27 — hexafluorobenzene; 28 — 1-iodopropane; 29 — methyl propionate; 30 — ethyl nitrate; 31 — 1,2-dimetoxyethane; 32 — 1-butanethiol; 33 — 1-bromobutane; 34 — 1,4-dioxane; 35 — methanol; 36 — pentanone-2; 37 — pentanone-3; 38 — N-methylpyrrole; 39 — propyl acetat; 40 — piperidine; 41 — cyclo-propylmethyl ketone; 42 — 1,1-dichlorobutane; 43 — methyl butyrate; 44 — pyridine; 45 — dimethyl sulfite; 46 — chlorobenzene; 47 — ethanol; 48 — hexanone-3; 49 — hexanone-2; 50 — methyl pentanoate; 51 — 2,4-pentanedione; 52 — butyl acetat; 53 — bromobenzene; 54 — styrene; 55 — phenylacetylene; 56 — 1,1,2,2-tetrachloroethane; 57 — water; 58 — heptanone-4; 59 — anisole; 60 — allyl alcohol; 61 — 1.2-dichlorobenzene; 62 — propanol-1; 63 — heptanone-2; 64 — methyl trichloroacetate; 65 — thiophenol; 66 — benzonitrile; 67 — ethylchloro acetate; 68 — iodobenzene; 69 — benzaldehyde; 70 — ethyl trichloroacetate; 71 — octanone-2; 72 — butanol-1; 73 — benzonirtile; 74 — N,N-dimethylaniline; 75 — 1-chlorooctane; 76 — methylphenyl sulphide; 77 — nitrobenzene; 78 — nonanone-5; 79 — phenyl acetate; 80 — methyl benzoate; 81 — aniline; 82 — acetophenone; 83 — nonanone-2; 84 — pentanol-1; 85 — decanone-2; 86 — hexanol-1; 87 — iodine; 88 — 1.4-dichlorobenzene; 89 — heptanol-1; 90 — undecanone-2; 91 — phenol; 92 — octanol-1; 93 — naphthalene; 94 — 1-bromodecane; 95 — 1,3-dinitrobenzene; 96 — decanol-1; 97 — 1,2,4,5-tetrachlorobenzene; 98 — diphenyl; 99 — hexachlorobenzene; 100 — phenanthrene; 101 — cis-azobenzene; 102 — benzophenone; 103 — trans-azobenzene; 104 — benzyl; 105 — anthracene; 106 — 9-methoxyanthracene; 107 — 1,2-diphenylethylene; 108 — 9-chloroanthracene; 109 — diphenylmercury.

This method of estimation of vaporization enthalpy is very useful. Experimental determination of solution enthalpy in cyclohexane is much easier than that of vaporization enthalpy. The accuracy of experimental vaporization enthalpy determination is substantially reduced for the substances with low volatility. Calorimetric or vapor-pressure experiment for these substances must be performed at temperatures substantially higher than 298 K and recalculation to standard vaporization enthalpies is conjugated with additional inaccuracies. Such experiment is rather impossible for thermally labile substances. Vapor pressure experiment is extremely susceptible to the residual traces of volatile impurities. As a result, the difference in vaporization enthalpies obtained for the same substance by different researchers is often much more than the sum of inaccuracies reported by the authors. Unfortunately, it is just the fact that prevents more exact determination of limits for the method based on Eqn (24). The known limit is conjugated with the branching of carbon skeleton that can be taken into account using the increments to intercept [60]. It seems that Eqn (24) is inapplicable to perfluorinated hydrocarbons.

4.3. Solvation Enthalpies of Various Nonelectrolytes in Tetrachloromethane

Tetrachloromethane does not interact specifically with the overwhelming majority of solutes. Although this statement was challenged in some cases [67-69] it underlies practically all quantitative methods for determining the thermodynamic parameters of specific interactions [70] in so far as they use tetrachloromethane as the inert solvent. Dipolar interactions also should not be present because of zero dipole moment of tetrachloromethane. Thus, only inductive and dispersion interactions seem to exist.

As it is evident from previous section, dispersion interactions can be successfully analyzed using the correlation of solvation enthalpy with solute molar refraction. This correlation for tetrachloromethane [71. 72] is shown in figure 6.

The main conclusions drawn from this correlation [72] can be summarized as follows:

1. The overall picture of solvation enthalpies in tetrachloromethane is noticeably more complex than in cyclohexane. As a rough approximation all solute points at figure 6 are divided into two groups. Good linear correlations are observed within each group with approximately the same slope.

2. The difference between two groups (difference in intercepts) cannot be explained by the contribution of inductive interactions since the dipole moments of solutes within each group vary over a wide range.

Analysis of solvation enthalpies in another solvents (thoroughly selecting the solute-solvent systems without specific interactions) shows that division into the groups remains unchanged while the value of difference in intercepts depends on the solvent [71. 72]. As a particular case, this difference in cyclohexane does not exceed the experimental accuracy.

It was supposed that this difference arises from the different abilities of solutes to dispersion interactions.

In other words, it means that the volume of the solute molecule (molar refraction) is not the only solute parameter defining the value of dispersion interactions enthalpies.

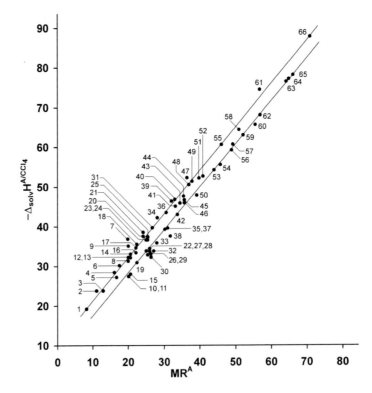

Figure 6. Correlation of solvation enthalpies in tetrachloromethane (kJ mol^{-1}) with molar refractions (cm^3 mol^{-1}) of solutes. Solutes: 1 — methanol; 2 — acetonitrile; 3 — ethanol; 4 — acetone; 5 — acrylonitrile; 6 — propanol-1; 7 — DMF; 8 — THF; 9 — DMSO; 10 — chloroform; 11 — cis-1,2-dichloroethylene; 12 — thiazole; 13 — pyrrole; 14 — butanone; 15 — trans-1,2-dichloroethylene; 16 — butanol-1; 17 — ethyl acetate; 18 — dimethyl sulfite; 19 — diethyl ether; 20 — 1,2-dimethoxyethane; 21 — pyridine; 22 — 1-chlorobutane; 23 — N-methylpyrrole; 24 — pentanone-2; 25 — phosphorus oxichloride; 26 — trichloroethylene; 27 — 1,4-difluorobenzene; 28 — fluorobenzene; 29 — benzene; 30 — tetrachloromethane; 31 — ethyl chloroacetate; 32 — n-butyl methyl ether; 33 — iodine; 34 — phenol; 35 — tetrachloroethylene; 36 — aniline; 37 — chlorobenzene; 38 — dipropyl ether; 39 — benzaldehyde; 40 — nitrobenzene; 41 — anisole; 42 — bromobenzene; 43 — heptanone-2; 44 — N-methylaniline; 45 — 1,2-dichlorobenzene; 46 — 1,4-dichlorobenzene; 47 — acetophenone; 48 — p-chlorobenzaldehyde; 49 — p-chloronitrobenzene; 50 — iodobenzene; 51 — thioanisole; 52 — N,N-dimethylaniline; 53 — naphthalene; 54 — 1,2,4,5-tetrachlorobenzene; 55 — 1-naphthol; 56 — 1-chloronaphthalene; 57 — 1,3,5-tribromobenzene; 58 — 1-nitronaphthalene; 59 — diphenyl; 60 — hexachlorobenzene; 61 — benzophenone; 62 — 1,3,4,5-tetrabromobenzene; 63 — trans-azobenzene; 64 — anthracene; 65 — trans-diphenylethylene; 66 — 9-anthraldehyde. $\Delta_{solv}H^{A/CCl_4}$ and MR^A values taken from Refs. [71;72].

5. Electrostatic Solute-Solvent Interactions: Estimation of the Contribution to the Solvation Enthalpy

According to Eqn (6) the enthalpy of polar interactions is the sum of dipolar and inductive contributions. They have the similar nature and are commonly described by various modifications of continuum model [73]. The values of static dipole (multipole) moments noticeably exceed the values of induced dipole (multipole) moments in the majority of cases. Therefore, we will consider the dipolar interactions first of all.

According to continuum models the solvation enthalpy is generally proportional to square of solute dipole moment (μ^2) and the functions of relative permittivity (ε_r) of the solvent (such as Kirkwood function $(\varepsilon_r - 1)/(\varepsilon_r + 2)$, or Onsager function $(\varepsilon_r - 1)/(\varepsilon_r + 1)$, or more simple function ($1/\varepsilon_r$). Classical electrostatic continuum models consider the solute as a point dipole (or multipole of higher order). This means that the distance between the positive and negative charges in solute molecule must be substantially smaller than the distance between the solute and solvent molecules. On the other hand the solvent is considered as the structureless medium with definite relative permittivity. It is evident that both assumptions are rather rough for real solute-solvent systems. Moreover, it can be noted that within the framework of continuum models there are no place for cavity formation term.

Despite wide usage and intensive development of continuum models it is quite difficult to prove definitely their applicability to description of experimental values of solvation enthalpy. Indeed, the correlations of solvation enthalpy for a wide series of solutes in certain solvent with square of solute dipole moment are rather unsuccessful because solutes with widely varied dipole moments vary in ability to specific interactions with the solvent. These correlations are absent at all for inert solvents (cyclohexane and tetrachloromethane) as it is shown in previous sections. More frequently, the correlations of solvation enthalpies for certain polar solute with Kirkwood or Onsager functions are considered as the confirmation of applicability of continuum models to solvation enthalpies. However, it was shown [51] that same correlations with these functions take place for solvation enthalpy of nonpolar n–hexane in a series of the solvents. In other words, the cavity formation enthalpy of the solvents depends on permittivity of a solvent.

There exist some attempts [74] to extract the electrostatic contribution to solvation enthalpy using the Eqn (7) (homomorph concept). We consider these attempts rather incorrect because they suppose the independency of dispersion interactions on any solute parameters except for molecular volume.

Our attempt to extract this contribution is based on comparing the solvation enthalpies in a series of solvents for certain geometrical isomers as solutes. Indeed, cis- and trans-disubstituted ethylenes or o-, m-, and p-disubstituted benzenes are the substances maximally similar one to another regarding their ability to intermolecular interactions with solvents. Isomers have approximately the same volume of molecules that results in the equality of cavity formation enthalpies. In addition to the equality of molecular volume, the identical group composition gives the solid argumentation for assuming the equality of dispersion interaction enthalpies. Even if specific interactions with a solvent are presented, as a rough approximation they should be the same for isomers. Consequently, the differences in solvation enthalpy for isomers with polar substituents must be the differences in dipolar interactions. The only difficulty is often the absence of vaporization enthalpies for highly polar solutes. In these cases the differences in solution enthalpies for a series of solvents must be examined because according to Eqn (1) they are equal to the differences in solvation enthalpies.

Comparison of solution enthalpies for isomers in a series of solvents was performed in Ref. [71]. The solutes examined were: cis- and trans-dichloroethylenes; cis- and trans-dicyanoehtylenes; o-, m-, and p-dichlorobenzenes; o-, m-, and p-dinitrobenzenes; o-, m-, and p-dicyanobenzenes The differences in dipole moment for isomeric solutes were up to 5.8 D. The solvents used for this study were highly various in polarity (relative permittivity was from 2.8 to 45 and dipole moment of solvent molecule was from 0 to 4.2 D). In all the cases it was found the linear correlations of solution enthalpies for isomers with the slope being close to unity. The examples of such correlation for m-, and p-dinitrobenzenes (DNB) and cis- and trans-dicyanoehtylenes (DCE) [71] is shown on figure 7.

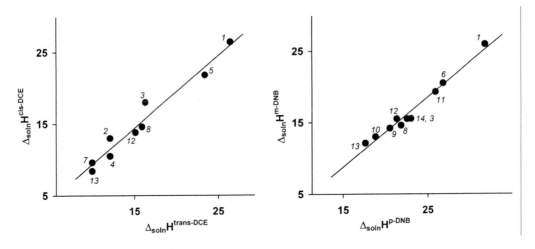

Figure 7. Correlations of solution enthalpies (kJ mol^{-1}) for cis-DCE vs. trans-DCE and m-DNB vs. p-DNB. The linear regression slopes are 1.01 and 0.98 respectively. Solvents: 1 — tetrachloromethane; 2 — 1,4-dioxane; 3 — benzene; 4 — ethyl acetate; 5 — 1-chloropentane; 6 — 1-chlorobutane; 7 — THF; 8 — 1,2-dichloroethane; 9 — acetone; 10 — benzonitrile; 11 — methanol; 12 — acetonitrile; 13 — DMF; 14 — DMSO.

Standard deviations for all correlations don't exceed 2 kJ mol^{-1}. Therefore, it can be concluded that the dipolar contribution to the solvation enthalpy caused by dipole moment of solute molecule (up to 5.8 D) either is absent or doesn't exceed 2 kJ mol^{-1}.

The similar result was obtained in Ref. [75] for solvation of cis- and trans-1,2-dihaloethylenes and in Ref. [76] for solvation of 1,3- and 1,4-dioxanes, but the authors interpreted the similarity of solvation thermodynamic parameters for these pairs of isomers by higher values of quadrupole moment for trans-1,2-dichloroethane and 1,3-dioxane. Taking into account the facts reported in current and two previous sections it seems as if compensation of electrostatic contributions derived by dipole moments and quadrupole moments take place in all cases without any exclusion. It seems very improbable.

We tested the role of quadrupole interactions [77] comparing the solvation enthalpies for three isomers (o-, m-, and p-dichlorobenzenes). Solvation enthalpies in a wide range of solvents are practically equal for these solutes. Dipole moments for these three isomers differ from one to another but quadrupole moments for o- and m-isomers are equal. So, the observed equality of solvation enthalpies can not be explained by the compensation of differences in dipole and quadrupole interactions.

But as it is well known, the multipole expansion is infinite and the authors of the paper [78] discovered that 'the small influence of the long-range interactions on the energetics of the equilibrium of cis-trans isomerization for dichloroethylenes can be only explained if electric multipole moments of higher order than quadrupole are considered'.

In such a way, two alternative conclusions can be drawn. (i) Electrostatic interactions don't contribute to the solvation enthalpy even for highly polar solutes within the accuracy of 2 kJ mol^{-1}. (ii) Following to the opinion of the specialists in continuum solvation models [75, 76, 78], we must conclude that the contribution of electrostatic interactions takes place. However the contribution from solute dipole moment is compensated by those from multipole moments of higher order.

In the latter case we must add that this compensation takes place practically always. For example, the solvation enthalpies for the series of a solutes in 17 solvents with various relative permittivity (from 2.3 for tetrachloromethane to 62.9 for propylene carbonate) were considered in Ref. [71]. The solutes were: benzene; naphthalene; anthracene; diphenyl; fluoro-, chloro-, bromo-, and iodo- benzenes; o- and p-dichlorobenzenes (m-dichlorobenzene can be added by the reader from Ref. [77]); and 1-chloronaphthalene. These solutes noticeably vary in its dipole moments and relative number of polar groups. Nevertheless, the excellent linear correlations with molar refraction of the solutes (with correlation coefficients from .0994 to 0.998 and standard deviations from 0.8 to 1.4 kJ mol^{-1}) were found for all the solvents. If contribution of dipolar interactions are presented it is compensated by a such successful manner that the enthalpy of electrostatic interactions with their multipole expansion must be linear to the simplest parameter which is the molar refraction! But where has polarity gone to? We think that these results show the groundlessness of any deduction about the polarity of transition state in chemical kinetics or excited state in electron transfer based on the high solvation enthalpy dependency on the permittivity of the solvent.

As long ago as in 1930 Hildebrand and Carter has shown that 'it is the number and polarity of the substituent groups rather than the electric moment of the whole molecule which determines deviations from Raoult's law' [79]. Probably, this conclusion might be altered to consider the role of dispersion interaction but the latter was discovered on the other continent some months later [80]. Nevertheless, up to now there are some researchers who think that solvent effects can be described in general by the simplest Kirkwood equation.

6. Specific Solute–Solvent Interaction Enthalpy

Solution calorimetry is often used for the determination of the enthalpies of donor–acceptor complex formation including the enthalpies of hydrogen bonding. In many cases, the values of complex formation enthalpies obtained by the calorimetric method are considered as more reliable than those obtained by spectroscopic (NMR-, IR-, UV-VIS) methods based on the temperature dependence of equilibrium constants. On the other hand, calorimetry gives the complex value which depends on variety of types of intermolecular interactions existing in solutions. So, the reliability of calorimetrically obtained complex formation enthalpy entirely depends on the correctness of specific interaction enthalpy extraction from the solution enthalpy. If only single type of complexes is present in solution then the specific interaction enthalpy $\left[\Delta_{int(sp)} H \right]$ is related with complex formation enthalpy ($\Delta_c H^{A..S}$) by simple Eqn (25).

$$\Delta_{int(sp)} H = \alpha \cdot \Delta_c H^{A..S} \tag{25}$$

where α is the degree of complex formation.

The solute-solvent systems with hydrogen bonding can be subdivided into four types. First, there are no intramolecular hydrogen bonds in the solute and solvent molecules and no intermolecular solvent-solvent hydrogen bonds. Second, there are no intramolecular hydrogen bonds in A and S molecules, but the solvent is associated via intermolecular hydrogen bonds. Third, intramolecular hydrogen bonds in A molecules are formed, but intermolecular hydrogen bonds in the solvent are absent . Fourth, both intramolecular hydrogen bonds in A and intermolecular hydrogen bonds in the solvent are present. Eqn (25) is applied to systems of first type only.

According to Eqn (4), solvation enthalpy is the sum of nonspecific solvation enthalpy ($\Delta_{solv(nonsp)} H^{A/S}$) and specific interaction enthalpy ($\Delta_{int(sp)} H^{A/S}$). The ratio of these two contributions widely varies with variation of solute and solvent that is demonstrated in table 2. Nevertheless, even if contribution of specific interactions is relatively small they are often of crucial importance for solvent effect on various physico-chemical processes. The reason is that nonspecific solvation enthalpy being the additive contribution is approximately the same for initial and final states of the process.

Taking into account Eqn (4) we must note that any method for determination of specific interaction enthalpy from the enthalpy of solvation includes (sometimes implicitly) the method of estimation of nonspecific solvation enthalpy.

Table 2. Values of nonspecific solvation enthalpy ($\Delta_{solv(nonsp)}H^{A/S}$) and specific interaction enthalpy ($\Delta_{int(sp)}H^{A/S}$) for some solute-solvent systems

Solute / solvent	$-\Delta_{solv(nonsp)}H^{A/S}$, kJ mol^{-1}	$-\Delta_{int(sp)}H^{A/S}$, kJ mol^{-1}
Phenol / benzene	44.3	4.6
Iodine / chlorobenzene	37.7	4.6
Pyrrole / DMF	37.2	13.4
Phenol / pyridine	44.1	30.3
Water / THF	18.3	20.2
Water / DMSO	16.4	32.6

The simplest, very old and very rough approach assumes that specific interaction enthalpy can be calculated as the difference in solvation (or solution) enthalpies for the solvent under consideration and for the inert solvent (I).

$$\Delta_{int(sp)}H^{A/S} = \Delta_{soln}H^{A/S} - \Delta_{soln}H^{A/I} \qquad (26)$$

Inert solvent is the solvent incapable of specific interactions with solute. Alkanes or tetrachloromethane are commonly used as the inert solvent. Some examples of application of this approach can be found in Refs [81;82]. Taking into consideration Eqn (4) it can be shown that Eqn (26) is correct if only $\Delta_{solv(nonsp)}H^{A/I} = \Delta_{solv(nonsp)}H^{A/S}$, that is, if nonspecific solvation enthalpy is independent on solvent. It is certainly very rough approximation.

Another approach is based on homomorph concept. It assumes that specific interaction enthalpy can be calculated as the difference in solvation enthalpies for the solute and its homomorph.

$$\Delta_{int(sp)}H^{A/S} = \Delta_{solv}H^{A/S} - \Delta_{solv}H^{h/S} \qquad (27)$$

Comparing the Eqns (27) and (7) shows that the difference in enthalpies of polar interactions for the solute and its homomorph is ignored. It is of little significance taking into consideration the previous section. It is more substantial that the use of Eqn (27) assumes that nonspecific solvation enthalpy depends only on the volume of solute molecule but not on its nature. We consider this supposition as erroneous.

The most widely used calorimetric method for determination of specific interaction enthalpy is the pure base method [83]. Specific interaction enthalpy is calculated from four experimental solution enthalpies:

$$\Delta_{int(sp)}H^{A/S} = \left[\Delta_{soln}H^{A/S} - \Delta_{soln}H^{M/S}\right] - \left[\Delta_{soln}H^{A/I} - \Delta_{soln}H^{M/I}\right] \qquad (28)$$

where I is the inert solvent and M is the model compound.

The pure base method can be considered as rather successful combination of the methods described by Eqns (26) and (27). Inert solvent (I) is the same in Eqns (26) and (28). The model compound in Eqn (28) is the compound which has the same enthalpy of nonspecific solvation as the solute under consideration but incapable to specific interactions with solvents. This definition is very similar to the definition of homomorph in Eqn (27). The choice of model compound in each case can be certainly the subject of discussion inasmuch as the nonspecific solvation enthalpies can not be measured directly for specifically interacting solutes. Nevertheless, Eqn (28) is more reliable than Eqn (26) because the former requires not the equality of nonspecific solvation enthalpies in any solvent but the equality of differences in nonspecific solvation enthalpies for solutes A and M in the solvents S and I. It is of course more probable situation.

The authors of the pure base method have shown that the use of methoxy-substituted derivatives as the model compounds for the hydroxyl containing solutes leads enthalpies of hydrogen bond formation which agree with values obtained by spectral methods. Nevertheless, it was shown in Ref [84] that replacement of the inert solvent (tetrachloromethane by cyclohexane) leads to the result that the specific interaction enthalpy determined by Eqn (28) depends on the choice of the model compound.

Fuchs et al have proposed so-called 'non-hydrogen bonding baseline' (NHBB) method [85] , the essential feature of which is the comparison of the difference in the enthalpies of the solution of the compounds A and M in the series of solvents with values of Kamlet–Abboud–Taft π^* solvatochromic parameter. The example of determination of $\Delta_{int(sp)}H^{A/S}$ by NHBB-method is shown in figure 8.

Dashed line in figure 8 is drawn through the points corresponding to inert solvents. It is assumed that nonspecific solvation in DMF must agree with this linear dependence. Therefore, the deviation of DMF point from the line is the specific interaction enthalpy.

NHBB-method use the model compounds. So, the problem of choice of model compound is inherent to this method as well as to pure base method. Besides, the choice of inert solvents is often very limited but this choice affects distinctly the resulted specific interaction enthalpy. For example, if we exclude the point of 1,2 dichloroethane from the plot in figure 8 (and draw the line through the points 1 and 2 only) the resulted specific interaction enthalpy increases noticeably.

Another method for determination of specific interaction enthalpy is the method of base solutes [92;93]. It is founded on the linear correlations of nonspecific solvation enthalpies with solute molar refraction. The examples of determination of $\Delta_{int(sp)}H^{A/S}$ for pyrrole and iodine with pyridine by method of base solutes are shown in figure 9. Base solutes are the substances which do not interact specifically with the solvent under consideration. The linear dependence of base solutes solvation enthalpies on their molar refractions is used to calculate the nonspecific solvation enthalpies for the specifically interacting solutes (in this case: pyrrole and iodine). Unfortunately, in any solvent except of saturated hydrocarbons, there is no the sole linear dependence for all bas solutes. So, it is required to analyze the corresponding dependences in tetrachloromethane for choosing the group of base solutes to which the solute under consideration must be referred.

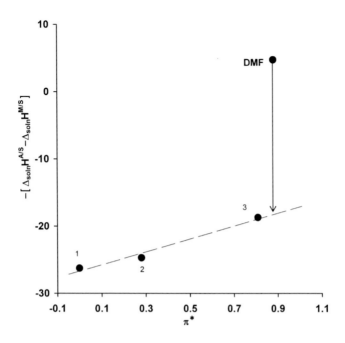

Figure 8. Determination of phenol-DMF specific interaction enthalpy by NHBB-method. Solute (A) – phenol. Model compound (M) – anisole; Inert solvents: 1 – cyclohexane; 2 – tetrachloromethane; 3 – 1,2-dichloroethane. Solution enthalpies (kJ mol^{-1} , 298.15 K) and π^* values taken from Refs.[86-90] and [91] respectively.

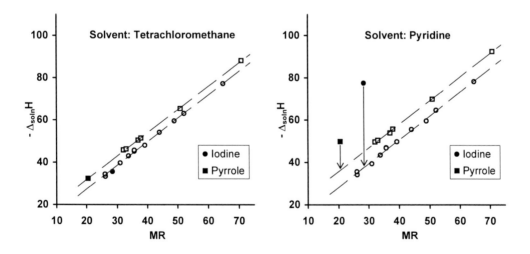

Figure 9. Determination of pyrrole-pyridine and iodine- pyridine specific interaction enthalpies by the method of base solutes. Base solutes used for these plots are listed below in the order of molar refraction increasing. First group (the lower line on the plots, circles): fluorobenzene; benzene; chlorobenzene; bromobenzene; 1,2- and 1,4-dichlorobenzenes; iodobenzene; naphthalene; 1-chloronaphthalene; anthracene . Second group (upper line, squares): benzaldehyde; nitrobenzene; p-chlorobenzaldehyde; p-chloronitrobenzene; 1-nitronaphthalene; 9-anthraldehyde. Solvation enthalpies (kJ mol^{-1} , 298.15 K) values taken from Refs. [27;68;86;93-97].

The disadvantage of this method is that it requires the analysis of a bulk of solvation enthalpy in each case. Furthermore, in contrast to pure base or NHBB methods, it requires the knowledge of vaporization enthalpies for each solute. The significant advantage is the absence of model compound. For example, the choice of model compound is rather undecidable problem for iodine and many other electron-acceptors. Moreover, this method helps to understand in same cases why the choice of model compound in pure base method effects on resulted value of specific interaction enthalpy.

Recently we proposed a new, very general method for the extraction of specific interaction enthalpy from the enthalpy of solvation [50;98]. It requires the minimum of experimental solution enthalpy data and does not require the choice of certain model compounds for a given solute. This method is based on our presupposition that the difference between the enthalpies of nonspecific interactions for some solvent S and cyclohexane (as solvent) is proportional to the same difference for tetrachloromethane and cyclohexane:

$$\Delta_{int(nonsp)}H^{A/S} - \Delta_{int(nonsp)}H^{A/C_6H_{12}} = q_S \cdot \left[\Delta_{int(nonsp)}H^{A/CCl_4} - \Delta_{int(nonsp)}H^{A/C_6H_{12}} \right] \quad (29)$$

where q_S is the solvent dependent proportionality factor. If solutes do not interact specifically with the solvents the differences between the enthalpies of nonspecific interactions can be calculated from experimental data by combining equations (2) written for each solvent and Eqn (12) for relative cavity formation enthalpy:

$$\Delta_{int(nonsp)}H^{A/S} - \Delta_{int(nonsp)}H^{A/C_6H_{12}} = \Delta_{solv}H^{A/S} - \Delta_{solv}H^{A/C_6H_{12}} - \left(\delta_{cav}h^S - \delta_{cav}h^{C_6H_{12}} \right) \cdot V_X^A$$

$$(30)$$

The values of proportionality factor q_S for 27 solvents were calculated by regression analysis using the experimental data of nonspecific solvation enthalpies for 59 solutes. The standard deviation of calculated solvation enthalpies from experimental ones varies from 0.28 to 2.88 kJ mol^{-1} (1.33 kJ mol^{-1} on average). The value of q_S depends on the solvent and reflects its ability to interact nonspecifically with solutes. So it would be reasonable to find the correlation of q_S with some solvent parameter such as Hildebrand solubility parameter, Kirkwood function, Dimroth–Reichardt or Kamlet–Abboud–Taft (π^*) solvatochromic parameters, etc. Indeed, some correlations with these parameters are observed but a substantially better correlation (correlation coefficient is 0.98) was found with the solvent parameter S_{vdW} calculated by Eqn. (15):

$$q_S = a + b \cdot S_{vdW} \quad (31)$$

where a and b values obtained by linear regression analysis are 0.34 and 0.61 respectively if the units for all the enthalpies in Eqns (29) and (12) are kJ mol^{-1} and the unit for V_X is cm^3 mol^{-1} 10^{-2}.

Although the correlation with S_{vdW} was found empirically, we think that it is not accidental. This parameter is to some extent the analogue of the Hildebrand solubility parameter because in regular solutions theory δ_H^2 characterizes the specific cavity formation energy. The Hildebrand parameter reflects the overall breaking of solvent – solvent interactions, being calculated from the vaporization enthalpy, whereas for cavity formation the breaking of only some part of such interactions is required. The parameter S_{vdW} probably reflects just this part of the interactions better.

The resulted equation for nonspecific solvation enthalpy is:

$$\Delta_{solv(nonsp)}H^{A/S} = \Delta_{solv}H^{A/C_6H_{12}} + \left(\delta_{cav}h^S - \delta_{cav}h^{C_6H_{12}}\right)\cdot V_x^A +$$
$$+\left(a+b\cdot S_{vdW}\right)\cdot\left[\Delta_{solv}H^{A/CCl_4} - \Delta_{solv}H^{A/C_6H_{12}} - \left(\delta_{cav}h^{CCl_4} - \delta_{cav}h^{C_6H_{12}}\right)\cdot V_x^A\right] \quad (32)$$

It should be stressed that it is an empirical equation. Despite some similarity of S_{vdW} and the Hildebrand parameter, Eqn (32) is not based on regular solution theory and certainly is not the modification or improvement of the latter. The above mentioned similarity is rather the result of the fact that both approaches are based on very old Berthelot rule (Eqn (14)).

Combination of Eqn (32) in a somewhat more common form and Eqn (4) gives the Eqn (33) for calculation of the specific interaction enthalpies:

$$\Delta_{int(sp)}H^{A/S} = \Delta_{soln}H^{A/S} - \Delta_{soln}H^{A/C_6H_{12}} - \left(\delta_{cav}h^S - \delta_{cav}h^{C_6H_{12}}\right)\times V_X^A -$$
$$-\left(a_R + b_R\cdot S_{vdW}\right)\times\left[\Delta_{soln}H^{A/R} - \Delta_{soln}H^{A/C_6H_{12}} - (\delta_{cav}h^R - \delta_{cav}h^{C_6H_{12}})\times V_X^A\right] \quad (33)$$

where $\Delta_{soln}H^{A/S}$, $\Delta_{soln}H^{A/R}$ and $\Delta_{soln}H^{A/C_6H_{12}}$ - are solution enthalpies of solute A in the solvent S, standard solvent R, and cyclohexane respectively; $\delta_{cav}h^S$, $\delta_{cav}h^R$ and $\delta_{cav}h^{C_6H_{12}}$ – are specific relative cavity formation enthalpies for each solvent (the values calculated by Eqn (12) slightly vary with length of n-alkane; therefore, the averaged values for all available solution enthalpies of n-alkanes in each solvent are used in our works); R is the reference solvent; a_R and b_R are intercept and slope in Eqn (31) and subscript R in this case means that these values depend on the choice of reference solvent. Reference solvent R is defined as a certain non-alkane solvent that does not interact specifically with the solutes. Reference solvent in Eqn (32) is tetrachloromethane but in Eqn (33) it can be changed by another solvent. This can be useful because tetrachloromethane can interact specifically with some electron-donor solutes [67-69] (e.g. triethylamine, pyridine, diethyl ether, 1,4-dioxane). For these solutes, another solvent (for example benzene) can be used as a reference (a_R and b_R for benzene as a reference solvent are equal to 0.20 and 0.38 respectively).

In Ref. [50], specific interaction enthalpies for 280 solute–solvent systems were calculated. For 82 of these 280 systems, the complexation enthalpy obtained by independent methods was documented in literature. Comparing the literature data with those determined via Eqn (33) gives the standard deviation of approximately 2 kJ mol^{-1}.

The main advantage of this method is its universality. Owing to the absence of model compounds it can be applied to a wider range of solutes (e.g. chloroform or iodine). This method, in contrast to pure base or NHBB ones, can be used for determination of specific interaction enthalpy of proton-acceptor solutes with proton-donor solvents (e.g. chloroform as a solvent [99]) including the determination of self-association enthalpy for the solvents whose molecules are proton-donor and proton-acceptor simultaneously (e.g. aliphatic alcohols [100]).Several examples of use of this method is shown below.

6.1. Enthalpies of Solvent Self-Association via Hydrogen Bonding

The important physical and chemical properties of self-associated solvents are due to the fact that a wide range of associated species of different stoichiometry and structure are formed, and these associated species are in thermodynamic equilibria with each other. One of the most significant parameters of such equilibria is their enthalpy. The enthalpy value obtainable from calorimetric measurements is that determined most directly but it is an average over all the associated species. In contrast, spectroscopic methods (e.g. IR or NMR) typically deal with particular associative complexes. However, information on particular complex species is obtainable only when the species are isolated in an inert medium (solvent, matrix or gas phase). Furthermore, even under this condition it is not always possible to account for all types of associations that may arise, therefore generally only several of the most significant species are considered. Thus, calorimetric and spectroscopic methods are mutually complementary.

The problem of determination of self-association enthalpy has a history more than a half-century long. Blaney and Reid [101] summarized the wide scatter of experimental values for H-bonding enthalpies in ethanol. They stated that reported enthalpies range from -10 to -40 kJ mol^{-1} and the majority of studies have found enthalpies in the range of -16 to -25 kJ mol^{-1}.

Eqn (33) is suitable for the determination of solvent self-association enthalpy. It must be noted that we mean by self-association namely the self-association via hydrogen bonding. From the another (trivial) point of view any liquid could be considered as associated (comparing to gas phase) and its self-association enthalpy could be equal simply to vaporization enthalpy. The enthalpy of self-association via hydrogen bonding is the average value of hydrogen bonding enthalpy for all associated species according to their molar fractions. It is the specific interaction enthalpy of solvent with itself. The latter value for aliphatic alcohols can be derived from Eqn (33) as follows:

$$\Delta_{int(sp)}H^{ROH/ROH} = -\Delta_{soln}H^{ROH/C_6H_{12}} - \left(\delta_{cav}h^{ROH} - \delta_{cav}h^{C_6H_{12}}\right) \times V_X^{ROH} -$$
$$-\left(a_{CCl_4} + b_{CCl_4} \cdot S_{vdW}\right) \times \left[\Delta_{soln}H^{ROH/CCl_4} - \Delta_{soln}H^{ROH/C_6H_{12}} - (\delta_{cav}h^{CCl_4} - \delta_{cav}h^{C_6H_{12}}) \times V_X^{ROH}\right] \qquad (34)$$

The enthalpies of self-association were determined [100] for seven aliphatic alcohols: methanol, ethanol, propanol-1, propanol-2, butanol-1, hexanol-1 and octanol-1. For all the studied alcohols except methanol the average hydrogen bonding enthalpies fall in the range from -16.9 to -17.7 kJ mol^{-1}. A slightly smaller value of -15.1 kJ mol^{-1} was observed for methanol. It can be noted that homomorph method gives the substantially overestimated values in the range from -23.5 to -27.1 kJ mol^{-1}.

6.2. Estimation of Aliphatic Alcohols Dimerization Enthalpies

The dimerization enthalpies of aliphatic alcohols can not be obtained directly from Eqn (33). Nevertheless, they can be estimated [100] by assuming that the proton-acceptor ability of an aliphatic alcohol relative to a certain standard proton-acceptor does not depend on the nature of the proton-donors.

If diethyl ether (DEE) and chloroform (CF) are chosen as the standard proton-acceptor and the second proton-donor, respectively, then the above assumption can be written as:

$$\frac{\Delta_{HB}H^{ROH...CF}}{\Delta_{HB}H^{DEE...CF}} = \frac{\Delta_{HB}H^{ROH...ROH}}{\Delta_{HB}H^{DEE...ROH}} \tag{35}$$

In this equation the dimerization enthalpy $\Delta_{HB}H^{ROH...ROH}$ is the unknown value whereas the other three values can be calculated from Eqn (33) using the calorimetric data. Chloroform is taken as the second proton-donor because it is a pronounced proton-donor but hardly exhibits proton-acceptor properties. Accordingly, chloroform as a solvent is not associated by H-bonding. The latter statement can be confirmed by the fact that the solvation enthalpy of chloroform in cyclohexane is relatively low (2.9 kJ mol^{-1}) [102]. This magnitude is not the self-association enthalpy of chloroform because it also contains the difference between the chloroform–chloroform and chloroform–cyclohexane non-specific interaction enthalpies, but the self-association enthalpy of chloroform does not exceed this magnitude. Moreover, the self-association enthalpy of chloroform calculated by Eqn (34) is -0.8 kJ mol^{-1}, thus the use of chloroform does not require the solvent reorganization effects to be taken into account (i.e. the breaking of the solvent–solvent H-bonds).

When considering possible diethyl ether–chloroform interactions, it must be kept in mind that the formation of 1:2 complexes is viable theoretically, because the oxygen atom of diethyl ether has two lone electron pairs. Nevertheless, it was shown [100] that the 1:1 complex is only formed.

For determining the H-bonding enthalpy of diethyl ether with aliphatic alcohols $\left(\Delta_{HB}H^{DEE...ROH}\right)$ it is more convenient to use the alcohol not as a solvent but as a solute, because in that case it is not necessary to account for the solvent reorganization effect (breaking of the solvent–solvent H-bonds). Thus, Eqn (35) is transformed into Eqn (36):

$$\Delta_{HB}H^{ROH...ROH} = \Delta_{int(sp)}H^{ROH/DEE} \times \frac{\Delta_{int(sp)}H^{ROH/CF}}{\Delta_{int(sp)}H^{DEE/CF}} \tag{36}$$

Dimerization enthalpies for six aliphatic alcohols were calculated by Eqn (36) [100]. It was found that the dimerization enthalpies are very close for all the studied aliphatic alcohols : -8.6 ± 0.7 kJ mol^{-1}. The results obtained were compared with IR-spectroscopy data using the Badger–Bauer rule.

6.3. Specific Interaction Enthalpies for Proton-Acceptors with Associated Solvents

Specific interaction enthalpies of several aliphatic alcohols (ROH) with pyridine (Py) are shown in table 3. These values are of two types: (i) ROH is a solute and Py is a solvent ($\Delta_{int(sp)} H^{ROH/Py}$); (ii) Py is a solute and ROH is a solvent ($\Delta_{int(sp)} H^{Py/ROH}$).

Table 3. Enthalpies (298.15 K, kJ mol^{-1}) of specific interaction for alcohols with pyridine ($\Delta_{int(sp)} H^{ROH/Py}$), pyridine with alcohols ($\Delta_{int(sp)} H^{Py/ROH}$) and enthalpies of hydrogen bonding determined in tetrachloromethane ($\Delta_{HB} H_{CCl_4}^{ROH..Py}$) [103]

Alcohol	$\Delta_{int(sp)} H^{ROH/Py}$	$\Delta_{int(sp)} H^{Py/ROH}$	$\Delta_{HB} H_{CCl_4}^{ROH..Py}$
Methanol	-16.2	-5.8	-16.3
Ethanol	-15.9	-3.2	-15.9
Butanol-1	-15.8	-1.9	-16.3
Hexanol-1	-15.5	-1.9	-
Octanol-1	-15.6	-1.0	-16.7

As it is evident from table 3 $\Delta_{int(sp)} H^{Py/ROH}$ values are dramatically lower than $\Delta_{int(sp)} H^{ROH/Py}$ values. This difference is not the result of differences in hydrogen bonding enthalpies for different media. It is confirmed by near coincidence of values $\Delta_{int(sp)} H^{ROH/Py}$ and $\Delta_{HB} H_{CCl_4}^{ROH..Py}$ which also shown in table 3. The later values are the enthalpies of hydrogen bonding determined using IR spectroscopic and calorimetric methods in tetrachloromethane as the solvent [70]. The decrease in $\Delta_{int(sp)} H^{Py/ROH}$ relative to $\Delta_{int(sp)} H^{ROH/Py}$ is the result of competition for the most acidic H-atom in the alcoholic solvent between the alcohol and pyridine molecules. This phenomenon is investigated in a series of papers [104-106]. It was established that the enthalpy of specific interaction with an associated solvent depends in a complex manner on the solvent association and on structural features of solute molecules. These two factors determine the energy required to shift the association equilibrium in the solvent during the formation of solute-solvent complex (solvent reorganization energy). There was developed an approach [105] that allows qualitative conclusions on the occurrence (or absence) of the solvent reorganization effect in the formation of solute-solvent complexes. This approach consists in comparing the numbers of lone electron pairs capable of hydrogen bonding and of active hydrogen atoms in the solvent molecule. The type of hydrogen bonding centers (active hydrogen atoms or lone electron pairs) present in excess determines the type of solutes with which the solvent reorganization energy should be manifested at a specific interaction. For example, in alcohols as solvents , the number of lone electron pairs is twice as much the number of active hydrogen atoms. This means that solutes specifically interacting with a solvent via own lone electron pairs (ketones, ethers, esters) should cause reorganization of an alcohol as solvent. With proton-donor solutes, for example, chloroform, the solvent reorganization should not be manifested. If the numbers of lone electron pairs and active hydrogen atoms are equal, the solvent reorganization should be manifested as solvation of both proton-donors and proton-acceptors. The studies carried out show that specific interaction enthalpies of some proton-acceptors with associated solvents can be not only exothermic but in some cases close to zero and even endothermic. It means that the formation of solute-solvent hydrogen bonds in some cases can not compensate the cleavage of solvent-solvent hydrogen bonds.

6.4. Cooperativity of Hydrogen Bonding

Let us denote by $\Delta_{HB(2)}H$ the enthalpy of linear dimer formation for some alcohol. The formation of higher order linear multimers can be described as follows:

$$ROH + ROH \rightleftarrows (ROH)_2, \quad \Delta_{HB(2)}H$$
$$(ROH)_2 + ROH \rightleftarrows (ROH)_3, \Delta_{HB(3)}H$$
$$(ROH)_3 + ROH \rightleftarrows (ROH)_4, \Delta_{HB(4)}H$$
$$(ROH)_4 + ROH \rightleftarrows (ROH)_5, \Delta_{HB(5)}H$$
$$\cdots \qquad \cdots$$
$$(ROH)_{k-1} + ROH \rightleftarrows (ROH)_k, \qquad \Delta_{HB(k)}H$$

The phenomenon of cooperativity of hydrogen bonding is manifested in the fact that the above listed enthalpies are not constant but increase (in absolute magnitude) in the order: $\Delta_{HB(2)}H < \Delta_{HB(3)}H < \Delta_{HB(4)}H < \Delta_{HB(5)}H < ... < \Delta_{HB(k)}H$. The reason of this increase is the higher 'acidity' of free hydroxyl group in dimer (or in multimers of higher orders) as compared with hydroxyl group of monomer owing to removal of electron density from oxygen atom by the first hydrogen bond. This increase can not be unlimited but seems to reach the saturation at certain size of multimer. Cooperativity of hydrogen bonds is attributed not only to associated species of alcohol but also to their complexes with various electron-acceptors (B) such as $B \cdots ROH$ and $B \cdots (ROH)_2$. The phenomenon of cooperativity is manifested apparently in IR-spectroscopy owing to dependence of hydroxyl stretching vibration frequency on the energy of hydrogen bond formed [53;107]. It is studied by the methods of quantum chemistry [108]. Although IR-spectroscopy is most frequently used experimental method for hydrogen bonding cooperativity, its most faithful applications (methods of matrix isolation) is limited by the trimolecular complexes [109]. IR-spectroscopy of alcoholic solutions in inert solvent can obtain information on several simplest associated complexes using some simplifications. Solution calorimetry and Eqn (33) give the most direct information on cooperativity of hydrogen bonding in real associated solvents such as alcohols, although it give the values averaged over the all associated species presented in the solution. For example, the comparison of above mentioned enthalpies of solvent self-association ($\Delta_{int(sp)}H^{ROH/ROH}$) and enthalpies of dimer formation ($\Delta_{HB}H^{ROH...ROH}$) for the aliphatic alcohols gives the value of cooperativity factor ($A_b = \Delta_{int(sp)}H^{ROH/ROH} / \Delta_{HB}H^{ROH...ROH}$) in the range from 1.6 to 2.2 [100].

New calorimetric method for the determination of cooperative hydrogen bonding for proton-acceptors with associated solvents was developed in Ref. [103]. If proton-acceptor is pyridine (Py) and associated solvent is some aliphatic alcohol (ROH) then specific interaction enthalpy can be presented as the difference:

$$\Delta_{int(sp)}H^{Py/ROH} = \Delta_{int(sp)}H^{(ROH)_n...Py} - \Delta_{int(sp)}H^{ROH/ROH} \tag{37}$$

The second value on the right-hand side of Eqn (37) is the average self-association enthalpy of the alcohol. The first value on the right-hand side of Eqn (37) represents the average specific interaction enthalpy of pyridine with associated species of the alcohol. It is likely that an overwhelming majority of pyridine molecules in alcohol reside in $(ROH)_n...Py$ complexes (the degree of complexation of pyridine is close to 1). The large difference between the hydrogen bonding enthalpies for alcohol dimer ($\Delta_{HB}H^{ROH...ROH}$ =-8.7±0.6 kJ mol^{-1} [100]) and for $ROH...Py$ complexes ($\Delta_{int(sp)}H^{ROH/Py}$ =-15.8±0.2kJ mol^{-1} [103]). proves this conjecture. Consequently, the value $\Delta_{int(sp)}H^{(ROH)_n...Py}$ represent the average enthalpy of cooperative HB of pyridine with associated species of alcohols.

In accordance with the work carried out by Kleeberg et al [107;110;111], not only the OH..N bond in the cooperative complex $(ROH)_n...Py$ becomes stronger, but also the OH..O bonds. This fact must be kept in mind when calculating the cooperativity factors from a comparison of $\Delta_{int(sp)}H^{(ROH)_n...Py}$ with the enthalpy of hydrogen bonding in the alcohol + pyridine complex obtained in pyridine or in an inert solvent. The average cooperativity factor for all alcohols studied amounts to 1.25±0.05 [103].

6.5. Intramolecular Hydrogen Bonds

The specific interaction enthalpy of a compounds with an intramolecular hydrogen bond in a proton-acceptor solvent can be represented as the difference in the contributions of intramolecular and intermolecular hydrogen bonds (intra-HB and inter-HB respectively).

$$\Delta_{\text{int}(sp)}H^{A/S} = \alpha_1 \times \Delta_{inter-HB}H^{A/S} - \alpha_2 \times \Delta_{intra-HB}H^{A} \qquad (38)$$

where α_1 and α_2 are the molar fractions of molecules involved in corresponding interactions. This equation was used for the determination of the enthalpies of intramolecular hydrogen bonds in ortho-substituted phenols [112;113]. The results obtained are in good agreement with literature data obtained by other methods.

7. Quantitative Description of the Hydrophobic Effect: The Enthalpic Contribution

It is well known that apolar substances are poorly soluble in water. This fact is usually attributed to their hydrophobicity. The importance of hydrophobicity studies is widely recognized. Hydrophobic effects play a significant role in various phenomena in aqueous solutions.

The differences between the thermodynamic functions of hydration and solvation in a reference solvent are often used as the quantitative characteristics of the hydrophobic effect. The reference solvent is supposed to model water 'in the absence of hydrophobicity'. For example, thermodynamic functions of transfer from liquid alkane into water are sometimes meant to be thermodynamic functions of the hydrophobic effect [114]. The most widely used parameter of hydrophobicity, the octanol – water partition coefficient (log P) [115], is related to the Gibbs energy of transfer from octanol into water phase. In these approaches it is tacitly assumed that the partial molar thermodynamic functions of nonspecific solvation in the reference solvent and in 'water in the absence of hydrophobicity' are equal. If we use transfer function as the measure of hydrophobicity, we should agree that there is no difference in thermodynamic functions of solvation for the same solute in different solvents when no specific interactions occur. Such assumption is not correct. For example, enthalpies of transfer of hexane from its own neat phase into DMF [38] and DMSO [40] amount, respectively, to 8.5 kJ·mol^{-1} and 13.9 kJ·mol^{-1}.

It was also proposed [116] to estimate the hydrophobic effect contribution from the temperature dependence of thermodynamic functions of hydration of the hydrophobic compounds. The main idea is that the hydrophobic effect contribution decreases as the temperature increases, and disappears at a certain temperature. Other contributions to the enthalpy and entropy of hydration are supposed to be nearly independent from the temperature. This statement is not seems evident.

Abraham suggested [117-119] that the hydrophobic effect contribution is absent in thermodynamic functions of hydration of noble gases. He showed that a linear dependence of the Gibbs energies and enthalpies of solvation for noble gases and alkanes from their molecular radius R is observed in many different solvents, but not in water. In Abraham works, thermodynamic functions of the hydrophobic effect of alkanes are considered as the differences between their experimental thermodynamic functions and thermodynamic functions of a hypothetic noble gas with the same R. However, the assumption regarding zero values of these functions for noble gases was not proven.

Mastroianni et al [120] and Somsen et al [121] proposed another method to estimate the hydrophobic effect enthalpy from the data on solvation enthalpies in binary water - organic solvent mixtures. In this method, the preferential solvation phenomenon and the specific interactions between water and organic cosolvent are both neglected

Another attempt to evaluate the thermodynamic parameters of the hydrophobic effect was made in a Refs [122;123]. Thermodynamic functions of hydration ($\Delta_{hydr} G^A$, $\Delta_{hydr} H^A$) for the solutes A not interacting specifically with water are regarded as the sum of the non-specific hydration thermodynamic functions ($\Delta_{hydr\ (nonsp)} G^A$, $\Delta_{hydr\ (nonsp)} H^A$) and the hydrophobic effect thermodynamic functions ($\Delta_{h.\ e.} G^A$, $\Delta_{h.\ e.} H^A$):

$$\Delta_{hydr} G^A = \Delta_{hydr\ (nonsp)} G^A + \Delta_{h.\ e.} G^A \tag{39}$$

$$\Delta_{hydr} H^A = \Delta_{hydr\ (nonsp)} H^A + \Delta_{h.\ e.} H^A \tag{40}$$

The values of $\Delta_{hydr\ (nonsp)} G^A$ and $\Delta_{hydr\ (nonsp)} H^A$ had been determined from a linear dependence between the Gibbs energy of solvation of A in a series of solvents and the corrected Hildebrand solubility parameter δ_H^{S*}. It can be calculated similarly to the Hildebrand parameter δ_H^S, but the difference between the solvent vaporization ($\Delta_{vap} H^S$) and self-association ($\Delta_{ass} H$) enthalpies is used in the numerator. Instead of

$\delta_H^S = \sqrt{\dfrac{\Delta_{vap} H^S - RT}{V_M^S}}$ we   have $\delta_H^{S*} = \sqrt{\dfrac{\Delta_{vap} H^S - \Delta_{ass} H - RT}{V_M^S}}$.   Thermodynamic

functions of solvation in water deviate from the universal linear correlation with δ_H^{S*} observed for other solvents, including self-associated. The values of $\Delta_{h.\ e.} G^A$ and $\Delta_{h.\ e.} H^A$ are the differences ($\Delta_{hydr} G^A - \Delta_{hydr\ (nonsp)} G^A$) and ($\Delta_{hydr} H^A - \Delta_{hydr\ (nonsp)} H^A$), respectively.

However, this method has two severe imperfections. First, there is no linear dependence between $\Delta_{solv} G^{A/S}$ ($\Delta_{solv} H^{A/S}$) and δ_H^{S*} for many apolar compounds. Second, a lot of experimental data are required to plot the correlation line.

In our recent work [124] we developed a method to determine the enthalpy of the hydrophobic effect.

We suppose that the feature of liquid water in comparison with other solvents is the presence of the hydrophobic effect term in solvation (hydration) thermodynamic functions. As in other models, we suppose the additivity of the hydrophobic effect contribution:

$$\Delta_{hydr} H^A = \Delta_{hydr\ (nonsp)} H^A + \Delta_{int\ (sp)} H^{A/H_2O} + \Delta_{h.\ e.} H^A \tag{41}$$

To determine $\Delta_{h.\,e.}H^A$, we should know the hydration enthalpy and be able to estimate the non-specific hydration enthalpy for systems without specific interactions and both non-specific and specific hydration enthalpies for solutes interacting specifically with water.

In the absence of the specific interactions, Eqn (41) can be rewritten as:

$$\Delta_{h.\,e.}H^A = \Delta_{hydr}H^A - \Delta_{hydr\,(nonsp)}H^A \qquad (42)$$

$\Delta_{hydr\,(nonsp)}H^A$ can be calculated by Eqn (32) as described above.

The solution enthalpies of liquid alkanes in water are close to zero or even negative (pentane) [125]. According Eqn (12), we receive a zero or negative value for $\delta_{cav}h^S$. It means water-water nonspecific interactions are even weaker than alkane-alkane interactions. It is easy to suppose that the solution enthalpy contains the hydrophobic effect contribution and we should subtract the hydrophobic effect enthalpy of alkane from the solution enthalpy of alkane in the numerator:

$$\delta_{cav}h^{H_2O} = \frac{\Delta_{soln}H^{C_nH_{2n+2}/H_2O} - \Delta_{h.\,e.}H^{C_nH_{2n+2}}}{V_X^{C_nH_{2n+2}}} \qquad (43)$$

We used $\Delta_{h.\,e.}H^{C_nH_{2n+2}}$ obtained previously [126] for calculation of $\delta_{cav}h^{H_2O}$. We calculated $\delta_{cav}h^{H_2O}$ from the solution enthalpies of $C_5 - C_8$ alkanes [125] using Eqn (43) and received an average value $\delta_{cav}h^{H_2O} = (9.5 \pm 1.0) \cdot 10^2$ kJ·cm^{-3}·10^2. This value is close to the dimethylformamide and acetonitrile $\delta_{cav}h^S$ values (8.6·10^2 and 10.7·10^2 kJ·cm^{-3}·10^2, respectively [50]) and indicates the closeness of the non-specific interaction parameters for water, dimethylformamide and acetonitrile.

In. Ref. [124] for the noble gases and alkanes the hydrophobic effect enthalpy is found to be negative and independent of the size of molecule. For aromatic hydrocarbons, it is positive and grows up with the size of the hydrocarbon.

The hydrophobicity of aliphatic alcohols, especially of the lowest homologues, can seem nonsense. Indeed, they mix with water in any proportion. But the solution entropy of alcohols in water is large negative [127], and the heat capacity of solution is large positive [128]. These anomalies allow to speak about the hydrophobicity of alcohols. According Eqn (41), we should know the specific alcohol-water interaction enthalpy as well as the non-specific interaction enthalpy to estimate the hydrophobic effect contribution to the solution enthalpy of alcohols in water.

It was shown [129-132] that the hydrogen bonding energy of water in itself is approximately -14 ± 1 kJ·mol^{-1} per bond. The hydrogen bonding enthalpy of methanol in itself is -15.1 kJ·mol^{-1} [100] This gives us the ground to use the hydrogen bonding enthalpies of alcohols in methanol to approximate the hydrogen bonding enthalpies of alcohols in water. Since we assume $\Delta_{int\,(sp)}H^{ROH/H_2O} = \Delta_{int\,(sp)}H^{ROH/CH_3OH}$, the hydrophobic effect enthalpy can be calculated by the following equation:

$$\Delta_{h.\ e.}H^A = \Delta_{hydr}H^A - \Delta_{hydr\ (nonsp)}H^A - \Delta_{int\ (sp)}H^{ROH/CH_3OH} \tag{44}$$

The hydrophobic effect enthalpies of considered (from methanol to octanol-1) alcohols, except methanol, fall in the range -10.0 ± 0.9 kJ·mol^{-1}, while the alkanes hydrophobic effect enthalpies are in the range -10.7 ± 1.5 kJ·mol^{-1}.

8. Conclusion

Solution calorimetry is currently an instrument of investigation which is widely used in different branches of science. Modern calorimetric instruments allow to obtain very accurate results. The main question now is how to interpret these results.

The authors conducted a consecutive study of the solvent effects basing on solution calorimetry data. The essence of this study is the analysis of experimental data with relation to various types of intermolecular interactions using the coherent transition from the simplest solute-solvent systems to more complex ones. Most significant results can be summarized as the following.

- *Simplest systems in which alkane is used as solute or solvent.* It is very probable that dispersion interactions are the only type of solute-solvent interactions in this case. Fuchs et al. [38] experimentally discovered the constancy of solute-solvent interaction energies for alkanes in different solvents. This constancy is not well-understandable from the 'physical' point of view, but as the experimental fact it was used to develop a method for determination of the relative cavity formation enthalpy [48, 49]. This value is extremely useful for the analysis of solvent effects. We tested whether the above mentioned constancy keeps for the case when an alkane is a solvent. The result was a linear dependence of the solvation enthalpies in alkane on the molar refractions of the solutes [57, 60]. This dependence is unique considering its simplicity and the diversity of solutes. It was used to develop the method for estimation of the vaporization enthalpies from the solution enthalpies in alkane.

- *Systems in which solvent is tetrachloromethane.* These are more complex systems because the inductive solute-solvent interactions are more probable and cannot be excluded a priori. Nevertheless, it is widely accepted that the specific interactions can be neglected in this case. It was found that linear dependencies of solvation enthalpies on solute molar refraction also take place in tetrachloromethane solutions [71, 72]. However, the picture is more complex than in alkane solvents. The points in the plot of solvation enthalpy vs. solute molar refraction fall into several groups (at least two as a rough approximation). The difference between these groups (difference in intercepts) cannot be explained by the contribution of inductive interactions. It was concluded that solvation enthalpies in tetrachloromethane are defined by dispersion solute-solvent interactions, but the volume of the solute molecule (molar refraction) is not the only solute parameter defining the value of dispersion interactions enthalpies.

- *Systems in which non-interacting-specifically solute is dissolved in any non-associated solvent.* Qualitatively, the overall picture is the same as in the previous case. The difference as compared with tetrachloromethane solvent consist in the differences in the values of intercept and slope for the corresponding dependences of the solvation enthalpy from solute molar refraction [71,72]. This result is, of course, surprising. It means that polar interactions (inductive, dipole-dipole etc.) are not manifested not only in tetrachloromethane, but also in other solvents such as benzene, acetone, ethyl acetate, acetonitrile, DMF, DMSO, etc. The negligible contribution of polar interactions was confirmed by comparison of solution enthalpies for some cis- and trans- disubstituted ethylenes and o-, m-, and p-disubstituted benzenes with the substituents of high polarity [71,77]. The unified equation (32) for calculation of the nonspecific solvation enthalpy in any solvent was derived empirically [50,71, 77, 98].
- *More complex systems.* As far as the nonspecific solvation enthalpies can be calculated, the solute-solvent specific interaction enthalpies can be obtained from the data on solution enthalpies [50, 71, 77, 98]. The specific interaction enthalpies of any solvent with itself (the enthalpy of solvent self-association) can also be found. This was made for some aliphatic alcohols [100]. The comparison of the behavior of aqueous solutions with other solvents allowed us to develop a quantitative method for description of the hydrophobic effect [124, 133]. We think that analyzing solution calorimetry data is the only way to determine these quantities from experiment.

We hope that after reading this chapter, researchers who use the calorimetry of infinitely diluted solutions in their studies, will consider fruitful the analysis of the intermolecular interactions, the example of which is given here.

Acknowledgement

This work was supported by the Russian Foundation for Basic Research, project no. 06-03-32734a.

References

[1]   Solomonov, B. N., Novikov, V. B., Solomonov, A. B. *Zh. Obshch. Khim.* 2002, *72*, 915.

[2]   Solomonov, B. N., Novikov, V. B., Solomonov, A. B. *Zh. Obshch. Khim.* 2002, *72*, 1126.

[3]   Sherman, S. R., Suleiman, D., Hait, M. J., Schiller, M., Liotta, C. L., Eckert, C. A., Li, J. J., Carr, P. W., Poe, R. B., Rutan, S. C. *J. Phys. Chem.* 1995, *99*, 11239.

[4]   Reiss, H., Frisch, H. L., Helfand, E., Lebowitz, J. L. *J. Chem. Phys.* 1960, *32*, 119.

[5]   Halicioglu, T., Sinanoglu, O. *Annals of the New York Academy of Sciences* 1969, *158*, 308.

[6]   Pierotti, R. A. *Chem. Rev.* 1976, *76*, 717.

[7]   Nguyen, V. P., Gander, B., Gentili, S., Sarraf, E., Ho, N. T. *J. Therm. Anal.* 1997, *48*, 697.

[8]   Fletcher, A. N., Heller, C. A. *J. Phys. Chem.* 1967, *71*, 3742.

[9]   Asprion, N., Hasse, H., Maurer, G. *Fluid Phase Equilibria* 2003, *208*, 23.

[10]   Sokolova, M., Barlow, S. J., Bondarenko, G. V., Gorbaty, Y. E., Poliakoff, M. *J. Phys. Chem. A* 2006, *110*, 3882.

[11]   Kwak, K., Park, S., Fayer, M. D. *Proc. Natl. Acad. Sci. U. S. A.* 2007, *104*, 14221.

[12]   Krishnan, C. V., Friedman, H. L. *J. Phys. Chem.* 1969, *73*, 1572.

[13]   Spencer, J. N., Wolbach, W. S., Hovick, J. W., Ansel, L., Modaress, K. J. *J. Solution Chem.* 1985, *14*, 805.

[14]   Benson, S. W. *J. Am. Chem. Soc.* 1996, *118*, 10645.

[15]   Dejaegere, A., Karplus, M. *J. Phys. Chem.* 1996, *100*, 11148.

[16]   Beglov, D., Roux, B. *J. Phys. Chem. B* 1997, *101*, 7821.

[17]   Best, S. A., Merz, K. M., Reynolds, C. H. *J. Phys. Chem. B* 1997, *101*, 10479.

[18]   Selves, J. L., Abraham, M. H., Burg, P. *Fluid Phase Equilibria* 1998, *148*, 69.

[19]   Silverstein, K. A. T., Haymet, A. D. J., Dill, K. A. *J. Am. Chem. Soc.* 1998, *120*, 3166.

[20]   Colominas, C., Luque, F. J., Teixido, J., Orozco, M. *Chem. Phys.* 1999, *240*, 253.

[21]   Arnett, E. M., Chawla, B., Bell, L., Taagepera, M., Hehre, W. J., Taft, R. W. *J. Am. Chem. Soc.* 1977, *99*, 5729.

[22]   Spencer, J. N., Berger, E. M., Powell, C. R., Henning, B. D., Furman, G. S., Loffredo, W. M., Rydberg, E. M., Neubort, R. A., Shoop, C. E., Slauch, D. N. *J. Phys. Chem.* 1981, *85*, 1236.

[23]   Madan, B., Lee, B. *Biophys. Chem.* 1994, *2-3*, 279.

[24]   Catalan, J. *J. Org. Chem.* 1995, *60*, 8315.

[25]   Luck, W. A. P., Klein, D. *J. Mol. Struct.* 1996, *381*, 83.

[26]   Kleeberg, H., Kocak, O., Luck, W. A. P. *J. Solution Chem.* 1982, *11*, 611.

[27]   Catalan, J., Gomez, J., Couto, A., Laynez, J. *J. Am. Chem. Soc.* 1990, *112*, 1678.

[28]   Nagata, I., Gotoh, K. *Thermochim. Acta* 1995, *258*, 77.

[29]   Mchale, M. E. R., Powell, J. R., Kauppila, A. S. M., Acree, W. E., Huyskens, P. L. *J. Solution Chem.* 1996, *25*, 1089.

[30]   Catalan, J., Palomar, J., Diaz, C., Depaz, J. L. G. *J. Phys. Chem. A* 1997, *101*, 5183.

[31]   Wormald, C. J. *Fluid Phase Equilibria* 1997, *133*, 1.

[32]   Goralski, P. *Fluid Phase Equilibria* 2000, *167*, 207.

[33]   Diaz, C., Barrio, L., Catalan, J. *Chem. Phys. Lett.* 2003, *371*, 645.

[34]   Brown, H. C., Barbaras, G. K., Berneis, H. L., Bonner, W. H., Johannesen, R. B., Grayson, M., Nelson, K. L. *J. Am. Chem. Soc.* 1953, *75*, 1.

[35]   Reichardt, C. *Solvents and Solvent Effects in Organic Chemistry*; Wiley-VCH: Weinheim, 2002.

[36]   Bakhshiev, N. G., Girin, O. P., Piterskaya, I. V. *Opt. Spektrosk.* 1968, *24*, 901.

[37]   Krishnan, C. V., Friedman, H. L. *J. Phys. Chem.* 1971, *75*, 3598.

Application of Solution Calorimetry of Nonelectrolytes...   137

[38] Saluja, P. S., Young, T. M., Rodewald, R. F., Fuchs, F. H., Kohli, D., Fuchs, R. *J. Am. Chem. Soc.* 1977, *99*, 2949.

[39] Fuchs, R., Peacock, L. A., Stephenson, W. K. *Can. J. Chem.* 1982, *60*, 1953.

[40] Fuchs, R., Stephenson, W. K. *Can. J. Chem.* 1985, *63*, 349.

[41] Fuchs, R., Chambers, E. J., Stephenson, W. K. *Can. J. Chem.* 1987, *65*, 2624.

[42] Solomonov, B. N., Antipin, I. S., Gorbachuk, V. V., Konovalov, A. I. *Zh. Obshch. Khim.* 1982, *52*, 2154.

[43] Abraham, M. H., McGowan, J. C. *Chromatographia* 1987, *23*, 243.

[44] Abraham, M. H., Whiting, G. S., Doherty, R. M., Shuely, W. J. *J. Chem. Soc. Perkin Trans. 2* 1990, 1451.

[45] Abraham, M. H., Green, C. E., Acree, W. E., Hernandez, C. E., Roy, L. E. *J. Chem. Soc. Perkin Trans. 2* 1998, 2677.

[46] Poole, C. F., Poole, S. K., Abraham, M. H. *J. Chromatogr. A.* 1998, *798*, 207.

[47] Antipin, I. S., Arslanov, N. A., Palyulin, V. A., Konovalov, A. I., Zefirov, N. S. *Dokl. Akad. Nauk SSSR* 1991, *316*, 925.

[48] Solomonov, B. N., Antipin, I. S., Gorbatchuk, V. V., Konovalov, A. I. *Dokl. Akad. Nauk SSSR* 1978, *243*, 1499.

[49] Solomonov, B. N., Antipin, I. S., Gorbachuk, V. V., Konovalov, A. I. *J. Gen. Chem. USSR (Engl. Transl.)* 1982, *52*, 1917.

[50] Solomonov, B. N., Novikov, V. B., Varfolomeev, M. A., Mileshko, N. M. *J. Phys. Org. Chem.* 2005, *18* , 49.

[51] Solomonov, B. N., Antipin, I. S., Gorbachuk, V. V., Konovalov, A. I. *Zh. Obshch. Khim.* 1982, *52*, 696.

[52] Berthelot, D. *C. R. Acad. Sci.* 1898, *126*, 1703.

[53] Solomonov, B. N., Varfolomeev, M. A., Novikov, V. B., Klimovitskii, A. E. *Spectrochim. Acta A* 2006, *64*, 405.

[54] Solomonov, B. N., Varfolomeev, M. A., Novikov, V. B., Klimovitskii, A. E. *Spectrochim. Acta A* 2006, *64*, 397.

[55] Fuchs, R., Young, T. M., Rodewald, R. F. *J. Am. Chem. Soc.* 1974, *96*, 4705.

[56] Saluja, P. S., Peacock, L. A., Fuchs, R. *J. Am. Chem. Soc.* 1979, *101*, 1958.

[57] Solomonov, B. N., Antipin, I. S., Gorbatchuk, V. V., Konovalov, A. I. *Dokl. Akad. Nauk SSSR* 1979, *247*, 405.

[58] Spencer, J. N., Gleim, J. E., Blevins, C. H., Garret, R. C., Mayer, F. J. *J. Phys. Chem.* 1979, *83*, 1249.

[59] Dellagatta, G., Stradella, L., Venturello, P. *J. Solution Chem.* 1981, *10*, 209.

[60] Solomonov, B. N., Antipin, I. S., Novikov, V. B., Konovalov, A. I. *Zh. Obshch. Khim.* 1982, *52*, 2681.

[61] Airoldi, C., Roca, S. *J. Solution Chem.* 1993, *22*, 707.

[62] Solomonov, B. N., Konovalov, A. I. *Usp. Khim.* 1991, *60*, 45.

[63] Hildebrand, J. H. *J. Am. Chem. Soc.* 1929, *51*, 66.

[64] Hildebrand, J. H., Scott, R. L. *The solubility of nonelectrolytes;* Reinhold: New York, 1950.

[65] Hildebrand, J. H., Prausnitz, J. M., Scott, R. L. *Regular and related solutions;* Van Nostrand: Princeton, 1970.

[66] Ioffe, B. V. Refraktometricheskie metody khimii (Refractometric Methods in Chemistry); Khimiya: Leningrad, 1983.

[67] Drago, R. S., Parr, L. B., Chamberlain, C. S. *J. Am. Chem. Soc.* 1977, *99*, 3203.

[68] Stephenson, W. K., Fuchs, R. *Can. J. Chem.* 1985, *63*, 2540.

[69] Spencer, J. N., Andrefsky, J. C., Grushow, A., Naghdi, J., Patti, L. M., Trader, J. F. *J. Phys. Chem.* 1987, *91*, 1673.

[70] Joesten, M., Schaad, L. *Hydrogen bonding;* Marcel Dekker: New York, 1974.

[71] Solomonov, B. N., Konovalov, A. I., Novikov, V. B., Vedernikov, A. N., Borisover, M. D., Gorbachuk, V. V., Antipin, I. S. *Zh. Obshch. Khim.* 1984, *54*, 1622.

[72] Solomonov, B. N., Konovalov, A. I. *Zh. Obshch. Khim.* 1985, *55*, 2529.

[73] Cramer, C. J., Truhlar, D. G. *Reviews in Computational Chemistry 6.* 1995, *6*, 1.

[74] Kamlet, M. J., Taft, R. W., Carr, P. W., Abraham, M. H. *Journal of the Chemical Society-Faraday Transactions I* 1982, *78*, 1689.

[75] Stien, M. L., Claessens, M., Lopez, A., Reisse, J. *J. Am. Chem. Soc.* 1982, *104*, 5902.

[76] Luhmer, M., Stien, M. L., Reisse, J. *Heterocycles* 1994, *37*, 1041.

[77] Solomonov, B. N., Chumakov, F. V., Borisover, M. D. *Zh. Fiz. Khim.* 1993, *67*, 1289.

[78] Pappalardo, R. R., Martinez, J. M., Marcos, E. S. *Chem. Phys. Lett.* 1994, *225*, 202.

[79] Hildebrand, J. H., Carter, J. M. Proceedings of the National Academy of Sciences of the United States of America 1930, 16, 285.

[80] London, F. Zeitschrift fur Physikalische Chemie-Abteilung B-Chemie der Elementarprozesse Aufbau der Materie 1930, 11, 222.

[81] Iogansen, A. V., Kurkchi, G. A., Levina, O. V. *Zh. Fiz. Khim.* 1969, *43*, 2915.

[82] Kurkchi, G. A., Iogansen, A. V. *Zh. Fiz. Khim.* 1967, *41*, 563.

[83] Arnett, E. M., Murty, T. S. S. R., Schleyer, P. V. R., Joris, L. *J. Am. Chem. Soc.* 1967, *89*, 5955.

[84] Duer, W. C., Bertrand, G. L. *J. Am. Chem. Soc.* 1970, *92*, 2587.

[85] Stephenson, W. K., Fuchs, R. *Can. J. Chem.* 1985, *63*, 342.

[86] Arnett, E. M., Joris, L., Mitchell, E., Murty, T. S. S. R., Gorrie, T. M., Schleyer, P. V. R. *J. Am. Chem. Soc.* 1970, *92*, 2365.

[87] Arnett, E. M., Carter, J. V. *J. Am. Chem. Soc.* 1971, *93*, 1516.

[88] Spencer, J. N., Sweigart, J. R., Brown, M. E., Bensing, R. L., Hassinger, T. L., Kelly, W., Housel, D. L., Reisinger, G. W., Gleim, J. E., Peiper, J. C. *J. Phys. Chem.* 1977, *81*, 2237.

[89] Stephenson, W. K., Fuchs, R. *Can. J. Chem.* 1985, *63*, 2529.

[90] Goralski, P., Tkaczyk, M. *J. Chem. Soc. Faraday Trans. 1* 1987, *83*, 3083.

[91] Abboud, J. L. M., Notario, R. *Pure Appl. Chem.* 1999, *71*, 645.

[92] Solomonov, B. N., Novikov, V. B., Gorbachuk, V. V., Konovalov, A. I. *Dokl. Akad. Nauk SSSR* 1982, *265*, 1441.

[93] Solomonov, B. N., Konovalov, A. I., Novikov, V. B., Gorbachuk, V. V., Neklyudov, S. A. *Zh. Obshch. Khim.* 1985, *55*, 1889.

[94] Hartley, B. K., Skinner, H. A. *Trans. Farad. Soc.* 1950, *46*, 621.

[95] Fuchs, R., Rodewald, R. F. *J. Am. Chem. Soc.* 1973, *95*, 5897.

[96] Arnett, E. M., Mitchell, E., Murty, T. S. S. R. *J. Am. Chem. Soc.* 1974, *96*, 3875.

[97] Kiselev, V. D., Mavrin, G. V., Korshin, E. E., Konovalov, A. I. *Zh. Obshch. Khim.* 1980, *50*, 1135.

[98] Solomonov, B. N., Novikov, V. B. *Zh. Obshch. Khim.* 2004, *74* , 758.

[99] Novikov, V. B., Abaidullina, D. I., Gainutdinova, N. Z., Varfolomeev, M. A., Solomonov, B. N. *Zh. Fiz. Khim.* 2006, *80*, 2011.

[100] Solomonov, B. N., Novikov, V. B., Varfolomeev, M. A., Klimovitskii, A. E. *J. Phys. Org. Chem.* 2005, *18*, 1132.

[101] Blainey, P. C., Reid, P. J. *Spectrochim. Acta A* 2001, *57* , 2763.

[102] Trampe, D. M., Eckert, C. A. *J. Chem. Eng. Data* 1991, *36*, 112.

[103] Solomonov, B. N., Varfolomeev, M. A., Novikov, V. B. *J. Phys. Org. Chem.* 2006, *19*, 263.

[104] Solomonov, B. N., Borisover, M. D., Konovalov, A. I. *Zh. Obshch. Khim.* 1986, *56*, 3.

[105] Solomonov, B. N., Borisover, M. D., Konovalov, A. I. *Zh. Obshch. Khim.* 1987, *57*, 423.

[106] Siegel, G. G., Huyskens, P. L., Vanderheyden, L. *Berichte der Bunsen-Gesellschaft-Physical Chemistry Chemical Physics* 1990, *94*, 549.

[107] Kleeberg, H., Luck, W. A. P. *Z. Phys. Chem. (Leipzig)* 1989, *270*, 613.

[108] Parra, R. D., Bulusu, S., Zeng, X. C. *J. Chem. Phys.* 2003, *118*, 3499.

[109] Maes, G., Smets, J. *J. Phys. Chem.* 1993, *97*, 1818.

[110] Kleeberg, H., Heinje, G., Luck, W. A. P. *J. Phys. Chem.* 1986, *90*, 4427.

[111] Kleeberg, H., Klein, D., Luck, W. A. P. *J. Phys. Chem.* 1987, *91* , 3200.

[112] Khafizov, F. T., Breus, V. A., Solomonov, B. N., Kiselev, O. E., Konovalov, A. I. *Dokl. Akad. Nauk SSSR* 1988, *303*, 916.

[113] Khafizov, F. T., Breus, V. A., Kiselev, O. E., Solomonov, B. N., Konovalov, A. I. *Zh. Obshch. Khim.* 1990, *60*, 713.

[114] Gill, S. J., Wadso, I. *Proc. Natl. Acad. Sci. U. S. A.* 1976, *73*, 2955.

[115] Leo, A., Hansch, C., Elkins, D. *Chem. Rev.* 1971, *71*, 525.

[116] Shinoda, K. *J. Phys. Chem.* 1977, *81*, 1300.

[117] Abraham, M. H. *J. Am. Chem. Soc.* 1979, *101*, 5477.

[118] Abraham, M. H. *J. Am. Chem. Soc.* 1980, *102*, 5910.

[119] Abraham, M. H. *J. Am. Chem. Soc.* 1982, *104*, 2085.

[120] Mastroianni, M. J., Pikal, M. J., Lindenbaum, S. *J. Phys. Chem.* 1972, *76*, 3050.

[121] Rouw, A. C., Somsen, G. *J. Chem. Thermodyn.* 1981, *13*, 67.

[122] Jozwiak, M., Piekarski, H. *J. Mol. Liq.* 1999, *81*, 63.

[123] Jozwiak, M., Piekarski, H. *J. Mol. Liq.* 2002, *95*, 313.

[124] Solomonov, B. N., Sedov, I. A. *J. Phys. Chem. B* 2006, *110*, 9298.

[125] Plyasunov, A. V., Shock, E. L. *Geochimica et Cosmochimica Acta* 2003, *67*, 4981.

[126] Borisover, M. D., Baitalov, F. D., Solomonov, B. N. *J. Solution Chem.* 1995, *24*, 579.

[127] Graziano, G. *Phys. Chem. Chem. Phys.* 1999, *1* , 3567.

[128] Makhatadze, G. I., Privalov, P. L. *J. Solution Chem.* 1989, *18*, 927.

[129] Eisenberg, D., Kauzmann, W. *The structure and properties of water;* Charendon Press: Oxford, 1969.

[130] Luck, W. A. P. *J. Mol. Liq.* 1986, *32*, 41.

[131] Luck, W. A. P. *J. Mol. Struct.* 1998, *448*, 131.

[132] Efimov, Y., Naberukhin, Y. Spectrochimica Acta Part A: Molecular and Biomolecular Spectroscopy 2005, 61, 1789.

[133] Solomonov, B. N., Sedov, I. A., Varfolomeev, M. A. *Zh. Fiz. Khim.* 2006, *80*, 763.

In: Pain Management: New Research
Editors: P. S. Greco, F. M. Conti

ISBN: 978-1-60456-767-0
© 2008 Nova Science Publishers, Inc.

Chapter V

Topically Applied Morphine Gel for Painful Ulcers

Quy N.H. Tran, M.D.[*]
Department of Internal Medicine
University of California at Davis, Medical Center
Sacramento, CA 95817, USA

Abstract

Although it has been well established that opioid analgesics relieve pain by acting on receptors in the central nervous system, research has suggested that similar analgesia can be achieved through peripheral opioid receptors. Basic science research has demonstrated that malignant or benign skin ulcers can expose peripheral sensory nerve terminals, while local inflammation within the ulcer up-regulates opioid receptors. Thus, one strategy to manage pain arising from these ulcers would be to apply topical opioid agonists, usually in the form of a gel. While systemic absorption likely varies with extent of ulceration, topical analgesics could reduce the need for systemic medications and the resultant adverse effects. However, research in the area has been slow; a few small randomized trials and case series suggest benefits from morphine gel. Whether it is a placebo effect or actual analgesia produced from peripheral receptors, many unfortunate patients suffer from difficult to treat ulcerative pain and may appear to benefit from a topical strategy. Larger studies are needed and, fortunately, are being conducted to help establish topical opioid therapy as a viable adjunct to systemic therapy in treating pain from ulcers.

[*] Corresponding Author: Dr. Quy Tran, University of California at Davis, Medical Center, 4150 V Street, PSSB Suite 3100, Sacramento, CA 95817, E-mail: quy.tran@ucdmc.ucdavis.edu.

Introduction

Opioid analgesics relieve pain by acting on receptors in the central nervous system, often at the expense of significant side effects. Research has suggested that similar analgesia can be achieved through peripheral receptors through a neuroimmune pathway. Light microscopic techniques have demonstrated opioid receptors in the periphery of fine cutaneous nerves and, depending on particular circumstances, sensory axons can be immunostained for mu-, delta-, or kappa-receptors [1, 2]. These opioid receptors are quiescent and are difficult to find in normal tissue, but are detectable after peripheral injury and onset of inflammation. With pronounced inflammation, the perineurium is disrupted, exposing the receptors to potential opioid agonists, while also creating an environment to enhance their efficacy. These activated receptors may be stimulated by mechanical, chemical, or thermal means. In addition, inflammation promotes distal transport of these receptors along the axon to the periphery further concentrating the number of available and active receptors [3]. Immune cells within inflamed subcutaneous tissue can synthesize and release endogenous opioid peptides that interact with these receptors. This interaction alters potassium and calcium currents within the neurons that can cause inhibition of neuronal excitation, action potential propagation, and release of proinflammatory peptides, thereby producing analgesia [4]. Interestingly, similar effects can be produced with exogenous opioid agonists and the analgesia can be reversed with naloxone.

Because of these findings, there has been interest in using opioid agonists in patients with benign or malignant ulcers. Pain arising from these ulcers is often difficult to treat and it is common for patients to continue to experience pain despite using systemic medications. The destructive nature of these ulcers exposes cutaneous nerves that could potentially be a target for locally applied opioid agonists. The strategy of using locally-acting analgesia has the advantage of low systemic bioavailability and potentially decreased related adverse effects. Patients could conceivably achieve greater analgesia while taking fewer or lower doses of oral medications and thus reduce the risk of sedation, respiratory depression, nausea and constipation. Several clinical trials and case series have reported good analgesia with few side effects using topical morphine in the treatment of painful ulcers. In this chapter, two patients with painful ulcers (one with malignant ulcers, the other with benign ulcers) treated with topical morphine gel are discussed followed by a review of the available literature regarding this modality of treatment.

First Case

A 52-year-old man with Stage IIb mycosis fungoides was admitted for pain control. His pain arose from skin lesions that were in varying stages of healing. As an outpatient, he was initially started on hydrocodone as needed and was quickly titrated up to long-acting morphine with liquid short-acting morphine as needed. About one month before his admission, his long-acting morphine was converted to methadone 30 mg orally three times a day. On the day of admission, he reported that he self-titrated his methadone dose to 50 mg orally three times a day and continued to use short-acting morphine for breakthrough pain.

This regimen did not provide significant relief. He also noted that the pain medications affected his concentration, were quite sedating, and caused severe dose-limiting constipation. In addition, prior treatment with diverse chemotherapy regimens offered minimal resolution of his primary disease, and so, he continued to experience considerable pain. Given the chronic and progressive nature of his disease, his physical exam was notable for widespread skin lesions, which ranged from mild erythematous patches to scaly plaques to open weeping ulcers, covering his entire body. To control his pain, he was continued on his previously prescribed dose of methadone at 30 mg orally three times a day and started on a patient controlled analgesia (PCA) pump to calculate his additional needs.

Despite increasing analgesic dosing with the PCA, he continued to experience pain. By the fifth day of his admission, his PCA was discontinued and he was started on oxycodone 5-20 mg orally every 6 hours as needed. His pain continued. On hospital day seven, the methadone was increased to 40 mg orally three times a day and oxycodone was increased to 5-30 mg orally every 4 hours as needed. Pain control remained inadequate. On the eighth day of his admission, with his consent, a trial of topical opioids was initiated. A mixture of 10 mg of morphine sulfate injection was combined with 8 grams of a neutral water-based gel. A test dose applied to a small patch of skin was well tolerated. The patient then applied the morphine gel to five or six of the larger (greater than 2.5 cm in diameter) and more painful lesions. Under the guidance of a wound care nurse, he liberally applied the morphine gel to each lesion 2-3 times per day as needed. Before the utilization of morphine gel, the patient's pain scores ranged from 5-10 (on a scale from 0-10 with 10 being the worse pain) with most scores around 7. With the addition of morphine gel, his pain scores ranged from 0-9 with almost half of his scores under 5. He was discharged with satisfactory pain relief two days later on a regimen of morphine gel applied 2-3 times daily as needed, methadone 40 mg orally three times a day for basal pain control and oxycodone 5-30 mg orally every 4 hours as needed for breakthrough pain. He was admitted several more times over the next several months and continued to require higher doses of narcotics. He died 5 months later due to his progressive, uncontrolled disease.

Second Case

A 55-year-old sedentary woman with diabetes mellitus type 2 and stage III-IV bilateral lower extremity and decubitus ulcers was admitted to the surgical team for debridement of these ulcers. The medicine service was consulted to assist in managing the patient's diabetes and to recommend a medication regimen to help control the pain arising from these ulcers. As an outpatient, she was started on hydrocodone as needed for pain. As her ulcerative disease progressed, the pain worsened, and she was titrated to a regimen of extended release oxycodone 20 mg orally two times a day with hydrocodone as needed for pain. When she was admitted, she was continued on her extended release oxycodone and given morphine sulfate injections every two hours as needed for pain. Her pain scores ranged from 5-10 (on a scale from 0-10 with 10 being the worse pain), with higher numbers corresponding to dressing changes.

Because of the localizing nature of her pain, it was felt that a topical strategy for pain control would benefit her. With her consent, a trial of morphine gel was initiated. A mixture of 10 mg of morphine sulfate injection was combined with 10 grams of a neutral water-based gel. A test dose applied to a small patch of skin was well tolerated, so the patient self-applied the morphine gel to all of her lesions. Under the guidance of a wound care nurse, she liberally applied the morphine gel to each lesion 2-3 times per day as needed. She continued to have pain with scores ranging from 3-6, but she noted that this range was tolerable for her. She was titrated off the extended release oxycodone and only used morphine gel and as needed hydrocodone during the hospital course. She was discharged in good condition on this regimen.

Conclusion

The management of pain due to malignant or benign skin ulcers is of great importance. The number of patients who suffer from benign ulcers, including those with pressure ulcers or ulcers that develop as a result of long-standing diabetes mellitus or peripheral vascular disease is tremendous. Approximately 26% of hospice patients[5] and as many as 40,000 patients per year suffer from pain due to pressure ulcers and thousands more suffer from ulcers due to chronic medical conditions.[6] In addition, ulcers that develop from malignant etiologies such as Kaposi's sarcoma, melanoma, breast cancer, rectal cancer or mycosis fungoides, cause pain and suffering to an unfortunate patient population. The issue of adequate analgesia in these patients is difficult and the strategy of using topically applied agents may provide another form of pain relief.

Most studies on topically applied opioids to treat pain that arise from ulcers use a mixture of 10 mg of morphine sulfate combined with 8 g of a neutral water based gel (typically Intrasite® gel, Smith and Nephew Healthcare Ltd, Middlesex, UK), although other doses of morphine, alternative narcotics (such as methadone powder[7]) and other gels and delivery systems (such as metronidazole gel[8], silver sulphadiazine cream[9], and Stomahesive® powder[7]), have been utilized. Systemic absorption of morphine gel likely varies with extent of ulceration. When applied to cutaneous ulcers, one study noted that morphine and its metabolites, morphine-6-glucuronide (M6G) and morphine-3-glucuronide (M3G), were undetectable in the plasma of most patients.[10] The same study also noted that in one patient with a large surface area ulcer, morphine, M6G, and M3G were all detected in the plasma. In this patient, morphine and M6G bioavailability were 20% and 21%, respectively, while M3G was below the lower limit of quantification. Thus, systemic absorption for the majority of patients is negligible, which would lead to the decreased likelihood of systemic adverse effects.

Several years after basic science research demonstrated analgesic actions of exogenous opioids in peripheral tissue, case series began to appear in the literature. Jepson reported a series of 17 patients with 30 ulcers and used topical benzydamine in an aqueous solution.[11] Within the first 24 hours, significant pain relief was reported in 29 of 30 ulcers. Pain relief was achieved in all ulcers by 48 hours. Back *et al.* reported using diamorphine in Intrasite gel in three patients with skin ulcers and was able to produce adequate analgesia in these patients within 72 hours.[12] In a descriptive case series, Twillman *et al.* reported on nine consecutive patients treated with morphine-infused gel dressing.[6] Eight patients had open ulcers: three patients with decubitus ulcers, three patients with ulcers arising from chronic medical conditions, and two patients with malignant ulcers. The ninth patient had colorectal cancer and pain due to swelling and inflammation of his scrotum, but had no open wounds. All patients were treated with either a 0.1% or a 0.15% weight-to-weight concentration of morphine gel and seven of nine patients experienced substantial pain relief, one patient experienced some pain relief, and the patient without an open wound did not experience any relief.

Based on these promising observational studies, two small randomized, double-blind, placebo-controlled, crossover pilot studies were conducted.[13, 14] Published simultaneously, the first study recruited 13 patients in a palliative care setting with painful grade II or III pressure ulcers to be treated with a 0.1% weight-to-weight mixture of a diamorphine gel.[13] The six patients that did not complete the study died either before or during the trial or developed confusion necessitating withdrawal from the trial. The patients were randomly assigned to either three days of placebo gel followed by diamorphine gel or vice versa. Pain scores improved significantly 1 and 12 hours after application of diamorphine gel as compared to placebo gel. In the other study, five patients with painful sacral ulcers were first treated with either morphine gel or placebo for two days.[14] After a two-day washout, patients were crossed over for a further two days of the alternative treatment. Patients completed a visual analogue scale (VAS) twice daily, with lower numbers indicating more pain relief. Mean VAS scores for patients during placebo was 47 ± 11 and during morphine was 15 ± 11. There was no difference in the use of rescue medications during either treatment arm. Adverse effects included itching, burning or discomfort, but these effects occurred in both arms and none could be directly attributed to the morphine. Intrasite gel is generally well tolerated, but it is also used for debridement of necrotic tissue, thus some of the adverse effects noted could be attributed to the natural action of the hydrogel. A larger, follow-up randomized, double-blind, placebo-controlled study included 16 patients, 13 with pressure ulcers and 3 with malignant ulcers.[15] Analgesia was rated using a numerical rating score (NRS) with lower numbers indicating more pain relief. Mean NRS scores during pretreatment, with morphine, and with placebo were 6.6 ± 1.6, 2.8 ± 1.3, and 5.5 ± 1.9, respectively. Similar adverse effects were noted in the larger study. Because of these results, Porzio *et al.* encouraged further research and reported their own case series of three patients with pressure sores and two patients with malignant ulcers treated with morphine gel and reported significant pain relief in all five patients.[16] Similarly, Abbas reported a series of 17 patients with grade 2+ pressure ulcers treated with diamorphine gel and mean VAS scores improved from 9.4 to 4.6 after treatment.[17]

Topical morphine gel is not limited to use in the adult population and small case series are beginning to appear in the pediatric literature. Use of morphine gel in the pediatric population with painful inflammatory skin lesions would prove advantageous since the use of systemic opioids are often limited by frequent side effects experienced by young patients. In one study, two pediatric patients with epidermolysis bullosa with painful denuded areas of skin resulting from recurring bullae formation were treated with morphine gel.[18] The morphine gel mixture consisted of 10 mg of morphine sulfate with 15 g of Intrasite gel with the dose of morphine at 0.2 mg/kg. One patient had a 40-55% reduction in pain scores; the other patient who was opioid naïve had a 66% reduction in the pain score. To date, both patients have not reported any adverse side effects.

Expanding on the data collected for the treatment of cutaneous ulcers using topically applied opioids, several researchers have utilized locally applied exogenous opioids to treat the pain associated with esophageal and mucosal damage due to chemoradiotherapy. Gairard-Dory et al. used a slightly modified morphine gel for patients suffering from esophagitis.[19] They reported on three patients with non-small cell lung cancer treated with 36 Gy of radiotherapy and all patients subsequently experienced at least grade III radiotherapy-induced esophagitis. Instead of using Intrasite gel, morphine sulfate was mixed with a ready-mixed Purilon gel, and the patients swallowed 2 to 10 mL of 0.1% of this morphine gel. All patients reported pain relief with the morphine gel. One patient reported nausea with the mixture, which was corrected by having the patient take small amounts. No other adverse effects were reported. Cerchietti et al. did not utilize a morphine gel mixture in their study of mucositis-associated pain from chemoradiotherapy, but used a morphine mouthwash and compared it to a magic mouthwash comprised of aluminum hydroxide, viscous lidocaine and diphenhydramine. All twenty six patients had either grade 2 or 3 mucositis. The 14 patients assigned to the morphine mouthwash arm reported a significant decrease in pain scores, a longer duration of pain relief and a shorter duration of severe functional impairment.[20] Only one patient in this arm experienced local side effects. Esophagitis and mucositis are often the dose limiting toxicity associated with chemoradiotherapy with few options to utilize in treating pain associated with these inflammatory conditions. Based on these studies, topical opioids provide an attractive alternative or adjunct to traditional therapy.

In Practice

These case series and randomized controlled trials have all suggested that morphine gel is beneficial and efficacious, but the studies are small and no large definitive trials have been conducted. It is likely that morphine gel will not supplant the use of oral analgesics in the treatment of pain arising from ulcers, but experience has shown that it can be used as a successful adjunct to such therapy. In these two sample patients, morphine gel provided additional pain relief and worked in conjunction with the primary strategy of oral analgesics. Both patients reported that the morphine gel allowed them to rest at night and made dressing changes more tolerable, but both relied on oral medications as their main form of analgesia. Given the lessons learned from these and other similar patients, some institutions have begun to use morphine gel in patients with ulcer pain that is not controlled with oral analgesics alone.

Despite the lack of large trials, these smaller studies do yield promising results for the large patient population that suffers from pain arising from ulcers. Morphine gel may provide an effective and relatively safe modality to relieve pain. Morphine gel can readily be prepared by any compounding pharmacy. The choice of hydrogel to use is dependent on the pharmacy's formulary, but should be one in which the hydrogel is chemically stable and inert. The morphine component of the compound has been shown to be stable for up to 28 days when mixed with a neutral water based hydrogel with no detectable break down products.[21] If mixed under sterile conditions, it can be used safely for 28 days. If morphine gel is mixed under non-sterile conditions, due to infection control concerns, the mixture should be used within seven days. A month's supply can conveniently be prescribed and safely used if stored below 25°C in a dry place. Few adverse effects have been reported, but care needs to be exercised in patients with sensitivities to any component of morphine gel. Common adverse events reported in our patients are similar to reported case series and include itching and skin irritation, likely due to debriding action of the hydrogel. Systemic side effects are very rare, so patient adherence is high. Some patients have noted that morphine gel can be messy, but this can be minimized with gauze wraps. Abuse potential is low because of the difficulty in separating the morphine sulfate from the gel once it is mixed, but vigilance is recommended in prescribing large quantities of morphine gel.

Basic and clinical research supports the use of morphine gel, but the widespread utilization in actual clinical practice has been slow. Based on these promising studies, any patient presenting with pain of primarily ulcer origin should be evaluated for morphine gel therapy. Many treatment algorithms exist for treating patients with painful ulcers and morphine gel should be a component of these algorithms. Usually, patients can be started on morphine gel as an adjunctive therapy when patients continue to have pain despite increasing doses of oral medications or experience significant side effects from those medications. A starting concentration of 10 mg of morphine sulfate with 10 gm of a hydrogel can be initially tried and although there is no known maximum dose, most studies report achieving an effect before reaching a concentration of 10 mg of morphine sulfate with 5 gm of a hydrogel dosed at three times a day. No studies have looked at the amount of gel to apply to each wound and the dwell time the mixture should stay on the wounds. Most patients apply either a thin film or the minimum amount of morphine gel necessary to just cover the wound, and leave the mixture on until the next dressing change. Nursing protocols to utilize morphine gel can be adapted from standard wound care protocols. Caution is advised with stage IV ulcers as a minimum amount of morphine or its metabolites may be absorbed systemically. A slow titration schedule is recommended for these large and deep ulcers. Morphine gel applied to exudative wounds may be diluted or flushed away due to the extremely moist environment and dosing amounts and schedules should be adjusted to account for this.

Future Directions

Many patients would likely benefit from morphine gel, and larger clinical trials are beginning to appear to definitively establish efficacy. Trials utilizing morphine gel to treat pain arising from benign ulcers are currently underway, and trials focusing on malignant ulcers are being designed. Results of these larger trials should start to appear within the next couple of years. Trials examining whether morphine or its metabolites affect wound healing have not been conducted, and would be important to patients with benign ulcers, such as pressure ulcers, where wound healing is paramount. Duration of pain relief from morphine gel has not been well-studied and trials examining this would help in establishing proper dosing protocols. Currently, protocols are based on anecdotal evidence.

The fact that peripheral opioid receptors are active in inflamed tissue makes topical opioid therapy an attractive option in treating pain caused by many acute and subacute clinical scenarios, such as in post-operative wounds, vaginal or rectal fistulae, traumatic injuries, and arthritis. Combining an opioid with an antibiotic gel and affixing the mixture to a mesh would provide an appealing adjunctive solution to treating ulcers, wounds and injuries that are often painful and infected. This multimodality treatment strategy would allow convenient and rapid placement of local therapy at the site of the lesion. Fortunately, these trials and product developments are progressing quickly, making gel therapy a more attractive and viable option for patients and clinicians.

Acknowledgements

This chapter was inspired by an article originally printed in The Journal of Supportive Oncology, parts of which are re-printed here with permission from Elsevier Science.

References

[1]   Coggeshall RE, Zhou S, Carlton SM. Opioid receptors on peripheral sensory axons. *Brain Research* 1997;764(1-2):126-32.

[2]   Truong W, Cheng C, Xu Q-G, Li X-Q, Zochodne DW. Mu opioid receptors and analgesia at the site of a peripheral nerve injury. *Ann. Neurology* 2003;53(3):366-75.

[3]   Hassan A, Ableitner A, Stein C, Herz A. Inflammation of the rat paw enhanced axonal transport of opioid receptors in the sciatic nerve and increases their density in the inflamed tissue. *Neuroscience* 1993;55(1):185-95.

[4]   Stein C. The control of pain in peripheral tissue by opioids. *NEJM* 1995;332(25):1685-90.

[5]   Galvin J. An audit of pressure ulcer incidence in a palliative care setting. *Int. J. Palliat. Nurs.* 2002;8(5):214-21.

[6]   Twillman R, Long TD, Cathers TA, Mueller DW. Treatment of painful skin ulcers with topical opioids. *J. Pain Symptom Manage* 1999;17(4):288-92.

[7]   Gallagher RE, Arndt DR, Hunt KL. Analgesic effects of topical methadone - a report of four cases. *Clin. J. Pain* 2005;21(2):190-2.

[8]   Flock P, Gibbs L, Sykes N. Diamorphine-metronidazole gel effective for treatment of painful infected leg ulcers. *J. Pain Symptom Manage* 2000;20(6):396-7.

[9]   Krajnik M, Zylicz Z, Finlay I, Luczak J, Sorge AAv. Potential uses of topical opioids in palliative care - report of 6 cases. *Pain* 1999;80(1999).

[10] Ribeiro MDC, Joel SP, Zeppetella G. The bioavailability of morphine applied topically to cutaneous ulcers. *J. Pain Symptom Manage* 2004;27(5):434-9.

[11] Jepson BA. Relieving the pain of pressure sores. The Lancet 1992;339(8791):503-4.

[12] Back IN, Findlay I. Analgesic effect of topical opioids on painful skin ulcers. *J. Pain Symptom Manage* 1995;10(7):493.

[13] Flock P. Pilot study to determine the effectiveness of diamorphine gel to control pressure ulcer pain. *J. Pain Symptom Manage* 2003;25(6):547-54.

[14] Zeppetella G, Paul J, Ribeiro MDC. Analgesic efficacy of morphine applied topically to painful ulcers. *J. Pain Symptom Manage* 2003;25(6):555-8.

[15] Zeppetella G, Ribeiro MDC. Morphine in Intrasite gel applied topically to painful ulcers. *J. Pain Symptom Manage* 2005;29(2):118-9.

[16] Porzio G, Aielli F, Verna L, Cannita K, Marchetti P, Ficorella C. Topical morphine in the treatment of painful ulcers. *J. Pain Symptom Manage* 2005;30(4):304-5.

[17] Abbas SQ. Diamorphine-Intrasite dressings for painful pressure ulcers. *J. Pain Symptom Manage* 2004;28(6):532-4.

[18] Watterson G, Howard R, Goldman A. Peripheral opioids in inflammatory pain. *Arch. Dis. Child* 2004;89(7):679-81.

[19] Gairard-Dory AC, Schaller C, Mennecier B, et al. Chemoradiotherapy-induced esophagitis pain relieved by topical morphine: three cases. *J. Pain Symptom Manage* 2005;30(2):107-9.

[20] Cerchietti LCH, Navigante AH, Bonomi MR, et al. Effect of topical morphine for mucositis-associated pain following concomitant chemoradiotherapy for head and neck carcinoma. *Cancer* 2002;95(10):2230-6.

[21] Zeppetella G, Joel SP, Ribeiro MDC. Stability of morphine sulphate and diamorphine hydrochloride in Intrasite gel. *Palliative Medicine* 2005;19:131-6.

In: Pain Management: New Research
Editors: P. S. Greco, F. M. Conti

ISBN: 978-1-60456-767-0
© 2008 Nova Science Publishers, Inc.

Chapter VI

Chronic Right Iliac Fossa Pain in Children: A Therapeutic Role for Laparoscopy with Appendicectomy

Paul Charlesworth[1] and Anies Mahomed[2]
1. Royal Alexandra Hospital for Sick Children, Brighton
2. Royal Alexandra Hospital for Sick Children,
Brighton, BN2 5BE, UK

Introduction

Non-specific abdominal pain is the commonest diagnosis for children presenting with abdominal pain to hospital [1]. Chronic right iliac fossa (RIF) pain has been described in the adult population [2]. The most common population subset to complain of this condition is women of childbearing age. This can be related to gynaecological or appendiceal pathology [3,4].

In children right iliac fossa or right lower quadrant pain lasting longer than one month is a common complaint. In many cases the symptoms resolve spontaneously. However a population exists where no pathology is identified and symptoms persist. Psychological pathology, stress or anxiety can manifest itself as functional abdominal pain syndrome [5,6]. Children with functional abdominal pain are more likely to take time off school and to have parents of increased anxiety[7]. Where psychological cause is not thought likely, routine investigations to exclude common conditions are performed.

In the acute setting the diagnosis that needs to be excluded is appendicitis. Acute appendicitis is a clinical diagnosis. This is not always accurate, and many surgeons use laparoscopy where doubt exists. In a series of 1,320 patients investigatory laparoscopy changed the diagnosis in 30% of cases [8]. Chronic pain emanating from the pelvis or right iliac fossa is a vague symptom in which a definitive diagnosis remains elusive. There are multiple radiological and serological investigations at hand, although often these are inconclusive [9]. Macroscopic assessment of the appendix at diagnostic laparoscopy is reliable and in the acute setting gynaecologists have a false negative rate of 0% in removing an inflamed appendix [10]. This investigation has been used routinely in patients with chronic abdominal pain where other modalities have failed [11]. Chronic pain emanating from the appendix can be due to one of two reasons, firstly chronic appendicitis/ recurrent appendicitis [12] and secondly appendiceal colic [13].

There is evidence to support the hypothesis that chronic appendicitis/ appendicael colic improves in children following appendicectomy [14]. This chapter presents original scientific work followed by a literature review of chronic right iliac fossa pain in children to define the patient demographics, natural history of this condition and assess the value of laparoscopic appendicectomy in its treatment.

Methods

A prospective spreadsheet is used as a database for all patients undergoing laparoscopic surgery at The Royal Alexandra Hospital for Sick Children. Intra-operative details, histology and outpatient follow-up are recorded routinely. Details of patients undergoing laparoscopic appendicectomy for chronic abdominal pain were obtained from the database and complemented with a retrospective case-note review. Inclusion criteria were all patients who had symptoms lasting greater than 4-weeks who presented acutely or to outpatient clinic. The notes and database were studied for patient profile, symptom duration, number of preoperative clinic visits/ attendances to acute medical services for the same condition and investigations including routine blood markers, radiological investigations and endoscopy. Additional data analysed were intra and postoperative outcomes and histology.

A correlation between symptoms before and after surgery and positive finding at laparoscopy or histology were investigated. Positive histology included signs of acute or chronic inflammation, pus within the wall of the appendix, presence of a faecolith, excessive mucus, lymphoid aggregates and congested appendix. Data is presented as median and range.

A literature search was undertaken on Pubmed and Medline and critical references of previous published literature were scrutinised.

Results

Between October 2003 and October 2007, sixteen children underwent laparoscopic appendicectomy for chronic right iliac fossa pain. All but one patient were referred to the paediatric surgery out-patient clinic and were investigated for chronic RIF pain before a diagnostic laparoscopy and appendicectomy was performed. One patient presented with acute symptoms but on further detailed questioning had a history of chronic pain for 6 months. Data is summarised in Table 1.

Thirteen (81%) were female. The median age was 12 years 2 months, range 9 years 6 months to 14 years 4 months. No patients had undergone previous abdominal surgery.

The duration of pre-operative symptoms was 10 (1-30) months. The number of clinic visits or admissions before definitive diagnosis was 4 (0-11).

Table 1. Summary of Data

Patient	Age at operation	M/F	Symptom Duration	Operative findings	Histology	Resolution of symptoms	Follow-up
SM	12 yrs 2 months	F	22 months	Tubal cyst	2 small para-ovarian cysts	Yes	2 months
CG	11 yrs 11 months	F	7 months	Normal	Lymphoid hyperplasia	Yes	47 months
JD	9yrs 8 months	F	12 months	Normal	Lymphoid aggregates and congested vessels	Yes	46 months
LW	12 yrs 3 months	F	20 months	Normal	Faecolith within lumen	Yes	45 months
LK	14 yrs 4 months	F	24 months	Normal	Mucus within lumen	Yes	42 months
EB	11 years	F	9 months	Overlying band	Normal	Yes	34 months
LD	13 yrs 10 months	M	1 month	Normal	Faecal matter within wall	Chronic fatigue syndrome	31 months
BS	11 yrs 11 months	F	9 months	Normal	Fibrous obliteration, giant cell granuloma	Yes	11 months
LM	14 yrs 7 months	F	7 months	Adhesions	Normal	Mild pain for 5 months	15 months
RC	11 yrs 8 months	F	13 months	Lateral pelvic bands	Large faecolith, inflammatory cells	Yes	19 months
MG	9 yrs 6 months	F	30 months	Normal	Normal	Yes	18 months
BC	10 yrs 2 months	M	9 months	Lateral pelvic bands	Normal	Yes	1 months
SP	13 yrs 9 months	F	13 months	Long pelvic appendix	Normal	Yes	12 months
DC	14 years 6 months	F	10 months	Paraovarian cysts	fimbrial cysts and fallopian tube with congested vessels	Yes	8 months
LH	14 yrs 7 months	F	3 months	Adhesions between caecum and anterior abdominal wall	Pus in appendix wall	Yes	2 months
KT*	12 yrs 1 month	F	6 months	Normal	Chronic inflammation of appendix	Scar pain	3 months

* Presented acutely to accident and emergency

The fifteen patients that were referred through clinic had routine bloods including full blood count, urea and electrolytes, liver function and C-reactive protein, all of which were within the normal range.

All 15 had an abdominal ultrasound, four patients underwent barium studies, 2 patients had abdominal radiographs, 1 patient had upper and lower endoscopy and 1 patient had a white cell scan. All preoperative radiological and interventional investigations were reported as normal.

All sixteen patients underwent a standard laparoscopic appendicectomy with the use of endoloops to secure the appendix base. Operative time was 40 (30 – 90) minutes. The appendix was macroscopically normal in 14/16 (88%) patients. Four patients were noted to have adhesions at operation, 2 of which had lateral pelvic bands and one between the caecum and anterior abdominal wall (Figure 1). There were no appendix masses, free fluid was only present in the patient presenting acutely. There were no instances of intraoperative bleeding or serious complications. There was one minor visceral injury, which had no post-operative sequelae.

Postoperative analgesia consisted of simple non-steroidal analgesics and paracetamol, with only 2 patients requiring morphine. Median time to full feeds was 6 (4-48) hours. Postoperative stay ranged from same day discharge to 2 days. Six patients underwent day-stay procedure, 7 patients stayed for one day and 2 patents stayed for 2 days. One of the patients that stayed for two days was the patient who was admitted acutely.

One patient experienced pain immediately postoperatively and was treated accordingly. There were no episodes of wound sepsis, or dehiscence.

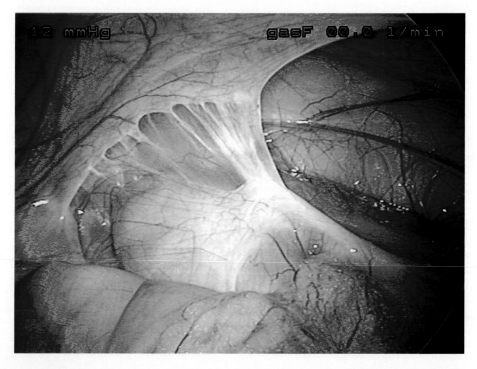

Figure 1. Adhesive bands between caecum and lateral abdominal wall in child presenting with chronic right iliac fossa pain.

There was immediate improvement in 14/16 patients, which is a correlation of 88% between procedure and symptom free post operatively. Median follow-up was 19 (1-47) months. One patient developed chronic fatigue syndrome secondary to a viral infection. This lasted for two years but he is currently well and discharged from medical follow-up. One patient experienced mild recurrent abdominal pain and nausea for five months post surgery, on last clinic appointment she was pain free at 15 months. The patient who presented acutely had two episodes of scar pain, which had resolved on recent follow-up of three months. Ultimately all patients got better.

Histology of the appendix was normal in seven patients. Of these seven patients; two had paraovarian cysts which were excised, two had macroscopic lymphoid hyperplasia noted at surgery, two were noted to have overlying bands which were divided and one had a faecolith removed at the time of surgery. The remaining nine had positive histology. The correlation between initial symptoms and positive finding on histology or at laparoscopy with ultimate clinical resolution was 100%.

Discussion

Chronic RIF, right lower quadrant or pelvic pain in the paediatric population is a common clinical entity. Despite this there have been few clinical series published. The current literature is summarised in Table 2. Gorenstein et al prospectively analysed 1,125 children presenting with abdominal pain, of these, 26 chlidren presented with recurrent right lower quadrant pain termed 'appendiceal colic'. These children underwent elective open appendicectomy[14]. The senior author has published a series of 16 children demonstrating the benefit of removal of the appendix at diagnostic laparoscopy in children with chronic RIF pain[15]. The message was repeated by Stringel et al although with a much higher complication rate[11]. Sylianos et al concluded that laparoscopy was an accurate technique for evaluation and treatment of children with recurrent abdominal pain[9]. Kolts et al described 44 children with chronic right lower abdominal pain who underwent laparoscopic exploration and appendicectomy. They demonstrated a resolution of symptoms in 70% of patients[16]. The largest series was by Stevenson. Fifty-two consecutive children undergoing open appendicectomy for appendicael colic were followed up for a mean of 4 years. There was a 98% resolution of symptoms[13].

In the paediatric population patients are mainly female. In the series presented in this text 14/16 (81%) were female - in our previous published series this was 9/11 (82%)[15]. This compares to a range between 53.8% and 87% in the literature. The age of patients varies between 10 and 17 years and symptoms persist for a period of between 2 and 12 months before laparoscopy is performed[13,14,16,9,11.]

There was an 88% instant resolution of symptoms in this series compared with 72% in our previous series. In the paediatric population the correlation between laparoscopic appendicectomy and resolution of symptoms ranges between 70% and 98%[13,14,16,9]. Kolts et al were able to demonstrate a higher statistical difference of resolution of symptoms in those who were not attending psychiatric clinic and those with positive histology [16].

Table 2. Paediatric Series of Chronic RIF pain

Author	Patients	Age Years	% Female	Symptom Duration (months)	Positive operative findings	Resolution of symptoms	Positive Histology	Follow-up
Kolts (2006)	44	13.3	61.4%	1.8	45.5%	56.8% - full 13.6% - partial	72.7%	2 years
Panchalingam (2005)	11	11.9	82%	12.1	0%	72%	82%	1 yr 4 mo
Stringel (1999)	13	13	53.8%	2	92.3%	76.9%	54%	6m – 3 yrs
Stevenson (1999)	50	12.3	75%	30	86% **	98%	86%**	4yrs 4mo
Stylianos (1996)	15	12	87%	11	73%	73%		
Gorenstein (1996)`	26	11.4	57.7%	12	92%	88.5%	30.8%	3 yrs 2 mo

** 14% patients deemed to have normal macroscopic and microscopic findings by surgeon and histologist respectively.

This finding is echoed in our original series with the patients with negative histology and intraoperative findings undergoing psychiatric evaluation [15], and other publications where those with positive histology were more likely to have an improved outcome [9].

The positive findings from radiological investigations remains low, and has been calculated at 5%[9], in this population. It is an important negative finding, occasionally diagnosing ovarian pathology [14]. The use of barium studies to diagnose appendiceal colic has also been employed although it's diagnostic accuracy is doubtful [14].

Our hypothesis is that chronic pain following inconclusive routine investigation warrants a diagnostic laparoscopy, and removal of the appendix, even if it is macroscopically normal. There is evidence to support incidental histological changes of the appendix in the background population. In a necropsy study, 22% of babies and newborns who died of unrelated causes showed signs of 'subacute appendicits'[17]. In both of our series and the paediatric literature the macroscopic appearance of the appendix is normal. In our series we had a positive correlation of histology in nine patients (56%). This included presence of pus within the appendix wall (figure 2), inflammatory cells, presence of granulomas, presence of a faecolith and lymphoid aggregates. Those patients without definitive histology all had alternate findings at laparotomy. In our earlier series 82% had positive histology.

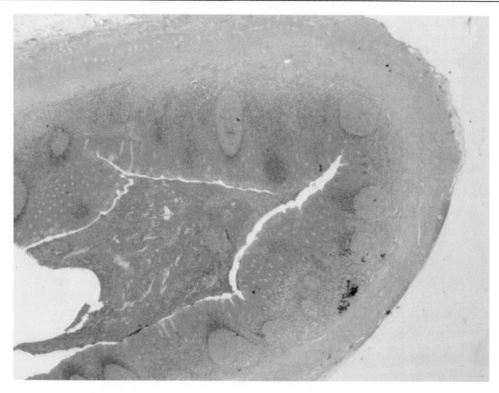

Figure 2. Pus in the lumen noted on histology in an otherwise macroscopically normal appearing appendix.

Positive histology in the literature ranges between 69.2% to 72% of patients [14,16] with similar histological findings to our series, that of chronic inflammatory changes or lymphoid hyperplasia.

Positive findings other than the appendix in our series were due to para-ovarian cysts in two patients, adhesional bands in two patients, the remaining three were noted to have appendix related macroscopic findings; lymphoid hyperplasia and a faecolith in one. In our previous series one patient had *Enterobius vermicularis* parasites and one patient had normal histology with unresolved symptoms at follow-up [15]. Macroscopic lymphadenopathy in the mesoappendix is a common finding in the paediatric literature and might well be related to chronic changes within the appendix. Stylianos et al reported three Meckel's diverticula, one inguinal hernia one urachal cyst and one parafallopian tube cyst in a series of 15 patients [9]. In a series of thirteen patients; Stringel reported inflammatory bowel disease in two, fallopian tube cysts in two, torsion of an ovarian cyst in one and salpingitis in one [11]. Gorenstein noted paraovairian cysts on ultrasound scan in three patients prior to appendiciectomy but doesn't note whether these were treated or whether symptoms persisted in these patients. Operative findings other than appendicael showed one ovarian cyst, one fimbrial cyst and one case of ileoileal intusssusception. One patient in this series was subsequently diagnosed with celiac disease [14]. In Kolts' series of 44 patients, six had Meckel's diverticulum, four had adhesions involving the caecum and two had hernias and one had an ovarian cyst. Histological differences in this series included on case of a carcinoid tumour and one case of Crohn's disease [16].

There are three distinct subset of patients that experience chronic right iliac fossa pain. The first is the paediatric population as presented. The second is adult patients and the third young women of child bearing age. Therapeutic laparoscopy has been employed in all groups with varying success.

In the acute setting there is a negative appendicectomy rate of 22% for laparoscopic and 15% for open procedure [10]. The question in the adult literature remains, whether a 'normal' appendix should be left at laparoscopy for acute appendicits [10,18,19]. Traditionally the appendix was always removed following a Grid-Iron incision to avoid diagnostic confusion in the future. Macroscopic assessment at laparoscopy has a false negative of 3% in a largely paediatric population according to a large meta analysis [10]. Laparoscopic appendicectomy has improved outcomes with increasing experience [20] and should be performed where diagnostic doubt arises. If a diagnostic laparoscopy is undertaken in the acute setting, it has been shown that patients benefit from removal of a 'normal' looking appendix with no increased morbidity or mortality [21]. However laparoscopic appendicectomy is not without risk and in some series has a reported 6.5% conversion and 4.7% complication rate [10].

The most common pathology seen at diagnostic laparoscopy for adults with chronic abdominal pain is adhesions. Symptomatic relief following laparoscopic division of adhesions varies between 71% and 90% [22,23,24,25,26,27], although one series reports it as low as 45% [28]. Morbidity is significantly related to age and symptom duration[29]. There is a mortality of 1% [30]. In a study of 41 patients undergoing diagnostic laparoscopy for chronic RIF pain symptom relief was significantly better in younger patients (median age 17 years) versus older patients (median age 30 years). They concluded that diagnostic laparoscopy and appendicectomy was a worthwhile procedure for adult patients [31].

In one centre diagnostic laparoscopy for chronic RIF pain made up 5% of all laparoscopic procedures. The most likely pathology was adhesions (56%) followed by hernias (19%) and appendiceal pathology (16%). At long term follow-up 71% of patients experienced pain relief. Of those patients specifically undergoing appendicectomy 81% experienced pain relief if histology was positive versus 57% with negative histology at a follow-up of 2 ½ years [23]. Fogli et el performed a laparoscopic appendicectomy on 131 patients, of which 97 had recurrent or acute non-specific abdominal pain. All 97 patients had appearances of chronic appendicitis. However follow-up is not stated [32]. A group in Slough in the United Kingdom has had limited experience at performing diagnostic laparoscopy under local anaesthetic and sedation in an attempt to map pain to the appropriate source. Accuracy and follow-up had not been established [33]. Rare causes for chronic RIF pain in adults includes ingestion of foreign bodies [34] chronic appendicitis causing intussusception [35] and digestive tract schwannoma [36]

In a study of women admitted with non-specific abdominal pain randomly assigned to laparoscopic assessment versus observation. The group assigned to laparoscopy had a higher rate of diagnosis 79% versus 45%, a shorter hospital stay and lower recurrence rate [37]. In a Croatian study of fertile women presenting with chronic RIF pain diagnostic laparoscopy demonstrated the appendix to be macroscopically abnormal in 51%. Removal of the appendix was performed in 77% of all women. The authors concluded laparoscopic appendicectomy to be of use in this population relieving symptoms and/or excluding the diagnosis of appendiceal pathology [3]. In a series of fifty five laparoscopic appendicectomies performed for chronic right lower quadrant pain 53 patients had symptom relief [38]. There is an 80% success rate in laparoscopic surgery for chronic pelvic pain in women, and an appendicectomy should be performed if right lower quadrant pain is part of the pain profile [4].

The evidence is conclusive for women investigated for chronic pelvic pain. In one study of 317 women, 269 had chronic pelvic pain. Laparoscopic appendicectomy was performed in 102 women, 93 of whom had symptomatic relief. Histology varied between endometriosis of the appendix tip (3.78%), obliteration of the appendix lumen (24.6%) and adhesions (6.93%). The authors concluded that the appendix is the key organ in management of chronic pelvic pain [39]. For cosmetic and improved diagnostic ability Laparoscopic appendicectomy is the preferred method of appendicectomy in young women [32,40].

Within the three distinct populations there is a clear role for diagnostic laparoscopy:

The paediatric population are predominantly girls of early teens. The senior author recommends that a diagnostic laparoscopy be performed for children presenting with right iliac fossa pain lasting longer than four weeks, where routine bloods and abdominal ultrasound scan have failed to produce a diagnosis. There is clear evidence to support a laparoscopic appendicectomy in all children, even if the appendix appears macroscopically normal. Following diagnostic laparoscopy and appendicectomy, between 70% and 98% of this population can expect symptomatic improvement in the short term with the figure rising to 100% over the longer term.

In fertile women, a diagnostic laparoscopy with proceed to treat, has an equally high symptom resolution, although the pathology is more variable.

In adults of varying ages that do not fit into the paediatric or fertile female population, adhesions are the most common pathology seen. If the patient is fit for surgery a diagnostic laparoscopy plus adhesionalysis should be performed.

The evidence from this text is that in all patients presenting with chronic pelvic or right iliac fossa pain a diagnostic laparoscopy should be performed, particularly when routine investigations prove inconclusive. If no other pathology is identified the appendix should be removed.

References

[1]   Driver CP, Youngson GG: Acute abdominal pain in children: a 25 year comparison. *Health Bull.* (Edinb) 53:167-172, 1995

[2]   Mattei P, Sola JE, Yeo CJ: Chronic and recurrent appendicitis are uncommon entities often misdiagnosed. *J. Am. Coll. Surg.* 178:385-389, 1994

[3]   Popovic D, Kovjanic J, Milostic D, et al: Long-term benefits of laparoscopic appendectomy for chronic abdominal pain in fertile women. *Croat. Med. J.* 45:171-175, 2004

[4]   Carter JE: Surgical treatment for chronic pelvic pain. *JSLS* 2:129-139, 1998

[5]   Clouse RE, Mayer EA, Aziz Q, et al: Functional abdominal pain syndrome. *Gastroenterology* 130:1492-1497, 2006

[6]   Ghanizadeh A, Moaiedy F, Imanieh MH, et al: Psychiatric disorders and family functioning in children and adolescents with functional abdominal pain syndrome. *J. Gastroenterol. Hepatol.* 2007

[7]   Ramchandani PG, Fazel M, Stein A, et al: The impact of recurrent abdominal pain: predictors of outcome in a large population cohort. *Acta Paediatr.* 96:697-701, 2007

[8]   Golash V, Willson PD: Early laparoscopy as a routine procedure in the management of acute abdominal pain: a review of 1,320 patients. *Surg. Endosc.* 19:882-885, 2005

[9]   Stylianos S, Stein JE, Flanigan LM, et al: Laparoscopy for diagnosis and treatment of recurrent abdominal pain in children. *J. Pediatr. Surg.* 31:1158-1160, 1996

[10] Kraemer M, Ohmann C, Leppert R, et al: Macroscopic assessment of the appendix at diagnostic laparoscopy is reliable. *Surg. Endosc.* 14:625-633, 2000

[11] Stringel G, Berezin SH, Bostwick HE, et al: Laparoscopy in the management of children with chronic recurrent abdominal pain. *JSLS* 3:215-219, 1999

[12] Chang SK, Chan P: Recurrent appendicitis as a cause of recurrent right iliac fossa pain. *Singapore. Med. J.* 45:6-8, 2004

[13] Stevenson RJ: Chronic right-lower-quadrant abdominal pain: is there a role for elective appendectomy? *J. Pediatr. Surg.* 34:950-954, 1999

[14] Gorenstin A, Serour F, Katz R, et al: Appendiceal colic in children: a true clinical entity? *J. Am. Coll. Surg.* 182:246-250, 1996

[15] Panchalingam L, Driver C, Mahomed AA: Elective laparoscopic appendicectomy for chronic right iliac fossa pain in children. *J. Laparoendosc. Adv. Surg. Tech.* A 15:186-189, 2005

[16] Kolts RL, Nelson RS, Park R, et al: Exploratory laparoscopy for recurrent right lower quadrant pain in a pediatric population. *Pediatr. Surg. Int* .22:247-249, 2006

[17] Schickedanz H, Giggel S: Appendicitis-eine Analyse nach 4000 *Appendektomien. kinderarzt.* 21:693-697, 1990

[18] Teh SH, O'Ceallaigh S, Mckeon JG, et al: Should an appendix that looks 'normal' be removed at diagnostic laparoscopy for acute right iliac fossa pain? *Eur. J. Surg.* 166:388-389, 2000

[19] Navez B, Therasse A: Should every patient undergoing laparoscopy for clinical diagnosis of appendicitis have an appendicectomy? *Acta Chir. Belg.* 103:87-89, 2003

[20] Bennett J, Boddy A, Rhodes M: Choice of approach for appendicectomy: a meta-analysis of open versus laparoscopic appendicectomy. *Surg. Laparosc. Endosc. Percutan Tech.* 17:245-255, 2007

[21] Greason KL, Rappold JF, Liberman MA: Incidental laparoscopic appendectomy for acute right lower quadrant abdominal pain. Its time has come. *Surg. Endosc.* 12:223-225, 1998

[22] Lavonius M, Gullichsen R, Laine S, et al: Laparoscopy for chronic abdominal pain. *Surg. Laparosc. Endosc.* 9:42-44, 1999

[23] Onders RP, Mittendorf EA: Utility of laparoscopy in chronic abdominal pain. *Surgery* 134:549-552, 2003

[24] Fayez JA, Clark RR: Operative laparoscopy for the treatment of localized chronic pelvic-abdominal pain caused by postoperative adhesions. *J. Gynecol. Surg* .10:79-83, 1994

[25] Swank DJ, Van Erp WF, Repelaer Van Driel OJ, et al: Complications and feasibility of laparoscopic adhesiolysis in patients with chronic abdominal pain. A retrospective study. *Surg. Endosc.* 16:1468-1473, 2002

[26] Swank DJ, Van Erp WF, Repelaer Van Driel OJ, et al: A prospective analysis of predictive factors on the results of laparoscopic adhesiolysis in patients with chronic abdominal pain. *Surg. Laparosc. Endosc. Percutan Tech.* 13:88-94, 2003

[27] Paajanen H, Julkunen K, Waris H: Laparoscopy in chronic abdominal pain: a prospective nonrandomized long-term follow-up study. *J. Clin. Gastroenterol.* 39:110-114, 2005

[28] Dunker MS, Bemelman WA, Vijn A, et al: Long-term outcomes and quality of life after laparoscopic adhesiolysis for chronic abdominal pain. *J. Am. Assoc. Gynecol. Laparosc.* 11:36-41, 2004

[29] Swank DJ, Van Erp WF, Repelaer Van Driel OJ, et al: Complications and feasibility of laparoscopic adhesiolysis in patients with chronic abdominal pain. A retrospective study. *Surg. Endosc* .16:1468-1473, 2002

[30] Swank DJ, Van Erp WF, Repelaer Van Driel OJ, et al: A prospective analysis of predictive factors on the results of laparoscopic adhesiolysis in patients with chronic abdominal pain. *Surg. Laparosc. Endosc. Percutan. Tech.* 13:88-94, 2003

[31] Chao K, Farrell S, Kerdemelidis P, et al: Diagnostic laparoscopy for chronic right iliac fossa pain: a pilot study. *Aust .N Z J. Surg.* 67:789-791, 1997

[32] Fogli L, Brulatti M, Boschi S, et al: Laparoscopic appendectomy for acute and recurrent appendicitis: retrospective analysis of a single-group 5-year experience. *J. Laparoendosc. Adv. Surg. Tech.* A 12:107-110, 2002

[33] Tytherleigh MG, Fell R, Gordon A: Diagnostic conscious pain mapping using laparoscopy under local anaesthetic and sedation in general surgical patients. *Surgeon* 2:157-160, 2004

[34] Hadi HI, Quah HM, Maw A: A missing tongue stud: an unusual appendicular foreign body. *Int. Surg.* 91:87-89, 2006

[35] Nyam DC, Davendran K, Seow-Choen F: An endoscopic diagnosis of appendicular intussusception in chronic appendicitis. *Singapore Med. J.* 38:131- 1997

[36] Khan AA, Schizas AM, Cresswell AB, et al: Digestive tract schwannoma. *Dig. Surg.* 23:265-269, 2006

[37] Morino M, Pellegrino L, Castagna E, et al: Acute nonspecific abdominal pain: A randomized, controlled trial comparing early laparoscopy versus clinical observation. *Ann. Surg.* 244:881-886, 2006

[38] Bryson K: Laparoscopic appendectomy. *J. Gynecol. Surg* .7:93-95, 1991

[39] Agarwala N, Liu CY: Laparoscopic appendectomy. *J. Am. Assoc. Gynecol. Laparosc.* 10:166-168, 2003

[40] Nana AM, Ouandji CN, Simoens C, et al: Laparoscopic appendectomies: results of a monocentric prospective and non-randomized study. *Hepatogastroenterology* 54:1146-1152, 2007

In: Pain Management: New Research
Editors: P. S. Greco, F. M. Conti

ISBN: 978-1-60456-767-0
© 2008 Nova Science Publishers, Inc.

Chapter VII

Current Trends in Pain Management in Paediatric Laparoscopic Surgery

Nathaniel Barber[1] and Anies Mahomed[2]
[1] Senior House Officer Paediatric Surgery,
Royal Alexandra Children's Hospital, Brighton, BN2 5BE, UK
[2] Consultant Paediatric and Minimally Invasive Surgeon,
Royal Alexandra Children's Hospital, Brighton, BN2 5BE, UK

Abstract

One of the major attractions of laparoscopic surgery in children is the reduced pain experience. However minimally invasive surgery is not painless and a significant number of patients suffer discomfort in the first few hours following intervention. This chapter highlights the multifactorial nature of the pain and summarises the current management options available to children.

Introduction

The feasibility of laparoscopic surgery was first demonstrated in children in 1971 by Gans and Berci[1]. Since that time there has been an exponential increase in its use in the paediatric population.

One of the most frequently cited benefits of laparoscopic surgery, and part of the reasoning for its increasing use is decreased postoperative pain. Other accepted advantages of laparoscopic surgery which may relate to the pain experience include improved visualisation of the operative field, decreased stress response to surgery and shorter recovery times[2]. Other potential reasons for decreased pain include smaller skin incisions and decreased manipulation of abdominal organs.

Attempts to reduce pain following laparoscopic surgery have resulted in a range of approaches further improving the pain experience for infants and children undergoing this form of intervention.

Uses of Laparoscopic Surgery in Children

Applications for laparoscopy have developed throughout paediatric surgery. In general paediatric surgery, common applications include its use for appendicectomy fundoplication and splenectomy. Additionally, the benefits of diagnostic laparoscopy compared to open surgery in establishing the cause of abdominal and pelvic pathology is now well established. In this context it has proved invaluable for a range of pathology including intussusception, Meckels diverticulum and malrotation[3].

Minimally invasive techniques are increasingly being employed for both diagnostic and therapeutic indications in the thorax. Lobectomy for congenital lung lesions, repair of oesophageal atresia and pleural lysis are now routinely offered in some paediatric surgical units[4].

In paediatric gynaecology applications include diagnosis and treatment of pelvic inflammatory disease and of addenexal pathology such as ovarian torsion and ovarian cyst.[5,6] In paediatric urology laparoscopic techniques have become progressively more widespread covering an increasing number of procedures[7]. These include; diagnosis and management of cryptorchidism, nephrectomy for both benign and malignant disease, ureteric reimplantation and for pyeloplasty. Laparoscopic surgery has been proposed as the optimal technique in right adrenalectomy[8].

Laparoscopic surgery in paediatric trauma has been promoted as a safe approach for diagnosis and treatment where patients are haemodynamically stable[9]. The principal benefit being reduced morbidity where there is a negative laparoscopy. In paediatric cancer surgery minimally invasive surgery has been found to be a safe diagnostic approach[10].

Whilst the use of paediatric laparoscopic surgery has been embraced enthusiastically, it is important to note that its use is not universally recognised as the optimal approach for every procedure[11].

Principles of Pain Experience
in Laparoscopic Surgery

Pain is defined by the International Association for the Study of Pain [12] as "an unpleasant sensory and emotional experience associated with actual or potential tissue damage or described in terms of such damage" Historically the importance of analgesia across paediatric surgery had been overlooked. However over the past 30 years, pain control has become increasingly recognised as being an integral part of good management in paediatric surgery. Acceptance of the need to pre-empt and adequately treat pain in the paediatric population comes not only from an ethical and humanitarian understanding [13] but also because of potential physiological and developmental consequences.

Pain occurs when a noxious stimulus (mechanical, thermal or chemical) causes tissue injury resulting in release of local neurotransmitters (bradykinin, substance P, histamine, prostaglandins, and leukotriene). The stimulus is then transmitted by one of two kinds of nerve fibres. Fast, myelinated A-delta fibres transmit sharp well localised acute pain sensation while unmyelinated slow conducting C fibres carry dull visceral pain sensation Impulses are then transmitted by the spinothalamic tracts to the thalamus where pain perception occurs. Modification of impulses is mediated by neurotransmitters which may attenuate or amplify signals. Different pharmacological interventions work at different levels within this system allowing multiple approaches to treating pain.

Physiology of Laparoscopic Surgery

Several physiological measures for reducing post-operative pain in laparoscopic surgery have been identified. The physiology of laparoscopic surgery presents both unique problems in terms of pain as well as unique solutions to surgery related pain.

Pneumoperitoneum

Essential to all laparoscopic surgery is the creation of the pneumoperitoneum; where gas is insufflated into the abdominal cavity allowing visualisation of the abdominal organs.

Generalised abdominal and referred shoulder tip pain resulting from the creation of the pneumoperitoneum is one of the major disadvantages of laparoscopic surgery.

Measures established to reduce the painful effects of the pneumoperitoneum include using heated gas, use of low pressure gas, use of nitrous oxide pneumoperitoneum as opposed to carbon dioxide, insertion of a gas drain and the use of intraperitoneal saline[14].

Ensuring that the abdomen is sufficiently deflated after surgery is one mechanism which has been identified to minimise post operative pain. Bisgarrd[15] et al studied pain after laparoscopic cholecystectomy. The study found that early pain after surgery could be reduced by minimising the residual pneumoperitoneum.

The mechanism by which the pneumoperitoneum causes pain is unclear. It may be that it is the result of trauma and phrenic nerve neuropraxia caused by air insufflation. Evidence from biopsies taken after laparoscopy shows peritoneal inflammation and capillary and nerve damage[16]. Another potential cause for post laparoscopic abdominal pain is a localized peritoneal acidosis. This has been demonstrated in a number of studies and may be a result of localised ischaemia[17].

Skin Incisions

Laparoscopic surgery allows significantly smaller skin incisions. As experience of laparoscopic surgery has increased modifications to surgical technique have allowed for smaller ports thus smaller incisions and fewer port sites. In a study of laparoscopic cholecystectomy in adults Gupta et al [18] found reducing the number of port-sites used was technically viable and significantly reduced pain and analgesic requirements. Port sites may account for the most severe pain after laparoscopic surgery[19] although this has not been a consistent finding. The site of placement of port sites has also been suggested as contributing to pain experienced after laparoscopic surgery[20].

Decreased Manipulation

The decreased manipulation of abdominal organs that occurs during laparoscopic surgery compared to open surgery may result in decreased surgical complications and therefore less pain. Studies relating to the implications of decreased manipulation have focused on the impact of manipulation on bowel obstruction. Tsao et al [21] studied adhesive small bowel obstruction after open and laparoscopic appendicectomy in children. This study suggested that small bowel obstruction was statistically less common after laparoscopic surgery. However the study also noted that the risk of small bowel obstruction is low in children and related to perforated appendicitis. Similar studies in adults have also found a decreased incidence of adhesion ileus after laparoscopic colorectal surgery[22].

Duepree et al [23] found both decreased bowel obstruction and ventral hernia after laparoscopic bowel resection compared to laparotomy.

A correlation between decreased intra-abdominal manipulation and therefore pain was also found in Garcia-Caballero and Vara-Thorbeck's [24] study of post-operative ileus after laparoscopic cholecystectomy in adults.

In adults it has been suggested that use of laparoscopic extra peritoneal repair of inguinal hernias is advantageous in that there is decreased manipulation of intra-abdominal organs with resultant decreased complications [25].

Studies of Pain and Laparoscopic Surgery

The majority of studies of pain and laparoscopic surgery in children have focussed on more commonly undertaken laparoscopic procedures in this group such as laparoscopic appendicectomy and fundoplication. Studies show both reduced pain after laparoscopic surgery and a resulting decrease in hospital stay.

Lintula et al's [26] study of children undergoing laparoscopic and open appendicectomy found better pain control with less need for 'rescue' analgesia after laparoscopic appendicectomy. The study also found a shorter hospital stay in patients undergoing laparoscopic surgery. This decreased length of stay may also be attributed to less need for strong, opiate analgesics.

Schmelzer et al [27] also found decreased duration of post-operative analgesia after laparoscopic appendicectomy. Laparoscopic appendicectomy was found in this study to be associated with fewer wound infections and intra-abdominal abscesses (not statistically significant). This decreased rate of complications could potentially decrease the pain experienced after surgery.

Less pain and faster recovery after laparoscopic appendicectomy in children was also reported by Canty [28] et al who found laparoscopic surgery to be equally safe and effective, even in perforated appendicitis.

Rowney et al report minimal analgesic requirements in children undergoing laparoscopic fundoplication. In this series there was no analgesic requirement after 48 hours in 95 percent of children. This represented a marked contrast to the author's experience of open fundoplication in children [29].

In adults same-day discharge after laparoscopic fundoplication has been found to be possible in selected patients with a close focus on analgesia and nausea.

Dick et al [30] also studied analgesic requirements following laparoscopic and open fundoplication in children. They found that the total amount of opiate analgesia required was similar for both open and laparoscopic surgery. However, the duration for which opiate analgesia was required was significantly shorter in the laparoscopic surgery group. A higher dose of opiate was needed over a shorter duration of time. It is unclear how this relates to overall pain as similar amounts of NSAIDs were used in both groups.

Studies of laparoscopic nephrectomy in children and adults have shown decreased use of opiate analgesia and associated shorter hospital stay [31,32]. Similarly, laparoscopic varicocelectomy has been shown to result in decreased anaesthetic requirement and decreased post operative length of stay [33].

Laparoscopic surgery may not be the best approach for minimising analgesic requirement in every circumstance. For example, laparoscopic pyloromyotomy was found to take longer and require equal amounts of analgesia to open pyloromyotomy[34]. Rudkin et al [35] report a higher analgesic requirement for laparoscopic inguinal hernia repair than open repair. Similarly, Beanes et al [36] found no advantage of laparoscopic splenectomy over open splenectomy in children. The authors found no benefit in postoperative pain, operative time, hospital stay and postoperative ileus.

Specific Pain Management

Multimodal Analgesia

A multimodal approach to analgesia describes the use of multiple (principally pharmacological) approaches to reduce and ideally eliminate pain. The approaches used in paediatric surgery include pre-operative sedation, regional anaesthesia and the use of paracetamol, non-steroidal anti-inflammatory and opioid analgesics as well as behavioural approaches.

Pre-operative Sedation

Preparing children for surgery involves a range of strategies from comfort and reassurance (of both child and parent) to the use of pharmacological approaches to reduce anxiety.

The appropriate approach in each case depends on the individual child and their circumstances. Benefits of using sedative pre-medication include increased cooperation with anaesthetic induction and improved parental satisfaction.

Benzodiazepines are the most frequently used anxiolytic used in sedating children undergoing procedures. The most often used benzodiazepines are midazolam and diazepam. Oral midazolam is regarded as having several benefits including rapid onset and minimal sedative effects [37].

Ketamine is another analgesic frequently used as a pre operative sedative in children.

Ketamine is an anaesthetic with both central and peripheral effects. It acts as a non competitive inhibitor at the N-methyl-D-aspartate (NDMA) receptor. Blocking this channel appears to be its principal mode of action although it also binds to μ opiate receptors. Ketamine may be used either on its own or with midazolam, with which it has a synergistic effect. Use of ketamine has been advocated in children who are particularly challenging to sedate for example older children/teenagers with developmental delay or urgent situations where delay to induction would be detrimental [38].

One benefit of Ketamine is its potential to be used intramuscularly in such situations.

Disadvantages of using ketamine include potentially prolonged sedation.

In many cases the use of pre-operative sedation is unnecessary.

Caudal Analgesia

Caudal anaesthesia and analgesia is achieved by inserting a needle through the sacrococcygeal membrane and instilling a local anaesthetic solution.

Caudal epidural block after laparoscopy in herniorraphy in children was found to have better pain outcomes by Tobias et al [39] with 82% of children not requiring any additional post operative analgesia. Conversely Borkar [40] et al found that combining rectal diclofenac with local anaesthetic infiltration resulted in analgesia comparable to caudal block in children undergoing diagnostic and therapeutic laparoscopy. They propose this is a significantly less traumatic approach than caudal anaesthesia with comparable results.

Side effects of epidural analgesia include: itching, nausea, sedation and hypoventilation, bowel dysfunction and urinary retention. Developments in caudal analgesia include the use of ketamine or Clonidine (a selective alpha-2 receptor antagonist with sedative effects) to prolong caudal block and the use of ultrasound imaging to aid in the positioning of the caudal needle [41].

Paracetamol

Non-opioid analgesics provide a first-line in the treatment of mild to moderate post operative pain because of their lack of side-effects compared to opiate analgesics (e.g. nausea and vomiting, respiratory depression, bowel dysfunction) [42,43].

Paracetamol is a centrally acting analgesic which reduces spinally released prostaglandin E2. Benefits of paracetamol over non steroidal anti-inflammatory drugs are derived from it not inhibiting peripheral cyclo-oxygenase therefore not increasing bleeding or causing renal toxicity. Its main disadvantage is its potential to cause potentially fatal hepatic damage in overdose.

Using rectal paracetamol at induction of anaesthesia in paediatric day-case surgery has been shown to significantly reduce post-operative need for opiate analgesia in children as well as decreasing post-operative nausea.

There is some evidence to suggest that the dose of paracetamol may need to be higher after major surgery in children because of erratic absorption [42].

Non Steroidal Anti Inflammatory Drugs

Non steroidal anti inflammatory drugs inhibit cyclo-oxygenase-2 resulting in drecreased prostaglandin production. This results in decreased sensitisation of nociceptive nerve endings to inflammatory mediators.

The use of non-steroidal anti-inflammatory drugs in children for acute post operative pain is widespread, although there is limited data concerning laparoscopic surgery. A study of PCA pain control following appendicectomy in children aged 5-13 found that diclofenac significantly reduced morphine requirement compared to paracetamol [43].

Intramuscular diclofenac has been shown to reduce post laparoscopic surgery morphine requirements in adults. Wilson et al [44] found that intermittent IM diclofenac in adults following laparoscopic cholecystectomy reduced postoperative morphine requirements by as much as 25%, significantly reducing post operative pain. Rectal diclofenac has been suggested as a more appropriate alternative in a paediatric population [43].

Local Anaesthesia

Intra-peritoneal local anaesthetic instillation is one method noted to significantly reduce post-operative pain following laparoscopic surgery in adults.

Zullo et al [45] found intra-pertioneal sub diaphragmatic instillation of lidocaine and bupivicaine resulted in significant decrease in postoperative pain for approximately six hours.

Barczynski et al [46] found that more effective pain relief was achieved if a peritoneal instillation of bupivicaine was used before the creation of pneumoperitoneum. This study found that instillation of local analgesic after creation of pneumoperitoneum was also useful but significantly less beneficial than pre-emptive instillation.

Instillation of local anaesthetic superficially into the abdominal wound may also help reduce post operative pain [47,48]. Research in adults suggests no benefit in pre-emptive injection compared to postoperative injection of local anaesthetic.

Intra-Peritoneal Saline Instillation

Studies in adults report significantly decreased post operative pain with instillation of saline into the peritoneum, with or without local anaesthetic and left in or aspirated from the abdomen. The mechanism of this effect may be the dilution of peritoneal acidosis [49].

Opioid Analgesia

Morphine like analgesics work on opiate receptors, analgesia is predominately mediated by μ receptors, which are also responsible for major unwanted effects such as sedation and respiratory depression.

Most frequently opioid analgesics are used as part of nurse controlled analgesia in children, although they are also used in patient controlled analgesia

Patient Controlled Analgesia

Patient controlled analgesia (PCA) may be an appropriate method of post-operative analgesia in some children. Till et al studied PCA in children following laparoscopic and open appendicectomy [50]. The authors found PCA to be safe, effective with few complications. Interestingly, a lower total dose of opiate was required in the laparoscopic group. Advantages of PCA cited include acting as an alternative route to oral and intramuscular analgesia and enabling the patient increased control over their own postoperative care. PCA has also been found to be associated with greater patient satisfaction.

Specific disadvantages of PCA use in a paediatric population include age appropriateness and understanding as well as potentially increased nursing input.

Till et al [50] found that children from school age were able to use the PCA device appropriately.

Preventing unwanted effects of opiate analgesia is an important consideration in their use. Bolus use of anti-emetics at induction is one means of reducing these effects as is the use of other analgesics to reduce the total dose needed. Interestingly, in studies of adults, the use of Ketamine has been shown to reduced post operative nausea and vomiting [38].

Other approaches

Stergiopoulou et al [51] reported decreased less post operative pain in adult patients undergoing laparoscopic cholecystectomy who had been provided with additional pre-operative education on the procedure. Patients who were provided with a multimedia CD consisting of photos, animation and narration explaining the diagnosis, surgery and providing information on the post-operative period showed less post operative pain than patients receiving conventional preoperative counselling, however, there was no significant difference compared to groups receiving other forms of additional counselling.

Benefits of Reduced Pain

Laparoscopic surgery is associated with a less pronounced inflammatory response. The clinical implications of this reduced response are unclear possible implications are reduced pain and fatigue after surgery.

Shorter separation from home environment – separation from parents is a major concern for children in hospital. For patients to go home there must be a tolerable level of pain therefore approaches which decrease pain and therefore shorten stay in hospital have a double benefit for patients [52].

Conclusion

Laparoscopic surgical techniques have developed throughout paediatric surgery and for some techniques it is recognised as the gold standard for treatment.

One of the major benefits advanced for laparoscopic surgery is less post operative pain.

Pre-empting, recognising and treating pain is an important goal in itself, the decreased pain experienced with laparoscopic surgery also results in decreased length of stay in hospital, a particularly important consideration in treating children.

Pain after laparoscopic surgery is multifactorial. Laparoscopic surgery presents some unique causes of pain in particular the pneumoperitoneum. Approaches to reduce pain developed specifically for use in laparoscopic surgery include modifications of the pneumoperitoneum and efforts to reduce its effects.

Management of post operative pain involves multimodal approach. The exact management will depend on the surgery involved as well as the individual patient.

References

[1]   Gans, SL. Berci, G. Advances in endoscopy of infants and children. *Journal of Paediatric Surgery*. 1971. 6 : 199-234
[2]   Tobias, J. Anaesthesia for minimally invasive surgery in children. *Best Practice and Research Clinical Anaesthesiology*. 2002. 16;1 :115-130.
[3]   Mattei, P. Minimally invasive surgery in the diagnosis and treatment of abdominal pain in children. *Current Opinion in Pediatrics*. 2007 19: 338-343
[4]   Rothenberg SS. Thoracoscopic pulmonary surgery. *Semin. Pediatr. Surg.* 2007 Nov;16(4):231-7.
[5]   Laparoscopy in the Diagnosis and Management of a Complicated Paraovarian Cyst. Macarthur M, Mahomed AA. *Surg Endosc.*

[6]   Ovarian Reconstitution Following Laparoscopic Decapsulation of Congenital Cyst. Pawel Politylo, Khalid Khan, Anies Mahomed. *J. Laparoendosc. Adv. Surg. Tech.* In press.

[7]   Peters, C. Laparoscopy in pediatric urology. *Current Opinion in Urology.* 2004. 14;2. 67-73.

[8]   Pampaloni, E. Valeri, A. Mattei, R. Presenti, L Centronze, N. Neri, A. Salti, R. Noccioli, B. Messineo, A. Initial experience with laparoscopic adrenal surgery in children: is endoscopic surgery recommended and safe for the treatment of adrenocortical neoplasms? *La pediatria medica e chirurgica.* 2004. 26;4: 450-9.

[9]   Feliz, A. Schultz, B. McKenna, C. Gaines, B. Diagnostic and therapeutic laparoscopy in pediatric abdominal trauma. *J. Pediatr. Surg.* 2006. 41;1: 72-77.

[10] Spurbeck, W. Davidoff, A. Lobe, T. Rao, B. Schropp, K. Shochat, S. Minimally invasive surgery in pediatric cancer surgery. *Annals of Surgical Oncology.* 2004. 11;3: 340-343.

[11] Rangel, S. Henry, M. Brindle, M. Moss, L. Small evidence for small incisions: pediatric laparoscopy and the need for more rigorous evaluation of novel surgical therapies. *J. Pediatr. Surg.* 2003.38;10: 1429-33.

[12] Mersky, H. Bogduck, N. editors. " Part III: Pain Terms, A Current List with Definitions and Notes on Usage" IASP Task Force on Taxonomy Classification of Chronic Pain, Sencond editon. Seattle. *IASP Press.* 1994: 209-214

[13] Johr, M. Postoperative pain management in infants and children: new developments. *Current opinion in anaesthesiology.* 2000. 13: 285-289.

[14] Wills, V. Hunt, D. Pain after laparoscopic cholecystectomy. *British Journal of Surgery.* 2000. 87;3: 273-284.

[15] Bisgaard, T. Kehlet, H. Rosenberg, J. Pain and convalescence after laparoscopic cholecystectomy. *European Journal of Surgery.* 2001. 167;2 : 84-96.

[16] Papparella, A. Novicello, C. Romano, M. Parmeggiani, P. Paciello, O. Papparella, S. Local and systemic impact of pneumoperitoneum on prepubertal rats. *Pediatr. Surg. Int.* 2007.23; 5 453-7.

[17] Moehrlen, U. Schwoebel, F. Reichmann, E. Stauffer, U. Gitzelmann, C.A. Hamacher, J. Early peritoneal macrophage function after laparoscopic surgery compared to Laparotomy in a mouse mode. *Surg. Endosc.* 2005. 19;7:958-63.

[18] Gupta, A. Shrivstava, UK. Kumar, P. Burman, D. Minilaporoscopic versus laparoscopic cholecystectomy: a randomised control trial. *Tropical Gastroenterology.* 2005 . 26;3 : 149-51.

[19] Ure, B. Suepelmann, R.Metzelder, M. Kuebler. J. Physiological responses to endoscopic surgery in children. Seminars in paediatric surgery. 2007. 16: 217-223.

[20] Kum, C.K. Eypasch, E. Aljarizi, A. Trodil, H. Randomized comparison of pulmonary function after the 'French' and 'American' techniques of laparoscopic cholecystectomy. *Br. J. Surg.* 1996. 83;7: 938-41

[21] Tsao, K. St Peter, S. Valusek, P. Keckler, S. Sharp, S. Holcomb, G. Snyder, C. Ostlie, D. Adhesive small bowel obstruction after appendicectomy in children: comparison between the laparoscopic and open approach. *J. Pediatr. Surg.* 2007. 42;6: 939-942.

[22] Rosin, D. Zamora, O. Hoffman, A. Khalikin, M. Bar-Zakai, B. Munz, Y. Shabtai, M. Ayalon, A. Low incidence of adhesion-related bowel obstruction after laparoscopic colorectal surgery. *J. Laparoendosc. Adv. Surg. Tech.* 2007. 17;5: 1092-6429.

[23] Dupree, H. Senagore, A. Delaney, C. Fazio, V. Does the means of access affect the incidence of small bowel obstruction and ventral hernia after bowel resection. Laparoscopy versus laparotomy. 2003. *Journal of the American College of Surgeons.* 2003. 19;2: 177-181.

[24] Garcia-Caballero, M. Vara-Thorbeck, M. The evolution of postoperative ileus after laparoscopic cholecystectomy. A comparative study with conventional cholecystectomy and sympathetic blockade treatment. *Surg. Endosc.* 1993. 7;5: 416-9

[25] Cohen, R. Morell, A. Mendes, J. Alvarez, G. Garcia, M. Kawahara, N. Margarido, N. rodrigues, A. Laparoscopic extraperitoneal repair of inguinal hernias. *Surgical Laparoscopy and endoscopy.* 1998. 8;1 : 14-6

[26] Lintula, H. Kokki, H. Vanamo, K. Single-blind randomized clinical trial of laparoscopic versus open appendicectomy in children. *Br. J. Surg.* 2001. 88:4: 510-514

[27] Schmelzer, T. Rana, A. Walters, K. Norton, H. Bambini, D. Heniford, B. Improved outcomes for laparoscopic appendectomy compared with open appendectomy in the pediatric population. J Laparoendosc *Adv. Surg. Tech.* 2007. 17;5: 693-697.

[28] Canty, T. Collins. D. Losasso, B. Lynch, F. Brown, C. Laparoscopic appendectomy for simple and perforated appendicitis in children: The procedure of choice? *J. Pediatr. Surg.* 2000. 35;11: 1582-1585.

[29] Rowney, D. Aldridge, L. Laparoscopic fundoplication in children: anaesthetic experience of 51 cases. *Paediatr. Anaesth.* 2000; 10(3): 291-6.

[30] Dick, A.C. Coulter, P. Hainsworth, A.M. Boston, V.E. Potts, S.R. A comparative study of the analgesia requirements following laparoscopic and open fundoplication in children. J Laparoendosc *Adv. Surg. Tech. Part A* .1998. 8 ;6: 425-429

[31] Fornara, P, Doehn, C. Friedrich, H, Jocham, D. Nonrandomized comparison of open flank versus laparoscopic nephrectomy in 249 patients with benign renal disease. *Eur. Urol.* 2001. 40;1 :24-31

[32] A Two Centre Experience with the Exclusive Use of Laparoscopic Transperitoneal Nephrectomy for Benign Renal Disease in Children. Mahomed AA, Hoare C, Welsh Findlay, Driver CP. Surg Endosc.

[33] Podkamenev, V. Stalamkhovich, V, Urkov, P. Solovkev, A. Iljin, V. Laporoscopic surgery for pediatric varicoceles: Randomized controlled trial. *J. Pediatr. Surg.* 2002. 37;5 :727-9.

[34] Hall, N. Ade-Ajavi, N. Al-Roubaie, J. Curry, J. Kiely, E. Pierro, A. Retrospective comparison of open versus laparoscopic pyloromyotomy. *Br. J. Surg.* 2004. 91;10: 1325-9.

[35] Rudkin, G. Maddern, G. Peri-operative outcome for day-case laparoscopic and open inguinal hernia repair. *Anaesthesia.* 1995. 50;7: 586-9.

[36] Beanes, S. Emil, S. Kosi, M. Appelbaum, H. Atkinson, J. A comparison of laparoscopic versus open splenectomy in children. *Am. Surg.* 1995. 61;10: 908-910

[37] Bailey, P. Bastien, J. Preintroductory techniques for paediatric anaesthesia. *Current opinion in anaesthesiology*. 2005. 18:255-269

[38] Adriaenssens, G. Post operative analgesia with IV patient controlled morphine: effect of adding ketamine. *British Journal Anaesthesia*. 1998. 89: 761-763

[39] Tobias, J. Holcomb, g. Lowe, S. Hersey, S. Brock, J. Caudal epidural block for analgesia following herniorrhaphy with laparoscopy in children. *J. Lapaorendosc. Surg*. 1994. 4;2: 117-20.

[40] Borkar, J. Dave, N. Analgesic efficacy of caudal block versus diclofenac suppository and local ananesthetic infiltration following pediatric laporoscopy. *J. Laparoendosc. Adv. Surg. Tech. Part A*. 2005. 15; 4. 415-418.

[41] Tsui, B. Berde, C. Caudal analgesia and anaesthesia techniques in children. *Current Opinion anaesthesiology*. 2005. 18; 283-288.

[42] Anderson, B. Woolard, G. Holford, N. Pharmokinetics of rectal paracetamol after major surgery in Children. *Paediatric Anaesth*. 1995 5:237-42

[43]   Morton, N. O'Brien, K. Analgesic efficacy of paracetamol and diclofenac in children receiving PCA morphine. *British Journal of Anaestheisa*. 1999. 82;5: 715-7

[44] Wilson, Y Rhodes, M Ahmed, R. Daugherty, M. Cawthorn, S. Armstrong, C. 1994. Intramuscular Diclofenac Sodium for Postoperative Analgesia After Laporoscopi Cholecystectomy: A Randomised, Controlled Trial. *Surgical Lapaproscopy and Endoscopy*. 1994 .3;5: 340-344

[45] Zullo, F. Pellicano, M. Cappiello, F. Zupi, E. Marconi, D. Nappi, C. Pain control after microlaparoscopy. *Journal of American Association of Gynaecologic Laparoscopists*. 1998. 5; 2:161-163.

[46] Barczynski, M. Konturek, A. Herman, R. Superiority of pre-emptive analgesia with intraperitoneal instillation of bupivicaine before rather than after the creation of pneumoperitoneum for lapaoroscopic cholecystectomy: A randomized, double-blind, placebo-controlled study. *Surg. Endosc*. 2006, 20;1088-1093.

[47] Shaw IC, Stevens J, Krishnamurthy S. The influence of intraperitoneal bupivacaine on pain following major laparoscopic gynaecological procedures. *Anaesthesia*. 2001, 56:1041 -1044

[48] Paulson J, Mellinger J, Baguley W. The use of intraperitoneal bupivacaine to decrease the length stay in elective laparoscopic cholecystectomy patients. *Am. Surg*. 2003, 69: 275-278.

[49] Barczynski M, Herman RM. Low pressure pneumoperitoneum combined with intraperitoneal saline washout for reduction of pain after laparoscopic cholecystectomy: a prospective randomised study. *Surg. Endosc*. 2004, 18:1368-1373

[50] Till, H. Lochbuler, H, Kellnar, S. Bohm, R. Joppich, I. Patient controlled analgesia (PCA) in paediatric surgery: a prospective study following laparoscopic and open appendicectomy. *Paediatr. Anaesth*. 1996. 6;1: 29-32.

[51] Stergiopoulou, A. Birbas, K. Katostaras, T. Mantas, J. The effect of interactive multimedia on preoperative knowledge and postoperative recovery of patients undergoing laparoscopic cholecystectomy. *Methods Inf. Med*. 2007. 46: 406-409

[52] Banieghbal, B. Beale, P. Day case Nissen Fundoplication in Children. *J. Laparoendosc. Adv. Surg. Tech*. A.2007. 17 ; 3. 350-352

In: Pain Management: New Research
Editors: P. S. Greco, F. M. Conti

ISBN: 978-1-60456-767-0
© 2008 Nova Science Publishers, Inc.

Chapter VIII

Rehabilitative Analgesia for Major Surgery

P. Brustia[1], L. Gramaglia[3], A. Renghi[3], and R. Cassatella[2]

1. Head of Vascular and Endovascular Unit, "Maggiore della Carità"
University Hospital – Novara, Italy
2. Vascular and Endovascular Unit, "Maggiore della Carità"
University Hospital – Novara, Italy
3. Anaesthesia and Intensive Care Unit, "Maggiore della Carità"
University Hospital – Novara, Italy

Abstract

Pain control is an indisputable human act, but alone it doesn't enhance the postoperative recovery nor decrease the adverse effects. The failed organization of Acute Pain Services may be due to their lack of cost-utility, because of high costs that aren't followed by reduction of hospitalization and adverse effects. When analgesia is integrated in a multimodal perioperative program there is an enhancement of early and long term outcome. We achieved a pathway for abdominal aortic surgery, aimed to reduce the postoperative pain and perioperative stress. The team work chose: transversal left subcostal incision, continuous epidural thoracic analgesia [48 hours], immediate transfer to the surgical ward, opiates-free perioperative analgesia, early feeding and deambulation. This pathway resulted from interaction between surgeons, anesthesiologists and nurses, aiming to improve not only best postoperative comfort, but also outcome and early resumption of daily living. For instance, although opiates are excellent analgesic drugs, we chose an opiates-free analgesia, in order to avoid nausea, vomiting and delay bowel movement, critical feature in this kind of surgery. From 2000 to 2007 we treated on this program more than 600 non selected patients. During the postoperative time we obtained a good pain control (Visual Analogical Scale: 0-2) without adverse effects analgesic therapy related. Conversely, this technique helped the postoperative rehabilitation; in particular postoperative morbidity was low, without any respiratory complication. Almost all patients had deambulation and took food on the day of surgery. The median hospital stay was 3 days. We observed an excellent recovery of the quality of life at the sixth month and twelfth month postoperatively [Short Form 36]. An optimum analgesic strategy integrated with mini-invasive surgery and rehabilitative perioperative program improves short and long term outcome, reducing perioperative length of stay and costs.

Introduction

Controlling pain while managing patients who are undergoing surgical procedures is certainly a humane gesture; perhaps it is effective, but it is not always efficient. Particular emphasis has been placed, for example, on the use of epidural analgesia after major surgical operations. Nonetheless, while it undisputedly does help in controlling pain [1], its efficacy seems controversial with regards to improving postoperative outcome [2]. Furthermore, nowadays, it is fundamental to also deal with the "social" requirement of optimizing therapies by providing high quality standards while using limited resources. In the surgical sphere, this does not simply mean good technical execution and low morbidity rates, but it also implies decreasing the length of convalescence and allowing patients to fully recover their physical, professional, and social roles, both in the short and long term. In the light of this, it can be postulated that submitting patients to surgical procedures may fall within the sphere of preventive medicine [3]. The failed implementation of the Acute Pain Services is partly associated with the fact that their cost-utility was not proven. As a matter of fact, despite their significant costs, they did not bring about a reduction either in the length of hospital stays or in adverse effects [4]. Furthermore, the absence of pain is not the main priority for the surgical patient; his or her rapid physical and mental recovery is [5]. In this regard, we are aware that the patient's satisfaction is undermined as much by pain as by the side effects of painkillers [6]. The guidelines of the American Society of Anesthesiologists provide a good summary of acute pain management in the perioperative setting: optimal pain management with a minimum of adverse effects in an effort to maintain both functional and psychological abilities [7]. If the objective is general well-being [no pain, no fatigue, appetite] [8], then the anesthesiologist is involved not only as a pain specialist, but also as a perioperative physician [9]. Thus, he or she may contribute to improving the postoperative outcome, not only meant as a decrease in morbidity [10] but also as optimum and rapid postoperative recovery and hence an improvement in the quality of life [11]. It is well known that postoperative recovery is influenced by a number of variables which, together with pain, determine postoperative disease. These variables include the patient's conditions and his or her co-morbidity, the degree of surgical trauma, the endocrine-metabolic and inflammatory response to stress, and the perioperative program chosen by the operating team [which ranges from the type of enteral preparation, to the postoperative stay in bed ...] [12,13]. It is evident that controlling one single variable does not suffice, and that pain management must be part of the team's strategy. A meeting between the anesthesiologist and the surgeon may give rise, for example, to the choice to do without opioids in an effort to decrease adverse effects and to favor gastrointestinal function, mental state, and oxygenation [14]. This means that multidisciplinary pathways must be created for the perioperative phase that would allow all the persons involved [surgeon, anesthesiologist, nurses, and patient] to express their own requests and to share the team's choices in terms of the instruments to be used and the goals to be reached. There are currently several reports of "fast track surgery" in which optimum pain control is matched with mini-invasive surgical approaches and quickened feeding and deambulation programs [15]. Within a multidisciplinary program, pain management leads to improved short and long-term outcome, and therefore to a consequent reduction in costs as well [169]. In the immediate postoperative period, it may help reduce ileus, thus favoring the immediate resumption of feeding, just as it may help with the implementation of early deambulation programs by controlling pain while avoiding over-sedation by opioids. After surgery, it may contribute to an improvement in both physical capacity and quality of life [17], as well as to preventing chronic postoperative pain [18]. Actually, it is impossible to provide the ideal analgesic "recipe", and despite the great number of guidelines [19], no single analgesic technique is definitely preferable [20]. Patients are often ill-suited to the "guidelines" [21], and proposing protocols does not automatically produce effects [22]. It is certainly more effective, in the differing scenarios, to promote discussion among the people involved in the perioperative period and to plan local pathways after having evaluated the available resources and the desired goals [23]. Therefore, this report concerns presents the current level of awareness with regards to perioperative physiopathology after major surgery , and it describes the strategies that we have implemented over time at our center. Our team was committed to studying early rehabilitation in abdominal aortic surgery in an effort to reduce not only pain, but also perioperative stress. This chapter sets out to describe this pathway, while focusing on rehabilitative analgesia, that is to say, on all the procedures that are implemented to ensure that the patients are protected from perioperative stress, thus allowing them to rapidly resume their daily habits.

The Importance of the Preoperative Phase

The first step in this pathway is to meet with the patient, who must be told about the types of pathology [i.e. cardiac, pulmonary, renal…] he or she is suffering from and the therapeutic strategies that have been planned. On one hand, patients seem to be increasingly more "well-informed", while on the other hand, the information is often obtained by hearsay from TV or from acquaintances, the press and Internet [24]. It follows that the meeting with the physician, especially if it is hurried and not thoroughly explanatory, can be a difficult moment, a source of anxiety and hence of increased stress [25]. First of all, it is important to understand the patient's expectations: they are often frightened not so much by the pain as by other side effects, such as postoperative nausea and vomiting [26], and by the fear of losing their full physical faculties [5]. None of their fears should be seen as trite: in one interview, patients claimed that one of the most common factors in preoperative stress is thirst, owing to the ban on drinks and to the removal of their dentures [27]. Time must be spent on providing the patient with the information and insight that are needed to prepare for surgery. This will not only lead to a decrease in anxiety, but also to a drop in postoperative pain, meaning more rapid recovery and a reduction in the amount of time spent in hospital [28]. Special attention must be paid to the study and optimization of the patient's conditions. It is well-known in the sphere of abdominal surgery – and in particular with regards to aortic aneurysms – that the average age of the patients we treat is constantly on the rise, as is the number of co-morbidities. Several studies have attempted to classify the specific risk index for aortic surgery, but they basically only quantified the level of risk without diminishing the degree. Significant efforts have been made to optimize preparation times so as to prevent the patient from undergoing a not-always-fruitful succession of long clinical and instrumental investigations. According to the ASA [American Society of Anesthesiologists], there is no need to carry out any tests prior to the anesthesiological examination, and the anesthesiologist's task should be to request the most opportune tests, on the basis of both the patient's conditions and the management of the surgical risk [29]. The National Institute for Clinical Excellence also claims that a profusion of tests may sometimes conceal other shortfalls and they also point out that the tests and their results should be discussed with the patient [30]. Sometimes several tests and consultations are requested prior to surgery in order to clear the patient for the operation [31]. Besides being a waste of resources, this attitude pointlessly prolongs the patient's course and increases anxiety [32]. The anesthesiologist and the surgeon must collaborate in focusing on the most suitable procedures and therapeutic strategies for every single pathology and each individual patient. Fundamentally, they must identify the route that allows the best results to be obtained while causing the least amount of stress. A striking example is the current orientation in the management of perioperative cardiological risk. The in-depth testing and the "preparatory" operations not only proved to be useless, but were actually damaging, both for the risks inherent to the procedures themselves, and for the therapeutic delay and the stress the patient incurred because of them. These days, other factors are acknowledged as being fundamental in the prevention of perioperative cardiac adverse effects. They include the prophylactic administration of beta-blocker drugs, and non-interruption of the patient's usual therapy, especially with regards to cardiovascular drugs like statins and antiplatelets drugs [31]. The one "traditional" intervention of the preoperative phase that undoubtedly needs to be reviewed is fasting. In 1999, the ASA published its guidelines, which envisage the intake of a light meal 6 hours before the anesthesia and the intake of liquids until two hours before [33]. Nevertheless, in many cases the classic recommendation of "nil by mouth from midnight" is still followed, which in some patients may mean refraining from liquids for up to 20 hours and from solid food for up to 37 hours [34]. Considering that this is often associated with aggressive enteral preparation, which is not however justified [35], it not only leads to a state of dehydration, but it is also a further cause of stress and discomfort for the patient [36]. Nowadays an increasing number of authors emphasize the importance not just of avoiding fasting, but of actually boosting the patient's metabolism by administering carbohydrate-rich drinks in the preoperative stage in order to counteract postoperative insulin resistance [37]. Special care is taken to provide the necessary information and insight to patients who are scheduled to undergo aortic surgery, as well as to their families. A meeting is held with all the members of the team [surgeon, anesthesiologist and nurses] and the patients receive an instruction handbook. They continue all their customary therapy, including on the morning of the operation itself (with the exception of anticoagulant drugs). This therapy is immediately resumed upon the patient's return to the surgical ward. On the night before surgery, solid food is allowed until midnight, and liquids can be drunk until two hours prior to the operation. The enteral preparation consists in administering activated carbon and two senna tablets during the three days prior to surgery (no enemas).

The Importance of the Intraoperative Phase

The team's activity thus enters its second phase, during which the surgical and anesthesiologic components overlap and give rise to a mini-invasive process in order to modulate the consequences of the surgical aggression.

The Surgical Technique

The chosen surgical approach is of fundamental importance with regards to the analgesic strategy. In Viel's recent update on the postoperative treatment of pain, the determining factors of a surgical nature occupy a decidedly larger space than do those of an anesthesiologic nature [3]. Mini-invasive techniques, which have been extensively developed over the last few years, do not merely attempt to reduce the scale of surgical incisions, but they also try to decrease perioperative stress and pain by causing the least possible tissue trauma [38]. This may be done in several ways, including decreasing the use of orthostatic retractors, non-evisceration, maximum delicacy in the manipulation of the intestines, minimal dissections, minimal peritoneal exposure, accurate hemostasis, transverse incisions [39] involving a reduced number of metameres [40], without use of prophylactic drainage [41] and nasogastric tubes [41]. In order to gain access to the abdominal aorta, our team uses a left subcostal incision [40]. A curvilinear 10-15 cm long, left sub costal incision with the patient in the supine position (Image 1), is performed, parallel to the costal edge, for transabdominal approach to the aorta. The viscera are left in the abdominal cavity and manually displaced on the right side without using self-retaining retractors. The length of the incision is relative to the width of the rectus muscle itself, which is often proportional to the patient's body mass. The muscle is sectioned by means of electrocautery, a maneuver that has proven to be less traumatic and subject to a lower incidence of postoperative hematomas. There are several advantages to this procedure, such as rapid execution, a reduction in the loss of heat and liquids, no evisceration and a decrease in intestinal manipulation. All of this equates to less tissue and physiopathologic trauma, allowing for rapid intestinal re-canalization. On the pain-relieving front it must be kept in mind that a transverse incision, as compared to a vertical one, affects one – or at most two – sensitive metameres, thus leading to reduced traction of the wound [6 Kg for a transverse section of the rectus muscles as compared to 20 kg for a midline cut], with a positive impact on respiratory function and canalization, as well as on the patient's mobilization [40, 43]. Neither a nasogastric tube nor drains are used.

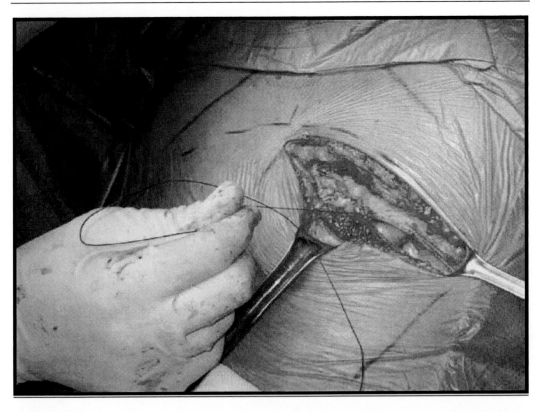

Image 1.

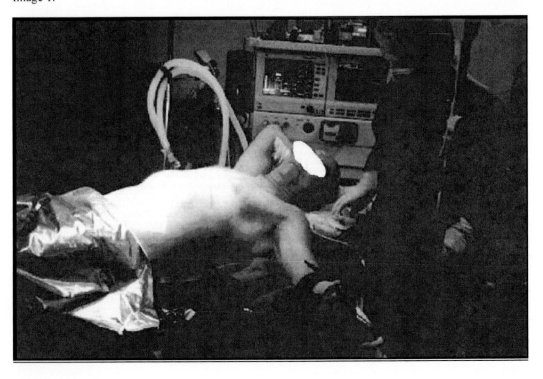

Image 2.

The Anesthesiological Technique

Within the sphere of the strategies aimed at fast track recovery after major surgery, several authors do agree on the importance of associating a peripheral block [for the intraoperative anesthesia and the subsequent postoperative analgesia] with a light general anesthesia [13,15]. In the last few years, the concept of "stress free" anesthesia has been developed. The goal of this strategy is to control the perioperative physiopathology; that is to say, to have a post-surgical patient who not only has no pain, but who rapidly returns to the physical and mental conditions he/she enjoyed before the operation. Epidural anesthesia-analgesia provides numerous advantages including: optimum pain control, decrease in metabolic endocrine afferences, a drop in postoperative insulin resistance, a reduction in pulmonary and thromboembolic adverse effects, and a decrease in postoperative ileus [2, 44, 45]. Thoracic epidural anesthesia appears to provide myocardioprotection and, by relieving pain without blocking the lower limbs, contributes to early deambulation [46]. However, should the postoperative recovery program not be modified, this technique is only "potentially" advantageous [16]. In fact, considering that it is not risk-free [47], Fisher claims that it must be used only by those who adopt the entirety of the courses oriented at improving the outcome of surgery [48]. Furthermore, it is necessary to bear in mind that inflammatory reaction is not controlled by epidural analgesia [49]. Therefore, the concept of a "multimodal" approach is important: besides acting on the inflammatory reaction to stress through surgical mini-invasiveness, non-steroidal anti-inflammatory drugs [NSAIDs] or glucocorticoids should be administered [50]. Mini-invasive aortic surgery can be performed using locoregional anesthesia alone [51]. Furthermore, it is a well-known fact that associating a light general anesthesia helps to decrease both the patient's anxiety, and hence also stress levels during the intraoperative period [52, 53]. Whenever optimal analgesic coverage is achieved in the surgical area, "mini-invasive" general anesthesia can be administered, guaranteeing faster re-awakening and avoiding over-sedation [54, 55]. Given that the local anesthetic determines a reduction in the minimum alveolar concentration [M.A.C.] of the gas, low doses of inhalatory anesthetic can be used [56]. The use of opioids can be avoided thanks to the good degree of analgesia that is obtained with the epidural analgesia associated with non-steroidal anti-inflammatory drugs [52]. The absence of opioids and of curares [which is possible for mini-invasive surgical techniques, especially in the case of transverse incisions] allows the patients to breathe spontaneously, thus benefiting the respiratory system [51, 52]. The use of a laryngeal mask, instead of a tracheal tube, allows for a further reduction in anesthesiologic aggressiveness, since it is less invasive and leads to quicker re-awakening [57]. On the basis of the aforementioned surgical approach, we chose to administer thoracic epidural anesthesia and analgesia [at the T6-T7 level] with only local anesthetics, associated with a light general anesthesia in spontaneous breathing by means of a laryngeal mask, and the perioperative administration of gas [sevoflurane 0.4 - 0.6% MAC] and NSAIDs. At the end of surgery the patient is awakened in the theatre, then is transferred to the surgical ward (Image 2).

Other Strategies for the Intraoperative and Immediate Postoperative Periods

In these moments, it is fundamental that the patient be protected from a series of factors that may contribute to perioperative illness. Hypothermia is a cause of discomfort and stress and tends to increase cardiac, metabolic, hemorrhagic and infectious morbidity [58]. Although not always easy, it is fundamental for the infusion of liquids to be properly managed, especially with regards to avoiding fluid overload [55, 59]. Preventing postoperative nausea and vomiting begins during surgery, by reducing intestinal manipulation, maintaining good oxygenation, limiting the use of opioids, and, if necessary, by using the prophylaxis in high-risk patients [60]. Invasive monitoring techniques must be limited to selected cases alone, since the well-known disadvantages are not outweighed by the limited amount of information they provide [61, 62]. The same holds for admission to the Intensive Care Unit, which can be safely avoided by the majority of patients [53, 63]. This leads to a reduction in the postoperative stress that is caused by admission to a highly medicalized and unfamiliar environment, where every-day habits are disrupted, starting from the loss of the physiological sleep-wake rhythm.

The Importance of the Postoperative Phase

In the postoperative phase of major surgery, the use of epidural analgesia for at least 48 hours not only provides the best possible pain control, but it also contributes to mobilization [because of the analgesia] and to early feeding (by countering postoperative ileus) [2]. As mentioned above, associating non-steroidal analgesics may be advantageous, both for inhibiting the postoperative inflammatory reaction and for controlling the muscle pain that is observed, which is often linked with prolonged and uncomfortable positioning on the operating table. It is best to avoid opioid analgesics in this phase as well. Although they are very effective, they increase the incidence of nausea and vomiting, of postoperative ileus, of urinary retention, and of sedation [64]. Of course, this requires first-rate management of the epidural analgesia: the infusion of local anesthetic must be monitored and adjusted with regards to the level of pain that is reported, to any variations in the hemodynamic parameters and according to the possible side effects (motor block, urinary retention...]. This is possible only by involving the nurses, since they are in constant contact with the patient. Like all "advanced" techniques, epidural analgesia runs the risk of producing more drawbacks than benefits whenever the ward nurses are not adequately up-to-date and trained [65]. Surgeons and anesthesiologists must hence spend a great deal of their time, in particular in the preliminary stages, creating protocols that are also shared by nurses. We must join together to choose the way to measure pain, as well as to identify the scoring system that is deemed most useful to safely modify the epidural infusion and to monitor any adverse events [66]. In our experience, for example, adopting integrated doctor-nurse clinical records proved to be highly effective. Involving the nurses in the choice of the goals [rapid postoperative recovery] and the means that are needed to reach them [epidural analgesia, immediate feeding and deambulation] is an essential requisite not only because it improves pain management

[67], but because it allows the entire therapy plan to be reviewed [15]. Postoperative well-being does not merely require the absence of pain. In the first nights after surgery, hypoxia contributes heavily towards adverse effects, primarily to cardiac and infectious ones [68]. In the postoperative period, the importance of pain control [in order to achieve valid respiratory function], as well as of early mobilization and of nocturnal oxygenotherapy must be highlighted [50]. The occurrence of postoperative mental confusion not only obstructs recovery programs, but it also augments the adverse effects [69]. Preventing confusion depends on several factors including: controlling pain and states of hypoxia, prescribing sedatives with care, having nurses favor the normal sleep-wake rhythm [by limiting stimulants during the nocturnal hours], encouraging diurnal mobilization, collaborating with family members, and resuming routine daily habits [13,70]. In the postoperative stage, the patients' well-being is reduced by postoperative fatigue, which reaches its peak in the first seven days and persists for up to a month in approximately one third of patients [71, 72]. This is particularly relevant in elderly patients, for whom hospital admission itself may lead to a decline in their functional state [73]. Combining mini-invasive surgery, pain control, and early rehabilitation reduces this state of discomfort [74]. Good pain control in the absence of sedation allows the nurses to adopt programs to encourage early mobilization and deambulation [75], both of which are favored by the absence of impediments such as tubes, drains, and intravenous infusions. Early mobilization protects patients from the many risks of bed rest [76] and favors the resumption of daily activities, thus contributing to the patients' well-being [77]. Postoperative ileus is another source of discomfort and possible adverse effects for the patient [78]. It can be prevented through mini-invasive surgery, epidural anesthesia, absence of opioids, and early feeding and deambulation [79]. This also involves the immediate resumption of postoperative nutrition by mouth, which is not only safe, but improves postoperative recovery and the patient's well-being, since they often complain of postoperative hunger and – especially – thirst [80,81]. Surgeons and anesthesiologists must "emerge" from the operating theaters and transfer the same level of alertness to the wards. It is well known that adverse effects usually present in the first few days following surgery [82], when the medical staff does not always receive important information, such as problems concerning the administration of therapy [83]. In our experience, the figure of the surgeon in charge of the ward and the daily visit by the anesthesiologist proved to be extremely effective. As a matter of fact, we found that the majority of elderly patients did not eat dinner, since they were not accustomed to the food that was offered to them. Adding bread and coffee with milk to their choices resolved the problem. In our department, epidural analgesia by continuous infusion of a local anesthetic is maintained for 48 hours in the postoperative stage, and is supplemented with anti-inflammatory drugs [ibuprofen] twice a day. After surgery, the patients are transferred directly to the surgical ward. They are immediately allowed to intake clear fluids and, approximately two hours later, they are given solid food. After two or three hours, the patients are helped to their feet for the first deambulation. The program comprises: immediate resumption of the patients' habitual therapy, oxygenotherapy during the first two nights, the administration of a tablet of senna the night after the operation, and the removal of the urinary catheter the morning after the operation. Nurses make a special effort to encourage patients to intake liquids and solids by mouth, as well as to begin moving, both by exercising in bed and by deambulation.

Table 1. Perioperative program

Preoperative	◆Precise instructions are given to the patients about the perioperative program ◆Patient's drug therapy : no interruption (except warfarin/coumarin) ◆Bowel preparation: active carbon and 2 senna tablets for 2 days ◆Preoperative fasting: 6 h for light meals, 2 hours for clear fluids ◆Premedication with morphine 0.1 mg/kg two hours before surgery
catheter	◆Sedation with midazolam 0.02 mg/kg ◆T6-T7 interspace level ◆Levobupivacaine 0.5%: 15-25 ml ◆Sensory block (pin prick) between T3 and S2
Anesthesia	◆Induction with propofol ◆ProSeal laryngeal mask and spontaneous ventilation ◆Maintenance with sevorane (0.4-0.8 MAC), O2 80%, air ◆Epidural infusion of bupivacaine 0.5% at 4-5 ml/h
Surgery	◆No nasogastric tube ◆Left sub costal incision ◆Transperitoneal access ◆No self-retaining retractors ◆No evisceration ◆No drains ◆Thermal blanket on the upper body ◆Standard surgical instruments
At the end of surgery	◆Flumazenil 1 mg i.v. ◆Removal of laryngeal mask ◆Administration of clear fluids per os ◆Transfer to the surgical ward once conditions are stable
Postoperative	◆Epidural infusion of bupivacaine 0.25% at 3-6 ml/h for 48 hours ◆Oral ibuprofen 600 mg every 8 hours for 48 hours ◆Oral metoclopramide 10 mg every 8 hours for 24 hours

Main Results

The team that currently works at the Novara "Maggiore della Carità" Hospital treated more than 700 abdominal aortic aneurysms between June 2000 and December 2007. In 2000 the team took a new approach to the perioperative care of patients undergoing elective abdominal aortic surgery. At that time, we introduced a multidisciplinary protocol for abdominal aortic surgery based on left subcostal minilaparotomy, thoracic epidural anaesthesia and analgesia and aggressive postoperative rehabilitation, including early mobilization and feeding. The perioperative program is summarized in Table 1.

The patients were provided with details (both spoken and in writing) regarding the course of postoperative care during their hospital stay and were given precise instructions to be followed when discharged home. We analyzed the data of all the patients who followed the whole multidisciplinary protocol. In particular, we excluded patients who were operated on between December 2003 and June 2004 due to a change in the hospital's surgical-anesthesiological team and therefore a period of nurses' training was necessary in the new Unit.

Table 2.Patients' characteristics

Age (median, range)	71 (41-88)
Weight (median, range)	75 (38-152)
Body Mass Index (median, range)	25.4 (15.26-36.79)

Table 3. Surgical features and numbers

Graft (number)	aorto-aortic	290
	aorto-iliac	47
	aorto-bifemoral	116
	aorto-iliac-femoral	32

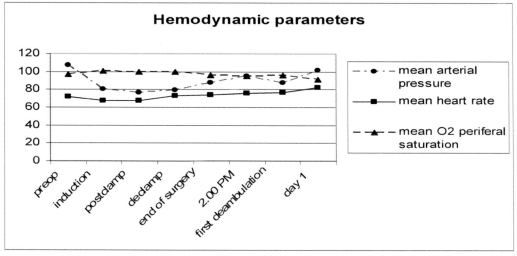

(preop: preoperative evaluation; postcalmp: five minute after clamping aorta; declamp: five minute after declamping aorta; 2.00 PM at day of surgery: parameters recordered in surgical ward; day 1: after day of surgery: parameters recordered in surgical ward)

Figure 1. Haemodynamic parameters.

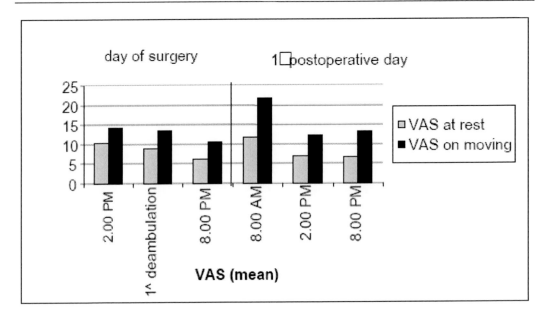

Figure 2. Visual analog scale evaluation.

Four hundred and eighty-five patients followed the whole protocol including 433 (89.3%) who were treated for aortic or aortic-iliac aneurysm and 52 (10.7%) who were treated for aortic or aortic-iliac obstructive disease. There were 439 males [90.5%] versus 46 females [9.5%]. A considerable number were high-risk patients of whom 348 (71.8%) were ASA 3-4.

The patients' characteristics are shown in Table 2. The surgical approach involved a left sub-costal minimal incision in all patients except 38 (7.8%), who required an extension in the bilateral sub-costal incision, due to either technical troubles or anatomical difficulties. The surgical features are shown in Table 3. Mean duration of surgery was 157.9 minutes (SD =53.9); mean blood loss was 722.7 ml (SD =714.8); the amount of intraoperative intravenous fluid administration was 1912 ml (SD=1275); 276 (56.9%) patients received autologous transfusions [cell saver]; allogeneic blood transfusions were necessary in 63 (13%) patients. Hemodynamic parameters were stable (see Figure 1). Pain relief at rest and on walking, as assessed by the visual analogue scale (VAS) on a scale of 0 to 100, proved optimal, as Figure 2 shows. On the day of surgery there were 41 requests for additional analgesia, while there were 31 requests on the first postoperative day. Residual motor block, requiring optimization of epidural infusion, was present in 20 (4.1%) patients in the postoperative period. Postoperative data are shown in Table 4. All of our patients were able to tolerate clear fluids within 1 hour post surgery, and ate solid food within 6 hours after surgery. Thirty five patients (7.2%) suffered from nausea or vomiting on the day of surgery as well as on the first postoperative day, though not severe enough to require discontinuation of oral intake (there was no need for nasogastric tube). All patients but 39 (8%) agreed to intake food on the day of surgery, while the remaining ones did so within the first postoperative day; 77.4% of patients passed stools within the second postoperative day and 95.9% did so within the third postoperative day.

Table 4. Postoperative data

Time of first solid food intake, minutes (median, range)	180 (30-360)
Time of first deambulation, minutes (median, range)	125 (35-2880)

Table 5. Morbidity

		number	%
Complications	pulmonary	0	0
	cardiac	9	1.9
	renal (extemporary dialysis for 3 pts, definitive dialysis for 1 pt)	18	3.7
	Embolectomy at the end of surgical procedure	5	
	peripheral by pass	2	
	digital foot embolism	2	
	wound dehiscence	2	
Readmission	gastritis	1	
	grip	1	

Most patients started to ambulate the same evening surgery was performed, and were out of bed for a mean period of two hours, except for 26 patients (5.4%) who were, however, able to walk the day after surgery. The day of surgery patients were able to ambulate on average 200 meters (range 5-1810). Mobilization time on the first postoperative day increased to a mean seven hours. Mortality rate was 2.3% (11 patients) and morbidity is shown in Table 5. Median discharge was 3 days post-surgery (range 2-21). A considerable number of patients (75.8 per cent) were discharged at home within the third postoperative day. Most of the discharges between the 4th and 7th days were connected to difficulties related to home care or to the considerable distance from the hospital. Readiness for discharge from hospital to home was determined according to standard criteria (tolerance to solid food, passage of stool, absence of infection and ambulation without assistance). Consultation with the medical team was scheduled for 6 days after surgery. Quality of life, as assessed by the SF 36 Questionnaire, was evaluated at the end of the first and sixth postoperative months revealed an overall improvement as compared to preoperative data. First month data are shown in Figure 3.

We conclude by saying that the multidisciplinary and mini-invasive approach to abdominal aortic surgery allows for good therapeutic standards, shortens hospital stay and recovery, and is cost effective. The Bocconi University of Milan performed a study regarding costs, which revealed a 44.7% reduction as compared to the traditional approach. Between December 2003 and June 2004 we studied the learning curve of the nursing management of epidural postoperative analgesia, as shown in Figure 4. We may comment that:

- Analgesia was good during medical management, but there were peaks that meant poor direct control
- During the first period of nursing management, there were many settlements of local anesthetic drug infusion, pain exacerbation, and episodes of hypotension
- Nursing management improved after 35 patients, thanks to the assiduous presence of a nurse in the ward, and fewer pain peaks were noticed because of continuous local anesthetic drug settlements.

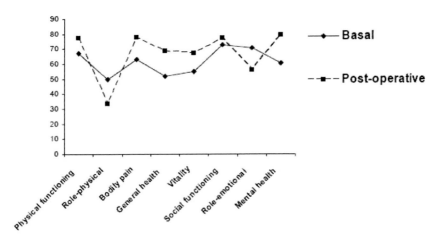

Figure 3. SF 36 Questionnaire: postoperative first month .

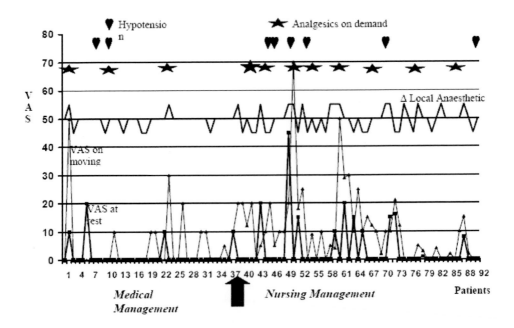

Figure 4. Learning curve of nursing management of epidural postoperative analgesia.

Conclusion

Currently, a great deal of information is available which allows us to improve postoperative well-being and at the same time to reduce perioperative costs [84]. Undoubtedly, the first step consists in being aware of and adopting the perioperative interventions that have proven to be effective [85]. This is not easy to implement since it requires significant organizational efforts by all the people involved in the perioperative phase, and hence support from the administrators [86]. We can surely further reduce our invasiveness: the availability of new analgesics may allow us to free ourselves from epidural anesthesia [49], just as non-invasive monitoring may provide fundamental support [62]. Treatment of perioperative illness is based on new clinical pathways more than on new techniques or new drugs [87]. Analgesia must take on its responsibilities in terms of improving surgical outcome [88]. Not feeling pain does not automatically equate to feeling well.

References

[1]   Block BM, Liu SS, Rowlingson AJ, Cowan AR, Cowan JA, Wu Cl. Efficacy of postoperative epidural analgesia: a meta-analysis. *JAMA* 2003 Nov 12; 290[18]:2455-63.

[2]   Liu SS, Wu CL. Effect of postoperative analgesia on major postoperative complications: a systematic update of the evidence. *Anesth Analg.* 2007 Mar; 104[3]: 689-702. Review.

[3]   Viel E, Jaber S, Ripart J, Navarro F, Eledjam J.J. Analgésie postoperatoire chez l'adulte [ambulatoire exclue] EMC [Elsevier Masson SAS, Paris], Aneshésie- Reanimation, 36-396-A-10, 2007.

[4]   Stadler M, Schlander M, Braeckman M, Nguyen T, Boogaerts JC. A cost-utility and a cost-effectiveness analysis of an acute pain service. *J. Clin. Anesth.* 2004May;16[3]:159-67.

[5]   Nies C, Celik I, Lorenz W, Koller M, Plaul U, Krack W, Sitter H, Rothmund M. Outcome of minimally invasive surgery. Qualitative analysis and evaluation of the clinical relevance of study variables by the patient and physician. *Chirurg.* 2001 Jan;72[1]:19-28; discussion 28-9.

[6]   Gan TJ, Lubarsky DA, Flood EM, Thanh T, Mauskopf J, Mayne T, Chen C. Patient preference for acute pain treatment. *Br. J. Anaesth.* 2004 May;92[5]:681-8.

[7]   American Society of Anesthesiologists Task Force on Acute Pain Management. Practice guidelines for acute pain management in the perioperative setting: an updated report by the American Society of Anesthesiologists Task Force on Acute Pain Management. *Anesthesiology* 2004Jun;100[6]:1573-81.

[8]   Bisgaard T, Støckel M, Klarskov B, Kehlet H, Rosenberg J. Prospective analysis of convalescence and early pain after uncomplicated laparoscopic fundoplication. *Br. J. Surg.* 2004 Nov;91[11]: 1473-8.

[9]   Rock P. The future of anesthesiology is perioperative medicine. *Anesthesiol. Clin. North America* 2000 Sep;18[3]:495-513.

[10] Foss NB, Christensen DS, Krasheninnikoff M, Kristensen BB, Kehlet H. Post-operative rounds by anaesthesiologists after hip fracture surgery: a pilot study. *Acta Anaesth Scand* 2006 Apr;50[4]:437-42.

[11] Wu C, Naqibuddin M, Rowlingson AJ, Lietman SA, Jermyn RM, Fleisher LA. The effect of pain on health-related quality of life in the immediate postoperative period. *Anesth. Analg.* 2003 Oct;97[4]:1078-85.

[12] Carli F. Perioperative factors influencing surgical morbidity: what the anesthesiologist needs to know. *Can. J. Anesth.* 1999; 46 [5]: R70-9.

[13] Jin F, Chung F. Minimizing perioperative adverse events in the elderly. *Br. J. Anaesth.* 2001 Oct;87[4]:608-24.

[14] Wu CL, Caldwell MD. Effect of post-operative analgesia on patient morbidity. *Best Pract Res Clin Anaesthesiol.* 2002 Dec;16[4]:549-63.

[15] Wilmore DW, Kehlet H. Management of patients in fast-track surgery. *BMJ* 2001 Feb 24; 322[7284]: 473-6.

[16] Buggy DJ, Smith G. Epidural anaesthesia and analgesia: better outcome after major surgery? Growing evidence suggest so. *BMJ* 1999 Aug 28;319[7209]:530-1.

[17] Carli F, Mayo N, Klubien K, Schricker T, Trudel J, Belliveau P. Epidural analgesia enhances functional exercise capacity and health-related quality of life after colonic surgery. *Anesthesiology* 2002 Sep; 97[3]:540-9.

[18] Perkins FM, Kehlet H. Chronic pain as an outcome of surgery. A review of predictive factors. *Anesthesiology.* 2000 Oct;93[4]:1123-33.

[19] Steinbrook R. Guidance for guidelines. *N Engl J Med* 2007 Jan 25;356[4]:331-3.

[20] Smith G, Power I, Cousins MJ. Acute pain--is there scientific evidence on which to base treatment? *Br J Anaesth* 1999 Jun;82[6]:817-9.

[21] Boyd CM, Darer J, Boult C, Fried LP, Boult L, Wu AW. Clinical practice guidelines and quality of care for older patients with multiple comorbid diseases: implications for pay for performance. *JAMA* 2005 Aug 10;294[6]:716-24.

[22] Dy SM, Garg P, Nyberg D, Dawson PB, Pronovost PJ, Morlock L, Rubin H, Wu AW. Critical pathway effectiveness: assessing the impact of patient, hospital care, and pathway characteristics using qualitative comparative analysis. *Health Serv. Res.* 2005 Apr;40[2]:499-516.

[23] Dahl JB, Kehlet H. Perioperative medicine – a new sub-speciality, or a multi-disciplinary strategy to improve perioperative management and outcome?. *Acta Anesthesiol. Scand.* 2002 Feb;46[2]:121-2.

[24] Huang QR. Creating informed consumers and achieving shared decision making. *Aust. Fam Physician.* 2003; 32[5]:335-41.

[25] Wallace Pearson S, Maddern GJ, Fitridge R. The role of pre-operative state-anxiety in the determination of intra-operative neuroendocrine responses and recovery. *Br. J. Healt Psychol.* 2005 May;10[Pt 2]:299-310.

[26] Macario A, Weinger M, Carney S, Kim A. Which clinical anesthesia outcomes are important to avoid? The perspective of patients. *Anesth. Analg.* 1999 Sep;89[3]:652-8.

[27]   Cobley M, Dunne JA, Sanders LD. Stressful pre-operative preparation procedures. The routine removal of dentures during pre-operative preparation contributes to pre-operative distress. *Anaesthesia* 1991 Dec;46[12]:1019-22.

[28]   Wallace LM. Informed consent to elective surgery : the "therapeutic" value?. *Soc. Sci.Med.* 1986;22[1]:29-33.

[29]   American Society of Anesthesiologists. Task Force on Preanesthesia Evaluation. Practice advisory for preanesthesia evaluation: a report by the American Society of Anesthesiologists Task Force on Preanesthesia Evaluation. *Anesthesiology* 2002 Feb;96[2]:485-96.

[30]   National Institute for Clinical Excellence. Preoperative tests. The use of routine preoperative tests for elective surgery. 2003, http:// www.nhs.uk/ .

[31]   Fleisher LA, Beckman JA, Brown KA, Calkins H, Chaikof E, Fleischmann KE, Freeman WK, Froehlich JB, Kasper EK, Kersten JR, Riegel B, Robb JF, Smith SC Jr, Jacobs AK, Adams CD, Anderson JL, Antman EM, Buller CE, Creager MA, Ettinger SM, Faxon DP, Fuster V, Halperin JL, Hiratzka LF, Hunt SA, Lytle BW, Nishimura R, Ornato JP, Page RL, Tarkington LG, Yancy CW. ACC/AHA 2007 guidelines on perioperative cardiovascular evaluation and care for noncardiac surgery: a report of the American College of Cardiology/American Heart Association Task Force on Practice Guidelines [Writing Committee to Revise the 2002 Guidelines on Perioperative Cardiovascular Evaluation for Noncardiac Surgery]: developed in collaboration with the American Society of Echocardiography, American Society of Nuclear Cardiology, Heart Rhythm Society, Society of Cardiovascular Anesthesiologists, Society for Cardiovascular Angiography and Interventions, Society for Vascular Medicine and Biology, and Society for Vascular Surgery. *Circulation* 2007 Oct 23;116[17]:e418-99. Epub 2007 Sep 27.

[32]   Garcia-Miguel FJ, Serrano-Aguilar PG, Lopez-Bastida J. Preoperative assessment. *Lancet* 2003;362:1749-57.

[33]   American Society of Anesthesiologists. Task Force on preoperative fasting. Practice guidelines for preoperative fasting and the use of pharmacologic agents to reduce the risk of pulmonary aspiration: application to healthy patients undergoing elective procedures. *Anesthesiology* 1999;90.896-905.

[34]   Crenshaw JT, Winslow EH. Preoperative fasting: old habits die hard. *Am. J. Nurse* 2002 May:102[5]:36-44.

[35]   Guenaga K, Matos D, Castro A, Atallah A, Wille-Jorgensen P. Mechanical bowel preparation for elective colorectal surgery. *Cochrane Database Syst Rev.* 2005 Jan 25;[1]:CD001544.

[36]   Hyausel J, Njgren J, Lagerkranser M, Hellstrom PM, Hammarqvist F, Almstron C, et al. A carbohydrate-rich drink reduces postoperative discomfort in elective surgery patients. *Anesh. Analg.* 2001 nov;93[5]:1344-50.

[37]   Noblett SE, Watson DS, Huong H, Davison B, Hainsworth PJ, Horgan AF. Pre-operative oral carbohydrate loading in colorectal surgery: a randomized controlled trial. *Colorectal Dis.* 2006 Sep;8[7]:563-9.

[38]   Robinson TN, Stiegmann GV. Minimally invasive surgery. *Endoscopy* 2004 Jan;36[1]:48-51.

[39] Grantcharov TP, Rosenberg J. Vertical compared with transverse incisions in abdominal surgery. *Eur. J. Surg.* 2001 Apr;167[4]:260-7

[40] Brustia P, Porta C. Left sub costal minilaparotomy in aortic surgery. *Minerva Cardioangiol* 2001 Feb;49[1]:91-7.

[41] Petrowsky H, Demartines N, Rousson V, Clavien PA. Evidence-based value of prophylactic drainage in gastrointestinal surgery : a systematic review. *Ann. Surg.* Dec;2004[6]:1074-84.

[42] Nelson R, Edwards S, Tse B. Prophylactic nasogastric decompression after abdominal surgery. *Cochrane Database Syst. Rev.* 2005 Jan 25;[1]:CD004929.

[43] Becquemin JP, Piquet J, Becquemin MH, Mellière D and Harf A. Pulmonary function after transverse or midline incision in patients with obstructive pulmonary disease. *Intensive Care Med.* 1985 ; 11 : 247 – 251.

[44] Peyton PJ, Myles PS, Silbert BS, Rigg JA, Jamrozik K, Parsons R. Perioperative epidural analgesia and outcome after major abdominal surgery in high risk patients. *Anesth Analg* 2003; 96: 548-54.

[45] Carli F, Schricker T. Perioperative epidural analgesia and nutrition after upper abdominal surgery: unraveling the mechanisms of protein conservation. *Reg. Anesth. Pain Med.* 2002 Jan-Feb;27[1]:6-8.

[46] Carli F, Klubien K. Thoracic epidurals: is analgesia all we want? *Can. J. Anesth.* 1999; 46 [5]: 409-14.

[47] Wheatley RG, Schug SA, Watson D Safety and efficacy of postoperative epidural analgesia. *Br. J. Anaesth.* 2001 Jul;87[1]:47-61.

[48] Fisher B. Does regional anaesthesia improve outcome? *Anaesthesia and Intensive Care Medicine* 2006; 7:11: 414-7. Elsevier.

[49] Carli F, Kehlet H. Continuous epidural analgesia for clonic surgery--but what about the future? *Reg. Anesth. Pain Med.* 2005 Mar-Apr;30[2]:140-2

[50] Kehlet H. Multimodal approach to control postoperative pathophysiology and rehabilitation. *Br. J. Anesth.* 1997; 78: 606-17.

[51] Kalko Y, Ugurlucan M, Basaran M, Aydin U, Kafa U, Kosker T, Suren M, Yasar T. Epidural anaesthesia and mini-laparotomy for the treatment of abdominal aortic aneurysms in patients with severe chronic obstructive pulmonary disease. *Acta Chir. Belg.* 2007 Jun;107[3]:307-12.

[52] Brustia P, Renghi A, Gramaglia L, Porta C, Cassatella R, De Angelis R, Tiboldo F. Mininvasive abdominal aortic surgery. Early recovery and reduced hospitalization after multidisciplinary approach. *J. Cardiovasc. Surg. [Torino]* 2003 Oct;44[5]:629-35.

[53] Brustia P, Renghi A, Fassiola A, Gramaglia L, Della Corte F, Cassatella R, Cumino A. Fast-track approach in abdominal aortic surgery: left subcostal incision with blended anesthesia. *Interact. Cardiovasc. Thorac. Surg.* 2007 Feb;6[1]:60-4. Epub 2006 Nov 22.

[54] Kehlet H, Dahl JB. Anaesthesia, surgery, and challenges in postoperative recovery. *Lancet.* 2003 Dec 6;362[9399]:1921-8.

[55] Hannemann P, Lassen K, Hausel J, Nimmo S, Ljungqvist O, Nygren J, Soop M, Fearon K, Andersen J, Revhaug A, von Meyenfeldt MF, Dejong CH, Spies C. Patterns in current anaesthesiological peri-operative practice for colonic resections: a survey in

five northern-European countries. *Acta Anaesthesiol. Scand.* 2006 Oct;50[9]:1152-60. Epub 2006 Aug 25.

[56] Morley AP, Derrick J, Seed PT, Tan PE, Chung DC, Short TG. Isoflurane dosage for equivalent intraoperative electroencephalographic suppression in patients with and without epidural blockade. *Anesth. Analg.* 2002 Nov;95[5]:1412-8.

[57] Cook TM, Lee G, Nolan JP. The ProSeal laryngeal mask airway: a review of the literature. *Can. J. Anaesth.* 2005 Aug-Sep;52[7]:739-60.

[58] Leslie K, Sessler DI. Perioperative hypothermia in the high-risk surgical patient. Best *Pract. Clin. Anesthesiol.* 2003 Dec;17[4]:485-98.

[59] McArdle GT, Price G, Lewis A, Hood JM, McKinley A, Blair PH, Harkin DW. Positive fluid balance is associated with complications after elective open infrarenal abdominal aortic aneurysm repair. *Eir. J. Vasc. Endovasc. Surg.* 2007 Nov;34[5]:522-7. Epub 2007 Sep 6.

[60] Apfel CC, Korttila K, Abdalla M, Kerger H, Turan A, Vedder I, et al. A factorial trial of six interventions for the prevention of postoperative nausea and vomiting. *N. Engl. J. Med.* 2004 Jun 10;350[24]:2441-51.

[61] Boldt J. Clinical review: hemodynamic monitoring in the intensive care unit. *Crit Care* 2002 Feb;6[1]:52-9. Epub 2002 Jan 11.

[62] Cannesson N, Attof Y, Rosamel P, Desebbe O, Joseph P, Metton O, Bastien O, Lehot JJ. Respiratory variations in pulse oximetry plethysmographic waveform amplitude to predict fluid responsiveness in the operating room. *Anesthesiology.* 2007 Jun;106[6]:1084-5.

[63] Bertges DJ, Rhee RY, Muluk SC, Trachtenberg JD, Steed DL, Webster MW, Makaroun MS. Is routine use of the intensive care unit after elective infrarenal abdominal aortic aneurysm repair necessary? *J. Vasc. Surg.* 2000 Oct;32[4]:634-42.

[64] White PF. The changing role of non-opioid analgesic techniques in the management of postoperative pain. *Anesth. Analg.* 2005 Nov;101[5 Suppl]:S5-22.

[65] Coleman SA, Booker-Milburn J. Audit of postoperative pain control. Influence of a dedicated acute pain nurse. *Anaesthesia* 1996 Dec;51[12]:1903-6.

[66] Bird A, Wallis M. Nursing knowledge and assessment in the management of patients receiving analgesia via epidural infusion. *J. Adv. Nurs.* 2002 Dec;40[5]:522-31.

[67] Ravaud P, Keita H, Porcher R, Durand-Stocco C, Desmonts JM, Mantz J. Randomized clinical trial to assess the effect of an educational programme designed to improve nurses' assessment and recording of postoperative pain. *Br. J. Surg.* 2004 Jun;91[6]:692-8.

[68] Noble DW. Hypoxia following surgery - an unnecessary cause of morbidity and mortality? *Minerva Anestesiol.* 2003 May;69[5]:447-50.

[69] Franco K, Litaker D, Locala J, Bronson D. The cost of delirium in the surgical patient. *Psychosomatics.* 2001 Jan-Feb;42[1]:68-73.

[70] Meagher DJ. Delirium: optimising management. BMJ. 2001 Jan 20;322[7279]:144-9.

[71] Christensen T, Kehlet H. Postoperative fatigue. *World J. Surg.* 1993 Mar-Apr;17[2]:220-5.

[72] Hall GM, Salmon P. Physiological and psychological influences on postoperative fatigue. *Anesth. Analg.* 2002 Nov;95[5]:1446-50.

[73] Covinsky KE, Palmer RM, Fortinsky RH, Counsell SR, Stewart AL, Kresevic D,et al. Loss of independence in activities of daily living in older adults hospitalized with medical illnesses: increased vulnerability with age. *J. Am. Geriatr. Soc.* 2003 Apr;51[4]:451-8.

[74] Hjort Jakobsen D, Sonne E, Basse L, Bisgaard T, Kehlet H. Convalescence after colonic resection with fast-track versus conventional care. *Scand J Surg* 2004; 93 [1]: 24-8.

[75] Markey DW, Brown RJ. An interdisciplinary approach to addressing patient activity and mobility in the medical-surgical patient. *J. Nurs. Care Qual.* 2002 Jul; 16 [4]: 1-12.

[76] Harper CM, Lyles YM. Physiology and complications of bed rest. *J. Am. Geriatr. Soc.* 1988 Nov; 36 [11]: 1047-54.

[77] Siebens H, Aronow H, Edwards D, Ghasemi Z. A randomized controlled trial of exercise to improve outcomes of acute hospitalization in older adults. *J Am Geriatr Soc.* 2000 Dec; 48[12]:1545-52.

[78] Baig MK, Wexner SD. Postoperative ileus: a review. *Dis Colon Rectum.* 2004 Apr; 47[4]:516-26.

[79] Holte K, Kehlet H. Postoperative ileus: a preventable event. *Br. J. Surg.* 2000 Nov;87[11]:1480-93.

[80] Lewis SJ, Egger M, Sylvester PA, Thomas S. Early enteral feeding versus "nil by mouth" after gastrointestinal surgery: systematic review and meta-analysis of controlled trials. *BMJ* 2001 Oct;323 [7316]: 773.

[81] Soop M, Carlson GL, Hopkinson J, Clarke S, Thorell A, Nygren J, et al. Randomized clinical trial of the effects of immediate enteral nutrition on metabolic responses to major colorectal surgery in an enhanced recovery protocol. *Br. J. Surg.* 2004 Sep;91[9]:1138-45.

[82] Goldhill DR. Introducing the postoperative care team. BMJ 1997 Feb 8;314[7078]:389.

[83] Wyld R,Nimmo WS. Do patients fasting before and after operation receive their prescribed drug treatment? *Br. Med. J.* [Clin Res Ed] 1988 Mar 12;296[6624]:744.

[84] Abularrage CS, Sheridan MJ, Mukherjee D. Endovascular versus "fast-track" abdominal aortic aneurysm repair. *Vasc. Endovascular Surg.* 2005 May-Jun;39[3]:229-36.

[85] Meeran H, Grocott MP. Clinical review: Evidence-based perioperative medicine? *Crit. Care* 2005 Feb;9[1]:81-5. Epub 2004 Aug 19.

[86] Murphy MA, Richards T, Atkinson C, Perkins J, Hands LJ. Fast track open aortic surgery: reduced post operative stay with a goal directed pathway. *Eur. J. Vasc. Endovasc. Surg.* 2007 Sep;34[3]:274-8. Epub 2007 Jun 22.

[87] McQuay H, Moore A, Justins D. Treating acute pain in hospital. *BMJ.* 1997 May 24;314[7093]:1531-5.

[88] Yeager MP, Carli F. *Reg Anesth Pain Med.* Anesthesia and surgical outcomes: an orphean ambition. 2004 Nov-Dec;29[6]:515-9.

In: Pain Management: New Research   ISBN: 978-1-60456-767-0
Editors: P. S. Greco, F. M. Conti   © 2008 Nova Science Publishers, Inc.

Chapter IX

Utility of Assessing and Modulating Postoperative Peri-Incisional Hyperalgesia After Major Surgery

Patricia Lavand'homme [*]

Department of Anesthesiology, St Luc Hospital – Université Catholique de Louvain,
Av Hippocrate 10 – UCL1821, 1200 Brussels Belgium

Abstract

Surgical incision results in both peripheral and central changes in sensory processes. Postoperative pain features involve pain associated with mechanical stimulations, like mobilization and cough, and also hypersensitivity to light touch in tissues surrounding the wound, even in areas distant from the incision. Current research, both in animal models and in patients, indicate that the presence and the extent of punctate mechanical hyperalgesia in uninjured tissues surrounding the wound (*secondary mechanical hyperalgesia*) is a clinical expression of the changes occurring in the nervous system after injury, reflecting a state of central nervous system sensitization which manifests as an increase in the responsiveness of the sensory system. This mechanical hyperalgesia expressing central hyperexcitability is important for several reasons. First, hyperalgesia participates in the postoperative pain experience and might enhance pain for some patients. Second, severe and undertreated postoperative pain seems to contribute to the risk of developing persistent postsurgical pain.

Several analgesic drugs and techniques which are commonly used during the perioperative period are able to modulate peri-incisional mechanical hyperalgesia, either to enhance it (i.e. systemic opioids) or to decrease it (ketamine, intrathecal clonidine, intraoperative neuraxial analgesia). Interestingly, a reduction of the area of mechanical hyperalgesia surrounding the incision positively correlates with lesser risk for the patient to develop persistent pain after major abdominal surgery. Further studies are mandatory to assess the development of peri-incisional hyperalgesia in other procedures such as orthopedic and spinal surgeries. Clinical trials are also ongoing to evaluate the preventive

---

[*] Phone +32 2 764 18 21, Fax +32 2 764 36 99 , E-mail : Patricia.Lavandhomme@uclouvain.be.

antihyperalgesic effects of novel drugs like gabapentin, pregabalin and selective COX-2 inhibitors which are currently proposed as perioperative analgesic adjuvants.

Introduction

Efforts in the practice of anaesthesiology have been directed toward an increase in patient's safety and a reduction of the adverse events occurring in the immediate postoperative period. Pain should be considered one of these unwanted events because optimal pain management is mandatory for early rehabilitation after surgery and severe, poorly relieved, postoperative pain has been associated with an increased risk to develop persistent postsurgical pain [1,2]. Among the patients who consult in Pain Clinic, 30% mention a surgical procedure as the cause of their pain [3]. Besides the suffering for the patients, *Chronic PostSurgical Pain (CPSP)* represents a real problem because its management requires a different approach and represents a major cost for the society.

However, despite the obviously simple nature of a surgical incision, postoperative pain still remains underevaluated and poorly treated. Recent surveys suggest that 80% of patients experience pain after surgery [4], 11% suffering severe pain, and that pain delays recovery in 24% of patients undergoing ambulatory surgery [5]. Such an evidence is challenging and certainly questions our current understanding of the mechanisms which underly incisional pain [6,7]. After major surgical procedures, patients complain of ongoing pain at rest, usually moderate and well controlled with opioids and NSAIDs. In contrast, pain associated with movements, i.e. cough, mobilization, ambulation..., is severe, longer lasting and poorly relieved with opioids, at least at doses devoid of adverse effects. Pain can also be evoked by mechanical stimulation, i.e. touch and pressure, in tissues surrounding the wound, even in area distant from the incision. These observations are the clinical translation of changes occurring in the nervous system following incisional injury [8]. Any tissue lesion activates nociceptive pathways yielding to activity-dependent plasticity, *i.e. sensitization*, which manifests as an increase in the responsiveness of the sensory system to subsequent stimuli [9]. In postoperative patients, the hyperexcitability of pain processing is represented as an increased pain for a given stimulus, also called *hyperalgesia*. Postoperative hyperalgesia participates to, even increases, the pain experienced by the patient and is now considered as an important mechanism for the development of persistent pain after surgery [10].

Postoperative Pain and Plasticity in the Light of Experimental Models: Focusing on Secondary Mechanical Hyperalgesia

Recently, the development of specific experimental models has allowed to approach postoperative pain, highlighting the fact that incisional pain is a unique form of acute pain which possesses features different from pure inflammatory or neuropathic pain [6,11]. Surgical injury causes flare formation around the wound and results in two different types of hyperalgesia. *Primary hyperalgesia* occurs for both thermal and mechanical stimuli applied to damaged tissues close to the site of injury [12]. Underlying mechanism involves peripheral sensitization of primary afferent nociceptors by algogenic mediators locally released. Although inflammation may certainly be involved, ischemia plays an important role and local acidosis parallels postoperative pain behaviors and hyperalgesia [13]. Surgical injury also induces hypersensitivity in adjacent tissues, which is called *secondary hyperalgesia and* is *observed only for mechanical stimuli applied to unlesioned tissues surrounding the wound* [12,14].

In the literature, two forms of secondary mechanical hyperalgesia or exaggerated response to stimuli applied to undamaged tissue surrounding an injury have been described: hyperalgesia to light touch (referred as allodynia) and hyperalgesia to punctate stimuli [15]. Both result from altered pain processing in the central nervous system, from an enhanced neuronal excitability in the spinal cord dorsal horn and the brain, also called central sensitization [16]. Hyperalgesia to punctate stimuli is much more frequent and more pronounced than secondary hyperalgesia to light touch and is facilitated by C-fiber discharge but mediated by nociceptive A-delta fibers [15]. Further, the fact that secondary hyperalgesia appears within minutes after the application of a peripheral noxious stimulus rules out anatomical reorganization within the central nervous system and rather suggests a mechanism linked to the activation of existing neuronal pathways [16].

The development of experimental incisional pain models has allowed to gain greater insight into the phenomenon of secondary hyperalgesia occurring in postoperative patients.

The initial model developed by Brennan [17] was a 1-cm incision through the skin, fascia and muscle of the plantar hindpaw in the rat. The incision was made close to the heel. To assess secondary hyperalgesia, the authors measured median withdrawal thresholds to application of von Frey filaments between the distal tori, an area located approximately 1 cm from the intended incision at the heel [12]. Secondary hyperalgesia was apparent only with punctate mechanical stimulation and was of shorter duration (from 2h until 24h post-incision) than primary hyperalgesia (present until one week post-surgery). Withdrawal thresholds for secondary punctate hyperalgesia were higher (median value 200 mN or 20 g, 2 h after surgery) than those measured around the incision (primary hyperalgesia: median value 30 mN or 3 g). These results suggest that secondary hyperalgesia, i.e. hyperalgesia in uninjured surrounding tissues, requires nociceptors activation [12]. Further, no heat sensitization was present, what suggested that remote punctate hyperalgesia was not caused by a spread of inflammation to afferents fibers [12]. Secondary mechanical hyperalgesia should therefore be considered a consequence of central sensitization. Electrophysiological studies have demonstrated that nociceptive afferent inputs from the wound are required for both the initiation and the maintenance of dorsal horn neurons excitability [18]. Plantar incision induces a sustained enhanced response of dorsal horn neurons (mostly wide dynamic range neurons, WDR): approximately 40 to 50% of dorsal horn neurons show an increased background activity and an expanded receptive field [18]. This hyperexcitable state of WDR neurons, with reduced mechanical thresholds and increased responsiveness to suprathreshold stimuli, transmits the exaggerated behavior observed, i.e. mechanical hyperalgesia. More importantly, a local anesthetic infiltration of the wound blocks the hyperexcitability of dorsal horn neurons but when the effects of local analgesic treatment abate, the incision is able to reinitiate central sensitization [6].

To better approach the mechanisms and the role of secondary hyperalgesia after surgery, the same authors have developed a slightly different experimental model [14]. After incision of the gastrocnemius region of the rat hindlimb, application of both mechanical and thermal stimuli was realized in a remote area, i.e. were applied to the plantar aspect of the hindpaw. Persistent reduced withdrawal thresholds to punctate mechanical stimuli were observed from 2h until day 6 after surgery (initial mechanical thresholds of 522 mN or 53 g were decreased to an median value of 194 mN or 20 g). Neither secondary heat hyperalgesia nor blunt mechanical hyperalgesia developed [14]. This absence of secondary heat hyperalgesia supports the general finding that it does not occur outside the zone of injury. Further, the lack of exaggerated response to application of non-punctate or blunt mechanical stimuli suggest that spinal facilitation of sensory processes mediating secondary hyperalgesia is particularly sensitive to punctate mechanical stimuli and should be mediated by A-delta fibers [14-16]. Finally, in contrast with plantar incision where the development of secondary hyperalgesia was modest and shortlasting, the sustained secondary hyperalgesia observed after gastrocnemius muscle incision in the hindlimb demonstrates that the magnitude and the duration of secondary hyperalgesia are clearly related to the degree of tissue injury.

The aforementioned models have also yield to a better understanding to the mechanisms which underly postoperative central sensitization, and the expression of secondary hyperalgesia. The role of glutamatergic transmission at N-methyl-D-aspartate (NMDA) receptors has been well established in the gain of pain and cental sensitization consecutive to various tissue injury [9]. Activation of NMDA receptor causes a sustained elevation of intracellular Ca^{2+} in secondary order neurons of the dorsal horn, inducing a cascade of intracellular events which contribute to synaptic plasticity. Incisional pain models have shown that distinct type of injuries are uniquely sensitive to NMDA receptors activation and block. After incision, the profile of spinal excitatory aminoacids (glutamate and aspartate) release is reduced and very short-lasting [19]. Furthermore, nor NMDA receptors nor metabotropic glutamate (mGLU) receptors seem to be involved in increased responsiveness of dorsal horn neurons following incision [20]. Spinal mechanisms underlying secondary mechanical hyperalgesia require activation of Ca^{2+} permeable alpha-amino-3-hydroxy-5-methyl-4-isoxazole-propionic acid (AMPA)/kainate receptors, which block inhibits central secondary punctate hyperalgesia without affecting behaviors involved in primary hyperalgesia and ongoing pain [21]. Therefore, an NMDA receptor independent process in the spinal cord dorsal horn may amplify mechanical transmission to contribute to postoperative secondary punctate hyperalgesia. The authors presumed that spontaneous activity of nociceptive afferents induced by the incision activates spinal Ca^{2+} permeable AMPA/kainate receptors located postsynaptic to C-fibers and hence sensitizes dorsal horn neurons, that was recently confirmed by others [22].

Finally, descending facilitatory pathways which contribute to secondary hyperalgesia in a variety of persistent pain models are not involved in incisional pain sensitization [23].

A recent *experimental incision model in human skin* has brought more light on the different mechanisms involved in the development and the maintenance of postoperative hyperalgesia. A 4-mm-long incision through skin, fascia and muscle was made in the volar arm of human volunteers [24,25]. Secondary hyperalgesia to punctate mechanical stimuli with a rigid von Frey hair (151 mN or 15 g) was apparent at 30 min post-incision, persisted for 3 h then gradually disappeared over the next 3 h. The extent of secondary punctate hyperalgesia surrounding the 4-mm-long incision was around 10 ± 2 cm^2 [25]. Experimental incision did not produce secondary hyperalgesia to non-punctate stimuli (e.g. to stroking, using a paintbrush) in most subjects as previously reported in animal models . In a first experiment, the authors evaluated the effect of a subcutaneous injection of local anesthetic lidocaine into the incision site, either pre- or post-traumatically. While pre-incision block prevented the development of secondary punctate hyperalgesia, post-incision block did not significantly affect fully developed secondary hyperalgesia. They concluded that the spread of secondary hyperalgesia is mediated via peripheral nerve fibers but when secondary hyperalgesia has fully developed, it becomes less dependent on or even independent of peripheral neural activity originating from the injured site [25]. In a second experiment, using similar protocole for drug administration, the authors assessed the effect of systemic lidocaine [24]. Pre-traumatic infusion of lidocaine suppressed the development of secondary punctate hyperalgesia, an effect still present even after completion of lidocaine infusion. Post-traumatic lidocaine treatment only temporarily suppressed secondary hyperalgesia which had fully developed. The difference observed in lidocaine effect on the development or on fully developed hyperalgesia suggests that the development and the maintenance of post-incisional secondary hyperalgesia are caused by different mechanisms [24].

A summary of the principal features and mechanisms which characterize *postoperative secondary hyperalgesia in pre-clinical models* is provided in Table1.

Changes in Peri-Incisional Sensory Processing after Surgery: Pointing out Secondary Mechanical Hyperalgesia with the Use of Quantitative Sensory Testing

In contrast with animal studies which measure nociception using objective measures of neuroplasticity, most of the clinical trials only assessed the subjective experience of pain, either directly with evaluation of pain intensity (Visual Analog Scale) or indirectly with analgesics requirements. To date, only few clinical trials have used tools which allow an "objective" measure of postoperative sensory changes due to nociceptive inputs from the surgical wound [7,26].

Quantitative Sensory Testing (QST) quantifies nervous system input-response relations, thereby may permit to detect postincisional neuroplasticity and its modulation by perioperative drugs [27]. QST usually quantifies different thresholds: sensation (stimulation just felt), pain detection and pain tolerance. Measures are realized pre-operatively and post-operatively at several time intervals and at different sites including the wound (primary hyperalgesia), close to the wound (secondary hyperalgesia) and distant to the wound (generalized effects) [26].

Hyperalgesia is defined as a leftward shift of the stimulus-response function, resulting in a lowering of pain threshold and/or an increase in pain intensity to suprathreshold stimuli.

Table 1. Characteristics and mechanisms of post-incisional secondary hyperalgesia

Secondary hyperalgesia, an exaggerated response to noxious stimuli applied to undamaged tissue surrounding a surgical incision

1. is apparent only with punctate mechanical stimulation; does not develop with heat or blunt mechanical stimuli
2. requires nociceptors activation facilitated by C-fiber discharge but is mediated by nociceptive A-delta fibers
3. nociceptive inputs from the wound lead to the initiation of dorsal horn neurons excitability, i.e. a state of central sensitization
4. mechanical hyperalgesia relies on an NMDA receptor independent process in the spinal cord dorsal horn which amplifies mechanical transmission: the processing involves Ca^{2+} permeable AMPA/kainate receptors located postsynaptic to C-fibers
5. the development and the maintenance of post-incisional secondary hyperalgesia are caused by different mechanisms; thereby, when secondary hyperalgesia has fully developed, it becomes less dependent on or even independent of peripheral neural activity originating from the injured site
6. the magnitude and the duration of secondary hyperalgesia are clearly related to the degree of tissue injury

In other words, hyperalgesia is also defined as an increase in pain sensitivity to normally painful stimuli [16]. *Mechanical stimulation, with application of either a pressure algometer or von Frey filaments,* has been used to evaluate the changes in sensory processing after surgery. A strong decrease in mechanical thresholds close to the wound (primary hyperalgesia) is easily detected for 4 to 5 days but can persist up to three months after surgery [28]. The development of secondary hyperalgesia has been demonstrated as following:

1. *Decreased pressure pain threshold (PPT) in uninjured tissues surrounding the incision.* In patients after abdominal hysterectomy, PPT measured at 10 – 15 cm from the incision were significantly decreased (42% at 4 h and 55% after 24 h) and the reduction persisted up to 96 h post-surgery [29,30]. In the pre-clinical experimental model of gastrocnemius incision [14], paw withdrawal threshold reduction reached 63% at 2 h post-surgery and the effect lasted for 6 days. PPT measured at distance from the surgical site, either on the forearm [29] or on the thigh [30] did not show significant changes. However, after sub-costal incision for nephrectomy [31], a procedure involving greater tissue trauma (26 cm-length incision versus 15 cm for hysterectomy), the authors reported modified PPT on the unoperated side. The modified contralateral PPT were affected by an infusion of NMDA antagonist, ketamine, suggesting the presence of secondary hyperalgesia related to central sensitization [31].

2. *Mapping of an area of punctate hyperalgesia surrounding the wound.* Briefly, the technique involves a stimulation with a von Frey hair started from outside the hyperalgesic area where no pain sensation is experienced toward the incision until

the patient reportes a distinct change in perception. The first point where a "painful", "sore" or "sharper" feeling appears is marked and the distance to the incision is measured. If no change in sensation appears, the stimulation stoppes at 0.5 cm from the incision. The area of hyperalgesia is determined by testing along radial lines at a distance of 5 cm around the incision. All the observations are translated on a graph paper to calculate the surface area [28,31]. After nephrectomy (22-29 cm length surgical incision), an area of 200 cm^2 punctate hyperalgesia persisted up to 7 days after surgery [31]. Major digestive procedures (with xypho-pubic incision) induced the development of extended punctate secondary hyperalgesia, with an average area of 55 ± 20 cm^2 at 48h which reached 90 ± 27 cm^2 at 72h post-surgery [32]. After inguinal hernia repair, the area of punctate hyperalgesia was evaluated to an average of 55 cm^2 at 24h and 78 cm^2 after 48h [33]. Thereby it seems to be a trend for the spread of secondary hyperalgesia over the first postoperative days. Further, for a similar 15 cm-median length incision, at 48h post-surgery, abdominal hysterectomy [34] induced a secondary hyperalgesia of 57 (82) cm^2 while elective cesarean delivery [35] a shortlasting procedure involving lesser degree of tissue damage displayed a 9.5 (14) cm^2 area (values are median,IQR). Finally, according to several studies, secondary punctate hyperalgesia was still observed at day 15 and day 30 after thoracotomy [36], persisted up to 6 weeks post-cesarean delivery [37] and was still present at 3 months after abdominal hysterectomy [28]. By comparison, a 4-mm length incision in human volunteers induced an immediate (within 30 min post-trauma) but shortlasting (3 – 6 h) punctate secondary hyperalgesia, evaluated to 10 ± 2 cm^2 [24,25]. All the aforementioned findings in postoperative patients support pre-clinical observations which clearly show a correlation between the extent and the duration of secondary punctate hyperalgesia and the degree of tissue injury. Moreover, the extent of secondary hyperalgesia might also correlate with the level of central sensitization because the area was modulated by different antihyperalgesic treatments [31,38].

3. *The prevalence of punctate secondary hyperalgesia* is only mentioned in few clinical trials although it seems that some patients do not develop this postoperative feature. At 48 h after surgery, the average percentage of patients presenting with secondary hyperalgesia was 32% after colectomy [39], 40 % after lumbar laminectomy and spinal fusion surgery [40] and 35% after elective cesarean delivery [35]. Secondary hyperalgesia was still detected in more than 60% of patients at 3 months after abdominal hysterectomy [28] and in 10% of patients at 6 weeks after elective cesarean section [37]. The same treatments which were effective in modulating the extent of secondary hyperalgesia, and hence central sensitization, were also able to affect the prevalence of its development [39,40].

Interestingly, in all these studies using QST, the differences observed in mechanical sensory thresholds were not reflected in clinical measures of pain (VAS scores and analgesics use). Animal experiments had previously shown that mechanisms for central sensitization causing secondary hyperalgesia may be separated from those for ongoing pain and primary hyperalgesia [21]. This might explain the fact that clinical drugs which modulate punctuate secondary hyperalgesia do not necessarily affect pain scores and postoperative analgesics requirements in patients. The extent of secondary hyperalgesia, either its reduction by antihyperalgesic drugs [38] and neuraxial analgesia [32] or its enhancement by intraoperative opioids [41], was not positively correlated to changes of verbal pain ratings. Therefore, PPT and punctate hyperalgesia can not be exchanged for VAS ratings in the assessment of postoperative pain [30]. Objective measures of neuroplasticity and subjective pain scores provide different but complementary informations in postoperative patients [42].

Modulation of Incisional Secondary Mechanical Hyperalgesia by Peri-Operative Treatments

Sensitization of central pain pathways involves both facilitated excitatory synaptic responses and depressed inhibitions, thereby responses to both noxious and innocuous stimuli are amplified, leading to the expression of hyperalgesia [9].

By consequence, perioperative treatments able to reduce spinal hyperexcitability or to enhance spinal inhibitory controls might have an impact on central sensitization which should be translated to a reduction of postoperative secondary hyperalgesia .

A summary of the effect of different treatments on both the extent and the prevalence of postoperative secondary hyperalgesia is provided in Table 2.

Table 2. Effect of perioperative treatments on the development of postoperative punctate secondary hyperagesia

Perioperative treatment: Drug and dose	Type of surgery	SH Area	SH Prevalence
Ketamine intravenous 0.5 mg/kg ➔ 2 µg/kg/min during 24 h	Nephrectomy [31]	↓ 80 %	NA
PCA morphine:ketamine (ratio 1:2)	Abdominal hysterectomy [34]	↓ 26 %	NA
Dextromethorphan 150 mg single dose	Abdominal hysterectomy [28]	No effect	No effect
Magnesium sulfate 50 mg/kg ➔ 2 g/ h	Elective cesarean section [37]	No effect	No effect
Gabapentin 1200 mg single dose	Inguinal hernia repair [33]	No effect	NA
Pregabalin 150 mg, 2 doses at 12 h interval	Lumbar spine fusion [40]	↓ 81 %	↓ 35 %
Lidocaine intravenous 2 mg/kg ➔ 2 mg/kg/h for 40 min	Volar forearm incision in volunteers [24]	↓ 65 %	NA
NSAID celecoxib 400 mg ➔ 200 mg	Lumbar spine fusion [40]	↓ 52 %	↓ 25 %

Perioperative treatment: Drug and dose	Type of surgery	SH Area	SH Prevalence
after 12 h			
Intraoperative opioid High dose remifentanil	Major digestive [41]	↑ 50 %	NA
Epidural analgesia with epidural ketamine	Thoracotomy [36]	↓ 35 %	NA
Intrathecal analgesia with bupivacaine with clonidine 300 μg with clonidine 150 μg	Major digestive [32] Major digestive [32] Elective cesarean section [35]	↓ 65 % ↓ 90 % ↓ 70 %	↓ 80 % ↓ 80 % ↓ 25 %

SH area: area of secondary hyperalgesia; SH prevalence: prevalence of secondary hyperalgesia; NA: data not available.

Glutamatergic receptors underly most of the excitatory processes at different levels of the central nervous system. However, only few antagonists are clinically available to date and those available are NMDA receptor antagonists. The antihyperalgesic effect of ketamine, a non-selective NMDA receptor antagonist, in various pathological pain states prompted its evaluation in postoperative pain conditions. Stubhaug [31] was the first to demonstrate that low-dose parenteral infusion of ketamine during 48h significantly reduced secondary punctate hyperalgesia for 7 days after nephrectomy. De Kock et al [38] further demonstrated that the antihyperalgesic effect of ketamine was likely not mediated through antagonism of spinal NMDA receptors because epidural ketamine in contrast with the same dose parenterally administered did not affect the development of secondary hyperalgesia after colectomy. These results corroborate experimental findings where spinal NMDA antagonists did not reduce secondary hyperalgesia while spinal AMPA/kainate antagonists were effective. The combination of ketamine with morphine (ratio 2:1) in patient-controlled analgesia after hysterectomy also decreased the extent of secondary hyperalgesia by comparison with morphine alone [34]. The antihyperalgesic effect of a shortlasting perioperative ketamine administration largely outlasted the pharmacological effect of the drug because the reduction of peri-incisional secondary hyperalgesia, extent and prevalence, were still present at day 7 after nephrectomy [31] and at 3 months after radical mastectomy [43]. Other treatments acting as NMDA antagonists, oral dextromethorphan and magnesium sulphate, were ineffective in modulating secondary hyperalgesia post-hysterectomy and post-cesarean delivery.

Novel anticonvulsants such as gabapentin and its analog pregabalin, which are active in animal models of pathological pain but not in normal conditions, are now evaluated as alternative to ketamine [44]. The drugs bind to the α2-δ of the voltage-gated calcium channels and thereby decrease abnormal neuronal excitability through reduced neurotransmitters (e.g. glutamate) release [45]. Several meta-analysis support their analgesic and opioid-sparing effect in the postoperative period but their effect on incisional hyperalgesia remains unknown. Single dose of preoperative gabapentin did not reduce secondary hyperalgesia following inguinal hernia repair [33]. The negative result might be related to the dose used or more likely to the fact that a single pre-operative dose treatment was administered. In pre-clinical models, pre-incisional treatment does not differ from post-incisional one explaining the failure of preemptive analgesia administered as single dose treatment in clinical practice and the need for an effective analgesia covering the entire perioperative period [46]. In contrast, the repeated administration of pregabalin (before and 12 h after surgery) shaw a significant reduction of both the extent and the prevalence of secondary punctate hyperalgesia after lumbar laminectomy and spinal fusion surgery [40].

The use of a neuraxial analgesia, and more importantly the efficacy and the duration of treatment covering the entire perioperative period, also permits to modulate the postoperative development of secondary hyperalgesia [11,42]. An effective epidural block displayed greater superiority over an effective parenteral analgesia (including ketamine at antihyperalgesic dose) in decreasing both the extent and the prevalence of punctate secondary hyperalgsia after major abdominal surgery , that clearly demonstrates the major contribution of spinal sensitization in postoperative pain (Figures 1 and 2).

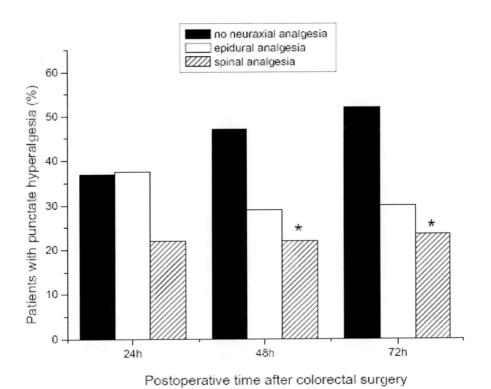

Figure 1. Percentage of patients presenting with postoperative punctate mechanical hyperalgesia after major abdominal surgery in relation to different intraoperative treatments. All the patients received general anesthesia (GA) combined to: no neuraxial analgesia (GA alone group), epidural analgesia (EPID group) or spinal analgesia (intrathecal, IT group). P <0.05 with the group without neuraxial analgesia at the same postoperative time. From Lavand'homme et al [39].

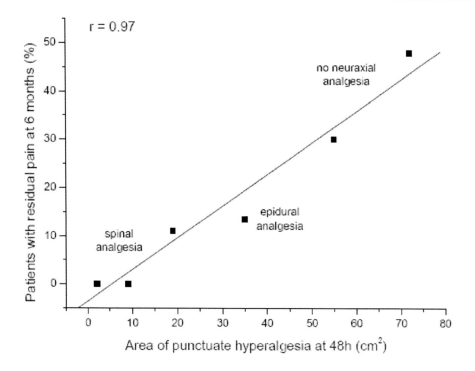

Figure 2. Relationship between the extent of punctate hyperalgesia surrounding the wound at 48 h and the percentage of patients presenting with chronic postsurgical pain at 6 months after major abdominal surgery according to the different intraoperative treatments. All the patients received general anesthesia (GA) combined to: no neuraxial analgesia (GA alone group), epidural analgesia (EPID group) or spinal analgesia (intrathecal, IT group).From Lavand'homme et al [39].

Similarly, the use of spinal analgesia with intrathecal bupivacaine which blocked nociceptive afferent inputs during the surgery significantly reduced secondary hyperalgesia after colectomy [32]. In pre-clinical trials, intrathecal, but not intravenous, clonidine possesses antihyperalgesic properties and a dose of 150 μg seems required to observe this antihyperalgesic effect, whereas 50 μg is ineffective [47]. After major abdominal surgery, intrathecal clonidine alone 300 μg effectively blunted the development of secondary punctate hyperalgesia [32]. A dose of 150 μg combined with bupivacaine reduced the incidence and the extent of peri-incisional punctate mechanical hyperalgesia at 48 h after elective cesarean delivery [35].

Finally, it is important to mention that certain intraoperative treatments may increase instead of reducing secondary hyperalgesia. Effectively, perioperative hyperalgesia is not only induced by sensory system sensitization consecutive to surgery (*nociception-induced hyperalgesia*) but also can occur as an effect of anesthetic drugs (*drug-induced hyperalgesia*) [10]. Recent findings have highlighted the fact that opioids, the most common perioperative analgesics, even after single administration, may paradoxically elicit an increased sensitivity to noxious stimuli by simultaneous activation of both pain inhibitory and pain facilitatory systems [48]. Acute pain sensitization by opioids results either from high doses administration or from abrupt changes in concentrations. In clinical setting, acute opioid-induced hyperalgesia has been demonstrated by increased postoperative pain (clinical expression) and morphine requirements (acute tolerance - pharmacological expression) following intraoperative administration of high doses of remifentanil, a potent and short-lasting μ-opioid agonist [49]. The concomitant use of a low dose of ketamine suppressed the phenomenon [50]. Exaggerated postoperative pain by opioids has been clearly demonstrated in animals [51] and more recently in humans [41]. Using QST with mechanical punctuate hyperalgesia after colonic surgery, the authors [41] found that intraoperative large doses of remifentanil extended by 50% the area of postoperative secondary hyperalgesia induced by the surgical injury itself. Sensitization by opioids added to incision-induced sensitization may reinforce pain memory and therefore contribute to pain chronicization [48].

Clinical Relevance of Postoperative Secondary Hyperalgesia: Prediction for a Risk to Develop Persistent Postsurgical Pain ?

The role and the clinical relevance of postoperative secondary hyperalgesia have been often questioned. On one hand, numerous clinical trials have clearly pointed out a relationship between the severity of acute postoperative pain and the risk for the patient to develop persistent pain after various surgical procedures [1,2]. By consequence, the degree of postoperative pain may appear as a surrogate measure for risk for chronic pain [52]. However, a high number of patients present with severe acute pain at one moment or another after surgery but only a small fraction of patients develops Chronic PostSurgical Pain (CPSP) [52].

On the other hand, the discrepancy between the objective measure of sensory processing by QST and the clinical expression of pain has caused us to seriously question the role played by hyperalgesia in postoperative pain [6,42]. Notwithstanding, hyperalgesia which reflects sensory system sensitization should clearly be part of the pain perceived by the patients after surgery [10].

Few clinical studies to date have considered late outcome, specifically persistence of pain, after a surgical procedure. Results from these trials however show that the presence and the extent of postoperative punctate secondary hyperalgesia, i.e. expression of central sensitization, highlights an increased risk for the patient to develop residual pain after the procedure [52]. Retrospective analysis of data in patients who underwent an elective cesarean section [53] revealed that patients with persistent pain at 6 months after the procedure presented with a higher prevalence of postoperative secondary hyperalgesia (56% at 48 h) than patients without chronic pain (14% at 48 h) (Figure 3).

Moreover, the effectiveness of perioperative treatments to modulate peri-incisional secondary hyperalgesia, i.e. reducing its extent or its prevalence, is positively correlated with a decrease of patients presenting with residual pain at 3 or 6 months after either major digestive surgery [32,38,54] or cesarean delivery [35]. CPSP after gastrointestinal surgery situates around 18% (95% CI: 13-23%) [55,56] at four to five years after surgery. Studies from De Kock and colleagues [32,38,54] are in agreement showing an incidence of 23% after one year which was significantly decreased to less than 5% by a perioperative combination of ketamine and epidural analgesia.

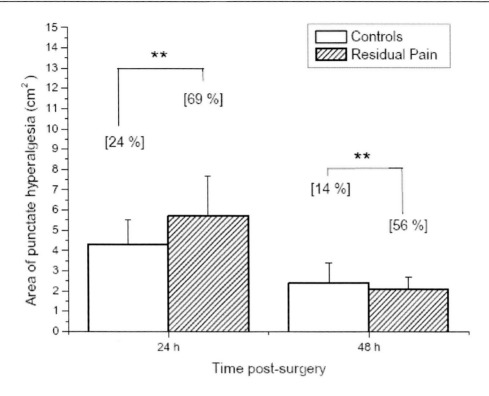

Figure 3. Area and prevalence (numbers in brackets) of punctate mechanical hyperalgesia at 24 h and 48 h after elective cesarean delivery in patients presenting with residual pain or without pain (controls) at 6 months after surgery. (**) P < 0.05 between the groups. From Genot et al [53].

Further, these studies have pointed out the superiority of neuraxial analgesia to block nociceptive inputs from the lesion from reaching the spinal cord, hence to prevent central sensitization [39] (Figure 2). This finding is supported by retrospective studies concerning cesarean section [57] and hysterectomy [58] which both mention general anesthesia alone as a risk factor for the development of persistent postoperative pain.

Conclusion

Progress in our understanding of incisional pain, thanks to the development of experimental models and to the use of Quantitative Sensory Testing in patients, have highlighted the complexity of incisional pain [42]. Recent developments have focused on postoperative secondary hyperalgesia, evoked by punctate stimuli in uninjured tissues surrounding the wound, which is the expression of central sensitization and which prevalence and spread may be indicative for the patients to the risk of developing persistent pain [42,52]. Several questions still remain unresolved: the relation between the area of secondary hyperalgesia and the intensity of acute and residual postoperative pain, the individual predisposition to develop secondary hyperalgesia , the apparent lack of secondary hyperalgesia expression for some surgical procedures, e.g. arthroplasty… but it is worthwhile to pursue. Effectively, regarding to the high number of patients still enduring severe postoperative pain and the reports concerning those who are presenting with chronic postsurgical pain, the management of postoperative pain remains a priority challenge. Objective measures of sensory processing plasticity and common subjective evaluation of postoperative pain experience by pain score ratings and analgesics requirements can provide different but complementary informations which should help to improve the quality of perioperative pain management and thereby benefit the patients.

References

[1] Kehlet H, Jensen TS, Woolf CJ: Persistent postsurgical pain: risk factors and prevention. *Lancet* 2006, 367:1618-1625.

[2] Perkins FM, Kehlet H: Chronic pain as an outcome of surgery. A review of predictive factors. *Anesthesiology* 2000, 93:1123-1133.

[3] Macrae WA: Chronic pain after surgery. *Br. J. Anaesth.* 2001, 87:88-98.

[4] Apfelbaum JL, Chen C, Mehta SS, Gan TJ: Postoperative pain experience: results from a national survey suggest postoperative pain continues to be undermanaged. *Anesth. Analg.* 2003, 97:534-540, table of contents.

[5] Pavlin DJ, Chen C, Penaloza DA, Polissar NL, Buckley FP: Pain as a factor complicating recovery and discharge after ambulatory surgery. *Anesth. Analg.* 2002, 95:627-634, table of contents.

[6] Brennan TJ: Frontiers in translational research: the etiology of incisional and postoperative pain. *Anesthesiology* 2002, 97:535-537.

[7] Lavand'homme P: Perioperative pain. *Curr Opin Anaesthesiol* 2006, 19:556-561.

[8] Dirks J, Moiniche S, Hilsted KL, Dahl JB: Mechanisms of postoperative pain: clinical indications for a contribution of central neuronal sensitization. *Anesthesiology* 2002, 97:1591-1596.

[9] Woolf CJ, Salter MW: Neuronal Plasticity: Increasing the Gain in Pain. *Science* 2000, 288:1765 - 1768.

[10] Wilder-Smith OHG, Arendt-Nielsen L: Postoperative Hyperalgesia. Its clinical importance and relevance. *Anesthesiology* 2006, 104:601-607.

[11] Pogatzki-Zahn EM, Zahn PK, Brennan TJ: Postoperative pain--clinical implications of basic research. *Best Pract Res Clin Anaesthesiol* 2007, 21:3-13.

[12] Zahn PK, Brennan TJ: Primary and secondary hyperalgesia in a rat model for human postoperative pain. *Anesthesiology* 1999, 90:863-872.

[13] Woo YC, Park SS, Subieta AR, Brennan TJ: Changes in tissue pH and temperature after incision indicate acidosis may contribute to postoperative pain. *Anesthesiology* 2004, 101:468-475.

[14] Pogatzki EM, Niemeier JS, Brennan TJ: Persistent secondary hyperalgesia after gastrocnemius incision in the rat. *Eur. J. Pain.* 2002, 6:295-305.

[15] Ziegler EA, Magerl W, Meyer RA, Treede RD: Secondary hyperalgesia to punctate mechanical stimuli. Central sensitization to A-fibre nociceptor input. *Brain* 1999, 122 (Pt 12):2245-2257.

[16] Cervero F, Laird JM, Garcia-Nicas E: Secondary hyperalgesia and presynaptic inhibition: an update. *Eur. J. Pain* 2003, 7:345-351.

[17] Brennan TJ, Vandermeulen EP, Gebhart GF: Characterization of a rat model of incisional pain. *Pain* 1996, 64:493-501.

[18] Vandermeulen EP, Brennan TJ: Alterations in ascending dorsal horn neurons by a surgical incision in the rat foot. *Anesthesiology* 2000, 93:1294-1302; discussion 1296A.

[19] Zahn PK, Sluka KA, Brennan TJ: Excitatory amino acid release in the spinal cord caused by plantar incision in the rat. *Pain* 2002, 100:65-76.

[20] Zahn PK, Pogatzki-Zahn EM, Brennan TJ: Spinal administration of MK-801 and NBQX demonstrates NMDA-independent dorsal horn sensitization in incisional pain. *Pain* 2005, 114:499-510.

[21] Pogatzki EM, Niemeier JS, Sorkin LS, Brennan TJ: Spinal glutamate receptor antagonists differentiate primary and secondary mechanical hyperalgesia caused by incision. *Pain* 2003, 105:97-107.

[22] Jones TL, Lustig AC, Sorkin LS: Secondary hyperalgesia in the postoperative pain model is dependent on spinal calcium/calmodulin-dependent protein kinase II alpha activation. *Anesth. Analg.* 2007, 105:1650-1656, table of contents.

[23] Pogatzki EM, Urban MO, Brennan TJ, Gebhart GF: Role of the rostral medial medulla in the development of primary and secondary hyperalgesia after incision in the rat. *Anesthesiology* 2002, 96:1153-1160.

[24] Kawamata M, Takahashi T, Kozuka Y, Nawa Y, Nishikawa K, Narimatsu E, Watanabe H, Namiki A: Experimental incision-induced pain in human skin: effects of systemic lidocaine on flare formation and hyperalgesia. *Pain* 2002, 100:77-89.

[25] Kawamata M, Watanabe H, Nishikawa K, Takahashi T, Kozuka Y, Kawamata T, Omote K, Namiki A: Different mechanisms of development and maintenance of experimental incision-induced hyperalgesia in human skin. *Anesthesiology* 2002, 97:550-559.

[26] Wilder-Smith OHG: Changes in Sensory Processing after surgical nociception. *Current Review of Pain* 2000, 4:234-241.

[27] Wilder-Smith OH, Tassonyi E, Crul BJ, Arendt-Nielsen L: Quantitative sensory testing and human surgery: effects of analgesic management on postoperative neuroplasticity. *Anesthesiology* 2003, 98:1214-1222.

[28] Ilkjaer S, Bach LF, Nielsen PA, Wernberg M, Dahl JB: Effect of preoperative oral dextromethorphan on immediate and late postoperative pain and hyperalgesia after total abdominal hysterectomy. *Pain* 2000, 86:19-24.

[29] Collis R, Brandner B, Bromley LM, Woolf CJ: Is there any clinical advantage of increasing the pre-emptive dose of morphine or combining pre-incisional with postoperative morphine administration? *Br. J. Anaesth.* 1995, 74:396-399.

[30] Moiniche S, Dahl JB, Erichsen CJ, Jensen LM, Kehlet H: Time course of subjective pain ratings, and wound and leg tenderness after hysterectomy. *Acta Anaesthesiol. Scand.* 1997, 41:785-789.

[31] Stubhaug A, Breivik H, Eide PK, Kreunen M, Foss A: Mapping of punctuate hyperalgesia around a surgical incision demonstrates that ketamine is a powerful

suppressor of central sensitization to pain following surgery. *Acta Anaesthesiol Scand* 1997, 41:1124-1132.

[32] De Kock M, Lavand'homme P, Waterloos H: The Short-Lasting Analgesia and Long-Term Antihyperalgesic Effect of Intrathecal Clonidine in Patients Undergoing Colonic Surgery. *Anesth. Analg.* 2005, 101:566-572.

[33] Bossard A, Guignard B, Attal N, Chauvin M: Evaluation de l'efficacité de la gabapentine versus placebo dans le traitement de l'hyperalgésie péricicatricielle. *Ann Fr Anesth Réan* 2007, SFAR Abstracts 2007:R299.

[34] Burstal R, Danjoux G, Hayes C, Lantry G: PCA ketamine and morphine after abdominal hysterectomy. *Anaesth Intensive Care* 2001, 29:246-251.

[35] Lavand'homme P, Roelants F, Waterloos H, Collet V, De Kock M: Evaluation of the postoperative antihyperalgesic and analgesic effects of intrathecal clonidine administered during elective cesarean delivery. *Anesth. Analg.* 2008, in press.

[36] Ozyalcin NS, Yucel A, Camlica H, Dereli N, Andersen OK, Arendt-Nielsen L: Effect of pre-emptive ketamine on sensory changes and postoperative pain after thoracotomy: comparison of epidural and intramuscular routes. *Br. J. Anaesth.* 2004, 93:356-361.

[37] Paech MJ, Magann EF, Doherty DA, Verity LJ, Newnham JP: Does magnesium sulfate reduce the short- and long-term requirements for pain relief after caesarean delivery? A double-blind placebo-controlled trial. *Am. J. Obstet. Gynecol.* 2006, 194:1596-1602; discussion 1602-1593.

[38] De Kock M, Lavand'homme P, Waterloos H: 'Balanced analgesia' in the perioperative period: is there a place for ketamine? *Pain* 2001, 92:373-380.

[39] Lavand'homme P, De Kock M: The use of intraoperative epidural or spinal analgesia modulates postoperative hyperalgesia and reduces residual pain after major abdominal surgery. *Acta Anaesthesiol. Belg.* 2006, 57:373-379.

[40] Tsao G, Reuben S, Buvanendran A: Celecoxib, pregabalin or their combination on punctuate hyperalgesia following spine fusion surgery. *Anesthesiology* 2007, ASA Abstracts 2007:A489.

[41] Joly V, Richebe P, Guignard B, Fletcher D, Maurette P, Sessler DI, Chauvin M: Remifentanil-induced postoperative hyperalgesia and its prevention with small-dose ketamine. *Anesthesiology* 2005, 103:147-155.

[42] Brennan TJ, Kehlet H: Preventive analgesia to reduce wound hyperalgesia and persistent postsurgical pain: not an easy path. *Anesthesiology* 2005, 103:681-683.

[43] Crousier M, Cognet V, Khaled M, Gueugniaud P, Piriou V: Effet de la ketamine dans la prévention des douleurs chroniques post-mastectomies, étude pilote. *Ann. Fr. Anesth. Réan.* 2007, SFAR Abstracts 2007:R313.

[44] Dahl JB, Mathiesen O, Moiniche S: 'Protective premedication': an option with gabapentin and related drugs? A review of gabapentin and pregabalin in in the treatment of post-operative pain. *Acta Anaesthesiol Scand* 2004, 48:1130-1136.

[45] Taylor CP, Gee NS, Su TZ, Kocsis JD, Welty DF, Brown JP, Dooley DJ, Boden P, Singh L: A summary of mechanistic hypotheses of gabapentin pharmacology. *Epilepsy Res.* 1998, 29:233-249.

[46] Moiniche S, Kehlet H, Dahl JB: A qualitative and quantitative systematic review of preemptive analgesia for postoperative pain relief: the role of timing of analgesia. *Anesthesiology* 2002, 96:725-741.

[47] Eisenach JC, Hood DD, Curry R: Relative potency of epidural to intrathecal clonidine differs between acute thermal pain and capsaicin-induced allodynia. *Pain* 2000, 84:57-64.

[48] Simonnet G, Rivat C: Opioid-induced hyperalgesia: abnormal or normal pain? *Neuroreport* 2003, 14:1-7.

[49] Guignard B, Bossard AE, Coste C, Sessler DI, Lebrault C, Alfonsi P, Fletcher D, Chauvin M: Acute opioid tolerance: intraoperative remifentanil increases postoperative pain and morphine requirement. *Anesthesiology* 2000, 93:409-417.

[50] Guignard B, Coste C, Costes H, Sessler DI, Lebrault C, Morris W, Simonnet G, Chauvin M: Supplementing desflurane-remifentanil anesthesia with small-dose ketamine reduces perioperative opioid analgesic requirements. *Anesth. Analg.* 2002, 95:103-108, table of contents.

[51] Richebe P, Rivat C, Laulin JP, Maurette P, Simonnet G: Ketamine improves the management of exaggerated postoperative pain observed in perioperative fentanyl-treated rats. *Anesthesiology* 2005, 102:421-428.

[52] Eisenach JC: Preventing chronic pain after surgery: who, how, and when? *Reg. Anesth. Pain Med.* 2006, 31:1-3.

[53] Genot S, Lavand'homme P, Roelants F, Waterloos H: Risk factors for chronic pain after elective cesarean section in healthy women. *J. Pain* 2005, 6 - Supplement 1:A695.

[54] Lavand'homme P, De Kock M, Waterloos H: Intraoperative Epidural Analgesia combined with Ketamine provides effective Preventive Analgesia in patients undergoing major digestive surgery. *Anesthesiology. In Press.* 2005.

[55] Boas R, Schug S, Acland R: Perineal pain after rectal amputation: a 5-year follow-up. *Pain* 1993, 52:67-70.

[56] Bruce J, Krukowski Z: Quality of life and chronic pain four years after gastrointestinal surgery. *Dis. Colon. Rectum.* 2006, 49:1-9.

[57] Nikolajsen L, Sorensen HC, Jensen TS, Kehlet H: Chronic pain following Caesarean section. *Acta Anaesthesiol Scand* 2004, 48:111-116.

[58] Brandsborg B, Nikolajsen L, Hansen CT, Kehlet H, Jensen TS: Risk factors for chronic pain after hysterectomy: a nationwide questionnaire and database study. *Anesthesiology* 2007, 106:1003-1012.

In: Pain Management: New Research
Editors: P. S. Greco, F. M. Conti

ISBN: 978-1-60456-767-0
© 2008 Nova Science Publishers, Inc.

Chapter X

An Ethical Approach to Neonatal Pain

C.V. Bellieni and G. Buonocore*

Department of Pediatrics, Obstetrics and Reproductive Medicine,
University of Siena, Italy
*Centre of Bioethics, University of Siena, Italy

Abstract

Neonatal pain has become a much discussed topic. Premature births are more and more frequent and consequently many more babies need long periods of intensive care; but most manoeuvres performed in neonatal intensive care units are stressful or painful. This paper wants to promote the awareness that not only physical pain, but also the lack of a comfortable baby-centred environment can be the cause of suffering. This awareness rises from recent data about neonatal suffering and neonatal pain treatment.

A distinction should be made between pain and suffering: the former is due to a physical harm, while the latter (which may also be provoked by pain) results from harm done to a person's desires. This difference explains why the struggle against pain cannot be overcome without the full recognition of babies' personhood, i.e. being subjects capable of desires and fears: we cannot only administer analgesics, but we must also promote the integral wellbeing of premature babies. Pain and suffering are still poorly understood in neonatal age. We argue that this has multiple causes: a] bad definition of pain and difficulty in recognizing it; b] lack of concern about newborns' suffering; c] lack of legal consequences for provoking unnecessary pain; d] diffidence towards newborns' vitality which leads to diffidence of their personhood; e] lack of empathy toward the preverbal patient. An ethical approach towards neonatal pain should consider the right of the babies to analgesia and relief to be as mandatory as it is in adults. An ethical treatment of pain should start from recognizing newborns' personhood and their need to be soothed, comforted and respected during painful treatment. Recent studies show that this approach not only respects newborns' personality, but also increases the analgesic effect of the resources we employ against pain.

Concern has been recently raised about the increase in pre-term births [1]: more than 500,000 per year in the U.S.A and approximately 50,000 in the U.K; this increase has several causes, among which delayed childbearing [2]. Being born prematurely is a public health emergency which even concerns the market of tools for intensive care [3], thanks to which premature babies' survival is increasing. However, intensive care can be painful since it includes many invasive (blood sampling, intubations, surgery) and stressful procedures (tracheal aspirations, mechanical ventilation, X-ray procedures). It has been calculated that a single newborn in an NICU undergoes 14 potentially painful interventions per diem [4]; are we using the correct approach for this potential pain?

Up to 30 years ago, neonatal pain was never really considered. The majority of anaesthesiologists in the '80s denied that newborns could feel pain and only few used opioids even for major surgical interventions [5]. K.J.S. Anand was a pioneer in this field; he described that newborns feel pain even more than older babies and showed the post-operative complications and long term effects in newborns who did not receive adequate analgesia [6]. Since then, the importance of neonatal analgesia has increased; but why is it still underused [7] and neonatal pain still scarcely recognized?

We have five possible causes:

a) *Difficulty in defining pain.* One of the reasons is the difficulty in accepting that patients who cannot describe what they are experiencing may actually feel pain. In 1979 the International Association for the Study of Pain (IASP) proposed the following definition of *pain*: "A sensory and emotional experience based on actual or potential tissue damage or described in terms of such damage" [8]. This definition implies introspection and expression by language not present in the neonate: as a consequence full pain would not be felt in neonatal age [9]. The limits of this definition led researchers to propose new definitions of pain to encompass the preverbal experience. Anand and Craig revised the above definition as follows: "Pain is an inherent quality of life itself, expressed by all viable living organisms and while influenced by life's events, it does not require prior experience in the first instance." [9] and the recently published *Encyclopedia of Pain* adds to the IASP's definition the following sentence: "The inability to communicate verbally does not negate the possibility that an individual is experiencing pain and is in need of appropriate pain-relieving treatment" [10]. We proposed to define pain as "the clash arising from an attack to our body's integrity" [11].

b) *underscore of suffering.* Although pain and suffering are closely connected in medical literature, they are phenomenologically distinct. Schopenhauer defined suffering as the gap between what we demand or expect from life and what we actually get. While pain is a fundamentally "physical" phenomenon - *the clash arising from an attack to our physical integrity* - suffering is something broader with pain as one of its possible sources. We can define it as *the clash arising from an attack to our person's integrity, i.e. to our needs and desires* [11]. Most of the stress a premature baby shows is provoked by suffering (e.g. due to isolation, continuous noise, lack of relaxation), which sometimes overlaps with pain, but is not pain;

analgesic drugs kill only physical pain and the observation that distress is still present though the use of analgesics may lead to doubt of their efficacy.

c) *lack of legal consequences*: the concern about legal consequences leads to do everything that can avoid liability [12], sometimes exceeding in unnecessary examinations; but when the risk for legal consequences lacks [13], misconducts may be more frequent. This is the case for pain: it can determine long term consequences in newborns, but, unlikely other harmful conditions, those who provoke unjustified pain are not at risk of legal consequences [14], because a correlation between painful procedure and harm is not demonstrable; so we may feel less obliged to use painkillers .

d) *diffidence unto newborns' vitality*: up to recent years most efforts in neonatal medicine have been devoted to promote newborns' survival more than their wellbeing [15]. The fear to invest too much in the care of babies with precarious vitality was a psychological barrier for neonatologists to treat them as persons (i.e. as owners of full human rights), instead than simple subjects worth of cures (but not of care).

e) *lack of empathy*. A baby-centred care [17], which considers newborns' attitudes and desires has two positive consequences: an enhancement of tha greater power of non-pharmacological analgesia [18] and a decrease of brain damage [19]. Babies express whishes and fears and they should be treated consequently: only considering this we might make an effective analgesia, because considering someone's deisires is the only way to overcome his/her suffering.

Thus, an ethical and effective approach to neonatal pain has a milestone: recognizing prematures' personhood, because empathy is fundamental to recognize their unclaimed rights and the hidden sources of their discomfort; and to give relief. It is hard to realize, because it seems a waste of time trying to soothe an irresponsive micro preemie. However, recent research showed that a mother's cuddles [20] and body contact [21] enhance the mild effectiveness of non classic pharmacological analgesic procedures [oral sugar or sucking] provoking an almost absolute analgesia [22]. Visual examples of this can be seen at the following URL: http://www.euraibi.com/analgesia.htm . Body contact, massage, smell, warmth and speech distract the baby and activate inhibitory responses to pain through the so-called gate-control; they can even improve the neurological outcome [23]. However, it is not easy to establish a relationship with a patient who cannot show his/her needs or interests, both in the case of newborns and of adult patients [24]. Nevertheless, it is that sort of challenge that produces clinical results and deep professional growth: "Nurses having more empathy are more likely to develop higher occupational commitment [and] higher levels of empathy and occupational commitment of nurses are associated with lower emotional exhaustion" [25].

Consequently, we should acknowledge that neonatal pain cannot be an actual reason to withhold treatments, because nowadays we have sufficient analgesic drugs and techniques to overcome it. Moreover, a modern neonatal care should consider two further "pains" that are usually underscored: caregivers' and parents' pain and suffering. Both may feel weary and impotent in the presence of a newborn who has to undergo many daily procedures, and they may suppose that suffering newborns' best interest is to die. This is an excess of empathy, which leads to put ourselves in newborns' shoes, often with the presumption of imagining their very feelings. But it is easy to be pray of sentimentalism and assess that a suffering is excessive only because we cannot bear to see it. In some cases this attitude has been described to be due to personal fears [26]. Our endeavour is to objectivise and to recall to a sane sense of realism: a baby submitted to intensive care evokes pity, but his/her resources are broader than what we can suppose; this means that we have a deeper responsibility: a serious engagement with him/her, a covenant not to provoke what we would not bear.

Premature babies are more and more numerous; this constitutes a severe medical emergency. So far it has been considered a big success to recognize *their pain,* which has not been fully recognised till the end of the '80s [27]. Now we should learn to overcome *their suffering* by establishing contact with these non-verbal patients, and thus approach their hidden humanity.

References

[1]   Richard E. Behrman, Adrienne Stith Butler, Editors, Committee on Understanding Premature Birth and Assuring Healthy Outcomes. Preterm birth: causes, consequences and prevention. 2007, National Academies Press - Washington, DC

[2]   Sutcliffe AG: Outcome of assisted reproduction *The Lancet* 2007; 370:351-359

[3]   Millennium Research Group: Premature births on the rise Accessed on August 5th 2007 at the following URL: http://www.mrg.net/news_newwin.php?news_id=245

[4]   Simons SH, van Dijk M, Anand KS, Roofthooft D, van Lingen RA, Tibboel D. Do we still hurt newborn babies? A prospective study of procedural pain and analgesia in neonates. *Arch. Pediatr. Adolesc. Med.* 2003;157[11]:1058-64.

[5]   DeLima J, Lloyd-Thomas AR, Howard RF, Summer E, Quinn TM : Infant and neonatal pain : anaesthetists' perceptions and prescribing patterns. *BMJ* 1996;313:787

[6]   Anand KJ. The stress response to surgical trauma: from physiological basis to therapeutic implications. *Prog. Food Nutr. Sci.* 1986;10[1-2]:67-132.

[7]   American Academy of Pediatrics Committee on Fetus and Newborn; American Academy of Pediatrics Section on Surgery; Canadian Paediatric Society Fetus and Newborn Committee, Batton DG, Barrington KJ, Wallman C. Prevention and management of pain in the neonate: an update. *Pediatrics.* 2006;118[5]:2231-41.

[8]   Merskey H. Pain terms: a list with definition and notes on usage. Recommended by the IASP subcommite of taxonomy. *Pain* 1979; 6: 249-252

[9]   Anand KJ, Craig KD.New perspectives on the definition of pain. Pain. 1996;67[1]:3-6

[10]   Schmidt, Robert F.; Willis, W.D. (Eds.) *Encyclopedia of Pain.* Springer, New York, 2007

[11]   Bellieni C. Pain definitions revised: newborns not only feel pain, they also suffer. *Ethics Med.* 2005 Spring;21[1]:5-9.

[12]   Cunningham W, Dovey S. Defensive changes in medical practice and the complaints process: a qualitative study of New Zealand doctors. *N Z Med J.* 2006 Oct 27;119[1244]:U2283.

[13] Brennan F, Carr DB, Cousins M: Pain Management: A Fundamental Human Right. *Anesth. Analg.* 2007;105:205-221

[14] Bentham J. In: Burns JH, Hart HLA, eds. *An Introduction to the Principles of Morals and Legislation.* Oxford: Clarendon Press, 1996:343.

[15] Shechter N: Evolution of Pediatric Pain Treatment. In: Schmidt RF, Willis WD (Eds.) *Encyclopedia of Pain.* Springer, New York, 2007:749-52

[16] Anand KJS, Craig, KD: New perspectives on the definition of pain. *Pain* 1996;67:3-6

[17] Als H, Duffy FH, McAnulty GB: Effectiveness of individualized neurodevelopmental care in the newborn intensive care unit (NICU). *Acta Paediatr* 1996 Suppl 416:21-30

[18] Shah PS, Aliwalas L, Shah V. Breastfeeding or breastmilk to alleviate procedural pain in neonates: a systematic review. *Breastfeed Med.* 2007;2[2]:74-82

[19] Als H, Duffy FH, McAnulty GB, Rivkin MJ, Vajapeyam S, Mulkern RV, Warfield SK, Huppi PS, Butler SC, Conneman N, Fischer C, Eichenwald EC. Early experience alters brain function and structure. *Pediatrics.* 2004;113[4]:846-57.

[20] Bellieni CV, Cordelli DM, Marchi S, Ceccarelli S, Perrone S, Maffei M, Buonocore G. Sensorial saturation for neonatal analgesia. *Clin. J. Pain.* 2007 Mar-Apr;23[3]:219-21.

[21] Carbajal R, Veerapen S, Couderc S, Jugie M, Ville Y. Analgesic effect of breast feeding in term neonates: randomised controlled trial. *BMJ.* 2003;326[7379]:13

[22] Bellieni CV, Cordelli DM, Marchi S, Ceccarelli S, Perrone S, Maffei M, Buonocore G. Sensorial saturation for neonatal analgesia. *Clin. J. Pain.* 2007;23[3]:219-21.

[23] Westrup B, Böhm B, Lagercrantz H, Stjernqvist K Preschool outcome in children born very prematurely and cared for according to the Newborn Individualized Developmental Care and Assessment Program (NIDCAP). *Acta Paediatr.* 2004 Apr;93[4]:498-507

[24] Raiziene S, Endriulaitiene A. The relations among empathy, occupational commitment, and emotional exhaustion of nurses. *Medicina* (Kaunas). 2007;43[5]:425-31.

[25] Blass, David M., The Physician-Patient Relationship in Dementia Care, *Neurotherapeutics* 2007; 4[3]:545-548

[26] Barr P: Relationship of neonatologists' end-of-life decisions to their personal fear of death *Arch. Dis. Child Fetal Neonatal Ed.* 2007 Mar;92[2]:F104-7.

[27] DeLima J, Lloyd-Thomas AR, Howard RF, Summer E, Quinn TM : Infant and neonatal pain : anaesthetists' perceptions and prescribing patterns. *BMJ* 1996;313:787

In: Pain Management: New Research
Editors: P. S. Greco, F. M. Conti

ISBN: 978-1-60456-767-0
© 2008 Nova Science Publishers, Inc.

Chapter XI

Enabling Pregnant Women to Participate in Informed Decision Making Regarding their Labour Analgesia

Camille Raynes-Greenow [1,*], Christine Roberts [1,†] and Natasha Nassar [2,‡]

[1] The Kolling Institute of Medical Research
Northern Clinical School, The University of Sydney, Australia
[2] The Telethon Institute for Child Health Research
Centre for Child Health Research, The University of Western Australia

Abstract

The pain of labour is a central part of women's experience of childbirth. Many factors are considered influential in determining women's experience of and her satisfaction with childbirth. Women's expectations of the duration and level of pain suffered, quality of her care-giver support, and involvement in labour decision making are the most commonly reported factors [1].

Significantly, there have been more clinical trials of pharmacological pain relief during labour and childbirth than of any other intervention in the perinatal field[2] however to what degree this evidence is available or discussed with pregnant women before labour is unclear.

---

[*] PhD MPH GradDip PopHlth BA, NHMRC Postdoctoral Research Fellow
[†] DrPH MPH FAFPHM MBBS, NHMRC Research Fellow
[‡] PhD MPH BEc, NHMRC Postdoctoral Research Fellow

Decision Making and Pain in Labour

The importance of discussing women's preferences for labour pain relief and their hopes and expectations in terms of pharmacological pain relief before labour begins is well established although it may not be well practiced [2, 3]. Women report fear of pain in childbirth and often lack complete information on analgesic options prior to labour [4]. Epidural consent (covering only the procedure and complications) is obtained by the anaesthetist at the time of the procedure by which time most women are already distressed [5]. There is some debate surrounding whether informed consent can truly be gained at that time [6]. Some clinical practice guidelines have acknowledged this and suggest asking each woman about her preferences before labour begins [7]. Further issues for women have become evident as a result of research which has shown that women wish to maintain personal control during labour and birth, participate fully in the experience, and are concerned about untoward effects of medications during labour [8]. Antepartum decisions about the use of pain relief are likely to be influenced by women's cultural background, friends, family, the media, literature and her antenatal caregivers [9]. Regardless of their plans most women want more detailed and specific information about pain relief in labour [10].

Patient Participation in Clinical Decision Making

Recently decision aids are emerging as an effective tool to assist practitioners and their patients in evidence-based decision making [11]. They assist consumers with informed decision making by presenting unbiased information which is based on current, high quality, quantitative research evidence, which can be tailored to an individuals personal preferences. Decision aids are "interventions designed to help people make specific and deliberative choices among options by providing (at minimum) information on the options and outcomes relevant to the person's health status" [11]. They are non-directive in the sense that they do not aim to steer the user towards any one option, but rather to support decision making which is informed, consistent with personal values and acted upon [12]. There is a growing body of research in this area in regards to women and labour analgesia decision making and this will be the focus of this chapter.

Pain in Labour and Childbirth

Childbirth is an important cultural event and has a significant social and emotional impact on the life of a woman and her family. It is also the most common reason for accessing health services [13]. and a major pain experience, and for most women the most extreme and memorable pain of their lives [14]. Managing women's labour and childbirth pain is an important element of childbirth preparation and also an important aspect of the care provided for labouring women. Many factors are considered influential in determining women's experience of and her satisfaction with childbirth. Satisfaction with the birth experience has been associated with a woman's preparation for childbirth, her confidence in her ability to handle labour, the physiological intensity of labour, and her role in decision making [2, 5]. Women's expectations of the duration and level of pain suffered, quality of her care-giver support, and involvement in labour decision–making are commonly reported factors [13]. The pain of labour in particular is a central part of women's experience of childbirth. Labour pain and pain relief choices have implications for not only women and their families as it impacts on women's health but also have important consequences on health services [13].

Historically childbirth pain, and pain relief or amelioration has been subjected to different fashions. In recent years the view of childbirth and labour pain has been seen more dichotomously, and the gap between "natural childbirth" and "right to a pain free birth" has widened [15]. Childbirth pain is viewed as either an expected and normal part of life [1], or to be avoided and be controlled. Some providers emphasize the advantages of pharmacological methods (pain control) and others focus on potential disadvantages, and unintended side-effects [16]. For example, the American College of Obstetricians and Gynecologists practice guidelines say "that there is no other circumstance in which it is considered acceptable for a person to experience untreated severe pain" and suggest labour pain should be treated upon maternal request [17], whereas the Royal College of Obstetricians and Gynaecologists recommend a framework that suggests "working" with the pain of normal childbirth [4]. Regardless of the view point, labour pain and analgesia are a constant feature of antenatal discussion groups [4]. Whether it is something to be avoided or employed, the experience of labour pain is acknowledged to be individual and a function of "women's emotional, motivational, cognitive, social and cultural circumstances" [15, pg S4].

Labour pain can be managed in many ways, but epidural analgesia is the most effective form of pain relief for labour [15]. In western countries most women use some methods of pain relief during labour whether it be pharmacological and or non-pharmacological analgesia. In the US the use of epidural analgesia is widespread, and approximately 50% or two million women receive an epidural for pain relief each year [18]. In 2005 in New South Wales, Australia (the most populous state of Australia) 96% of primiparas (women having their first baby) and 85% of multiparas (women having a subsequent baby) used some pharmacological analgesic agents for birth [19]. The use of epidural analgesia is influenced by factors at the patient level, the provider level, and at the institutional level [16]. For example in populations that have increased access and availability of epidurals the rate is strongly associated with this. In New South Wales, in hospitals with greater availability this rate could be as high as 74% [20]. Around the world other pharmacological methods of pain relief are also widely available and used. In New South Wales, for primiparas in 2005 this included 27% opioids and 52% nitrous oxide [21].

Significantly, there have been more clinical trials of pharmacological pain relief during labour and childbirth than of any other intervention in the perinatal field [2]. There are however very limited examples of research translation of these clinical trials for pregnant women and to what degree this evidence is available or discussed with pregnant women before labour is unclear.

Decision Making and Pain in Labour

There is considerable evidence that women want to be involved in their pregnancy decision making, and that their level of involvement is related to their overall satisfaction with their care which in turn has been related to the quality of subsequent mothering [22 - 26]. Enabling women to make informed decisions for their pregnancy and labour care is therefore important, and relevant to health care providers, administrators and policy makers. However a study found that women's most important source of labour analgesia information was experiential information from their family and friends, and not with their antenatal care providers [27].

The importance of discussing women's preferences for labour pain relief and their hopes and expectations before labour begins is well known although it may not be well practiced [2, 3]. Women report fear of pain in childbirth and often lack complete information on analgesic options prior to labour [4, 27]. For example the Royal Australian and New Zealand College of Obstetricians and Gynaecologists brochure on 'Epidural and Spinal Anaesthesia' reports the advantages of epidurals but does not mention any possible adverse outcomes or complications [28]. While written informed consent is required for epidural analgesia, it is not required for other analgesic options. Further, the epidural consent (covering only the procedure and complications) is obtained by the anaesthetist at the time of the procedure - by which time most women are already distressed [5]. There is some debate if informed consent can truly be gained at that time and whether it is ethical [6]. Some clinical practice guidelines have acknowledged this and suggest asking each woman about her preferences before labour begins [7]. Further issues for women have become evident as a result of research which has shown that women wish to maintain personal control during labour and birth, participate fully in the experience, and are concerned about untoward effects of medications during labour [29]. Antepartum decisions to use pain relief is likely influenced by women's cultural background, friends, family, the media, literature and her antenatal caregivers [9], Specifically a survey of Australian women found that antepartum information about analgesia was most commonly derived from hearsay and least commonly from health professionals [26]. Ranta found that prior to birth 82% of women wish to see how labour progresses and only want analgesia when pain becomes severe or intolerable [30], however definite plans for analgesia are strongly associated with use. One study found that 96% of women who definitely planned to have an epidural, received one [9]. Regardless of their plans most women want more detailed and specific information about pain relief in labour [10].

Patient Participation in Clinical Decision Making

Making evidence-based decisions in clinical practice is not always straightforward: patients and their healthcare providers must often weigh up the evidence between several comparable options, and the evidence for some treatments may be inconclusive. O'Connor suggests that to be useful the information needs to be tailored to each patient's clinical context and personal preferences [31]. The (Australian) National Health and Medical Research Council states that good medical decision making should take into account the best available evidence, along with patients' preferences and values [32]. And a paper arising from a symposium on the nature and management of labour pain writes "We are obligated to inform women … so they can make truly informed decisions about the use of pain relief in labor" [33]. However, finding effective and efficient mechanisms for doing this in the clinical setting is a challenge.

Decision Aids to Support Decision Making

The first efforts to provide information to patients were through leaflets and brochures. However these often become outdated and or inaccurate, omit relevant data, fail to give a balanced view and ignore uncertainties and scientific controversies [34-36]. Conversely, decision aids have been shown as an effective tool to assist practitioners and their patients in evidence-based decision making [37]. They assist health consumers with informed decision making by presenting unbiased information which is based on current, high quality, quantitative research evidence, which can be tailored to an individuals personal preferences.

Decision aids are "interventions designed to help people make specific and deliberative choices among options by providing (at minimum) information on the options and outcomes relevant to the person's health status" [37]. Decision aids differ from usual health education materials because of their detailed, specific, and personalised focus on options and outcomes for the purpose of preparing people for decision making. In contrast, health education materials are broader in perspective, helping people to understand their diagnosis, treatment, and management in general terms, but not necessarily helping them to make a specific, personal, choice between options [11]. Decision aids are non-directive in the sense that they do not aim to steer the user towards any one option, but rather to support decision making which is informed, consistent with personal values and acted upon [38]. Decision aids have been found to improve patient knowledge and create more realistic expectations, to reduce decisional conflict (uncertainty about the course of action) and to stimulate patients to be more active in decision making without increasing anxiety [12].

Decision Aid Formats

There is a wide variety of formats for decision aids. A Cochrane systematic review of decision aids identified 221 aids, for screening or treatment decisions, using an array of presentation designs. The traditional format of an aid is a booklet style, with or without the an audio guide, however formats include video presentations, brochures, analytical hierarchal processing via personal computers, poster board cards and on-line presentations [11]. Despite the evaluation of decision aids in clinical settings the style and presentation format has not be properly evaluated. The results of a randomised controlled trial evaluating two formats will provide the first evidence of the benefit or otherwise of using an audio guided book compared to a stand alone book [39].

Decision Aid Components

Regardless of the format there are common components included in decision aids. All decision aids include; information about the clinical problem, the management options, the probability of these options, examples of other people making the decision, and guidance in the steps of decision making. They may also include a values clarification exercise, which helps the user consider the outcomes in accordance to how important each outcome is to the user [40]. An important difference between decision aids and other patient information are that they are tailored as much as possible to the individual considering the options [38]. The probabilistic information are obtained from the highest quality research evidence available. These probabilities are presented in styles that are specifically designed to assist consumers understand complex risk data using graphics such as the 100 faces™ (Ottawa Health Research Institute) diagrams (with the number of shaded faces representing the probability of each outcome occurring) and indicate via a rating system (such as gold, silver or bronze medal) the quality of evidence supporting each probability estimate. These pictorial designs have been shown to be acceptable to women and helpful to understanding risk data [41].

Decision Aids for Pregnancy and Consumer Participation

Although there are many decision aids that have been developed and evaluated for a variety of health conditions there are only a few decision aids developed for pregnancy and birth issues [39, 42-45]. However this is an area in which consumers are known to want to actively participate in decision making [46]. A survey of 790 Australian women reported a tenfold increase in dissatisfaction among those who did not have an active say in decisions about pregnancy care [46]. Similarly in the UK, women rated the explanation of procedures, including the risks, before they are carried out and involvement in decision making as most important in satisfaction with care [47]. A recommendation from a US survey suggested that women, caregivers and administrators need access to results of the best available research about the effectiveness and possible side-effects of both pain medications and drug-free measures for labour pain relief, and further stated that women need full and complete information about these matters well in advance of labour and again during labour [48]. It is increasingly evident that the provision of patient and provider information alone, even if evidence-based, is not sufficient to influence health outcomes and behavior [49]. It is only when mechanisms are provided that tailor this information to the individual patient that health outcomes, related to treatment decisions, are positively effected [50].

Importantly satisfaction with childbirth is not necessarily contingent upon the absence of pain [30]. Many women are willing to experience pain in childbirth but do not want pain to overwhelm them. The Royal College of Obstetrics and Gynaecology makes the following evidence-based recommendations [51], midwives must involve women in decisions about analgesia and recognise the value of promoting personal control, maternity services should ensure access to written and verbal information on pain relief and should support women in their choices for pain relief, maternity services should respect women's wishes to have some control over their pain relief and there should be improved public information and data on labour pain and analgesia.

Intrapartum Labour Analgesia
Evidence of Effectiveness for Pharmacological Analgesia

There is a myriad of evidence assessing the effectiveness and outcomes of analgesia for labour. Randomised controlled trials have shown epidural analgesia provides the most efficacious pain relief for labour, but this must be balanced by the increase in risk of adverse consequences [33]. For epidural analgesia the immediate outcomes can include prolonged labour, restricted mobility, use of oxytocin augmentation, unsatisfactory analgesia, dural-puncture headache, hypotension, nausea and vomiting, fever, intermediate localised backache, shivering, pruritis and urinary retention and an increased incidence of instrumental delivery [48, 49]. The consequences of instrumental delivery in the longer term can include increased risk of continuing perineal pain, short-term urinary incontinence, and sexual problems [50]. Although not as effective for labour pain relief as epidural, randomised trials show inhalational analgesia (e.g. 50% nitrous oxide in oxygen) and systemic opioid analgesics (e.g. pethidine) can provide modest benefit to some patients during labour or supplement an unsatisfactory epidural, however also have increased risks, although different to epidural analgesia [52]. These risks include nausea, vomiting and dizziness, and additionally opioid side-effects may include hypotension, delayed stomach emptying and respiratory depression in the baby [51]. Although the risks and benefits of these analgesics are well studied they may not be fully understood by women who are choosing these options for labour pain relief.

Evidence of Effectiveness for Non-Pharmacological Analgesia

Non-pharmacological analgesic options has also been widely investigated and often have less adverse consequences, and considerable numbers of women prefer to avoid the pharmacological methods if possible [29]. Non-pharmacological methods of pain relief include maternal movement and position changes, superficial heat and cold, immersion in water, massage, acupuncture, acupressure, transcutaneous electrical nerve stimulation (TENS), aromatherapy, attention focusing, hypnosis, music or audio-analgesia and continuous caregiver support. Most of these methods have been assessed in randomised trials [53]. The results vary with regard to the effectiveness of the pain relief they provide however they are well liked by women and have few side effects.

Although there is a large amount of information of the effectiveness and outcomes of labour analgesia the availability of this evidence for women who are known to be interested in making informed decisions is limited.

Facilitating Labour Analgesia Decision-Making Suitability for a Decision Aid

Eddy 1992, suggests that when a clinical decision is modifiable by patients' values and preferences then it fulfils the criteria in which patients would benefit from a decision aid [54]. The management of pain in labour meets Eddy's criteria for a decision aid as the outcomes for analgesia options and women's preferences for the relative value of benefits compared to risks are variable. For such a clinical decision, a decision aid would be expected to improve patient knowledge and create realistic expectations, to reduce decisional conflict and to stimulate patients to be more active in decision making without increasing anxiety [54].

The availability of good evidence for labour analgesia coupled with the desire of women to participate in their decision making suggests that a decision aid may be an ideal tool for women choosing between a range of options for the management of labour pain. Such a tool may also benefit antenatal care-providers who are interested in practicing shared decision making. Ideally any such tool would need to present pain management in a positive and flexible way, acknowledging the unpredictability of events around childbirth, and would encourage flexibility in choices and create awareness of the unpredictability of childbirth that may change the appropriateness of some options. The success of decision aids thus far in a variety of health settings is encouraging and results of trials conducted in the perinatal setting [43, 45, 55] also suggest that a decision aid will be well received and useful for pregnant women interested in making informed decisions regarding labour analgesia. There is currently a trial of a decision aid for labour analgesia recently completed [39], and another in development [56]. The results of these will be an important step for enabling pregnant women to participate in informed decision-making regarding their labour analgesia.

References

[1]   McLachlan, H. and U. Waldenstrom, Childbirth experiences in Australia of women born in Turkey, Vietnam and Australia. *Birth*, 2005. 32(4).

[2]   Dickersin, K., Pharmacological control of pain during labour, in *Effective care in pregnancy and childbirth*, I. Chalmers, M. Enkin, and M.J.N. Keirse, Editors. 1989, Oxford University Press: Oxford. p. 913-945.

[3]   Enkin, M., Keirse, M.J.N.C., Neilson, J., Crowther, C., Duley, L., Hodnott, E., Hofmeyr, J., Control of pain in labor, in *A guide to effective care in pregnancy and childbirth*. 2000, Oxford Medical Publications: Oxford. p. 314-331.

[4]   Leap, N., Pain in labour: towards a midwifery perspective. *MIDIRS Midwifery Digest*, 2000. 10(1): p. 49-53.

[5]   Swan, H.D. and D.C. Borshoff, Informed consent--recall of risk information following epidural analgesia in labour. *Anaesthesia and Intensive Care*, 1994. 22(2): p. 139-41.

[6]   Siddiqui Meraj N, et al., Does labor pain and labor epidural analgesia impair decison capabilities of paturients. *The Internet Journal of Anesthesiology*, 2005. 10(1).

[7]   National Collaborating Centre for Women's and Children' Health, *Antenatal care: routine care for the healthy pregnant woman Royal College of Obstetrician and*

Gynaecologists. Commissioned by the National Institute for Clinical Excellence (UK). 2003.

[8] Simkin, P. and O.H. M., Nonpharmacologic relief of pain during labor: Systematic review of five methods. *Am J Obstet Gynecol*, 2002. 186(Suppl 5): p. S131 - S159.

[9] Goldberg, A.B., A. Cohen, and E. Lieberman, Nulliparas' preferences for epidural analgesia: their effects on actual use in labor. *Birth*, 1999. 26(3): p. 139-43.

[10] Stewart, A., et al., Assessment of the effect upon maternal knowledge of an information leaflet about pain relief in labour. *Anaesthesia,* 2003. 58(10): p. p1015-9.

[11] O'Connor, A., et al., Decision aids for people facing health treatment ot screening decisions. In: *The Cochrane Library*, Issue 1. Oxford: Update Software., 2004.

[12] O'Connor, A., et al., Decision aids for patients facing health treatment or screening decisions: systematic review. *BMJ*, 1999. 319(7212): p. 731-4.

[13] Hodnett, E.D.R.N.P., Pain and women's satisfaction with the experience of childbirth: A systematic review. *American Journal of Obstetrics and Gynecology.* May, 2002. 186(5)): p. S160-S172.

[14] Niven, C. and T. Murphy-Black, Memory of labour pain: A review of the literature. *Birth*, 2000. 27: p. 244-254.

[15] Caton, D., et al., The nature and management of labor pain. *American Journal of Obstetrics and Gynecology,* 2002. 186(5 Suppl): p. S1-15.

[16] Rust, G., et al., Racial and ethnic disparities in the provision of epidural analgesia to Georgia Medicaid beneficiaries during labor and delivery. *Am J Obstet Gynecol*, 2004. 191(2): p. 456-462.

[17] American College of Obstetricians and Gynecologists, ACOG practice bulletin no. 36. Clinical management Guidelines for Obstetrician-Gynaecologists. *Obstetric Analgesia and Anesthesia,* 2002. 100(1).

[18] Hawkins, J.L., B.R. Beatty, and C.P. Gibbs, *Update on anaethesia practices in the US*, in *Society for Anesthesia and Perinatology.* 1999.

[19] NSW Department of Health, *NSW Mothers and Babies 1998*, in *NSW Public Health Bulletin.* 2000, NSW Department of Health: Sydney.

[20] NSW Department of Health, *NSW Mothers and Babies 2000*, in *NSW Public Health Bulletin Supplement.* 2001, NSW Department of Health: Sydney.

[21] Laws P.J, et al., *Australia' mothers and babies 2005*, in *Perinatal Statistics series.* no.20 Cat.no.PER 40. 2007, AIHW National Perinatal Statistics Unit: Sydney.

[22] Brown, J.B., et al., Women's decision-making about their health care: views over the life cycle. *Patient Education and Counseling*, 2002. 48: p. 225-231.

[23] Fenwick J, et al., The childbirth expectations of a self-selecetd cohort of Western Australian women. Midwifery, 2005. 21(1): p. 23-35.

[24] Gibbins J and Thomson A.M, Women's expectations and experiences of childbirth. *Midwifery,* 2001. 17(4): p. 302-13.

[25] Mackay, M.C., Women's evaluation of the labour and delivery experience. *Nursing Connections,* 1998. 11(3): p. 19-32.

[26] Paech, M.J. and L.C. Gurrin, A survey of parturients using epidural analgesia during labour. Considerations relevant to antenatal educators. *Australian and New Zealand Journal of Obstetrics and Gynaecology*, 1999. 39(1): p. 21-5.

[27] Raynes-Greenow, C.H., et al., Knowledge and decision-making for labour analgesia of Australian primiparous women. *Midwifery*, 2007. 23(2): p. 139-145.

[28] Royal Australian and New Zealand College of Obstetricians and Gynaecologists. Epidural and spinal anasthesia. Patient information pamphlet. 1998 [cited 1998 Feb]; Available from: http://www.ranzcog.edu.au.

[29] Simkin, P., Non-pharmacological methods of pain relief during labour, in Effective care in pregnancy and childbirth, I. Chalmers, M. Enkin, and M.J.N. Keirse, Editors. 1989, Oxford University Press: Oxford. p. 1182-1195.

[30] Ranta, P., et al., Maternal expectations and experiences of labour pain--options of 1091 Finnish parturients. *Acta Anaesthesiologica Scandinavica*, 1995. 39(1): p. 60-6.

[31] O'Connor, A., et al., Decision aids for people facing health treatment or screening decisions. *Cochrane Library*, Issue 4., 2002.

[32] National Health and Medical Research Council, A Guide to the Development, Implementation and Evaluation of Clinical Practice Guidelines. 1999.

[33] Lieberman, E. and C. O'Donoghue, Unintended effects of epidural analgesia during labor: a systematic review. *American Journal of Obstetrics and Gynecology*. 2002. 186(5 Suppl Nature): p. S31-68.

[34] Coulter, A., Evidence based patient information. is important, so there needs to be a national strategy to ensure it. *BMJ*, 1998. 317(7153): p. 225-6.

[35] Coulter, A., V. Entwistle, and D. Gilbert, Sharing decisions with patients: is the information good enough? *BMJ*, 1999. 318(7179): p. 318-22.

[36] Paech, M.J., R. Godkin, and S. Webster, Complications of obstetric epidural analgesia and anaesthesia: a prospective analysis of 10 995 cases. *International Journal of Anesthesia*, 1998. 7: p. 5-11.

[37] O'Connor, A. and A. Edwards, The role of decision aids in promoting evidence-based patient choice, in Evidence based patient choice, A. Edwards and G. Elwyn, Editors. 2001, Oxford University Press: Oxford.

[38] O'Connor, A.M., et al., Decision aids for patients considering options affecting cancer outcomes: evidence of efficacy and policy implications. *Journal of the National Cancer Institute*. Monographs, 1999(25): p. 67-80.

[39] Roberts, C., et al., Protocol for a randomised controlled trial of a decision aid for the management of pain in labour and childbirth [ISRCTN52287533]. *BMC Pregnancy and Childbirth*, 2004. 4(1): p. 24.

[40] O'Connor, A., et al., Decision aids for people facing health treatment or screening decisions. *Cochrane Library*, Issue 4., 2001.

[41] Nassar, N., et al., Development and pilot-testing of a decision aid for women with a breech-presenting baby. *Midwifery*, 2007. 23(1):38-47.

[42] Karraz, M.A., Ambulatory epidural anesthesia and the duration of labor. *Int J Gynaecol Obstet*, 2003. 80(2): p. 117-22.

[43] Nassar, N., et al., Evaluation of a decision aid for women with breech presentation at term: a randomised controlled trial [ISRCTN14570598]. *BJOG: An International Journal of Obstetrics and Gynaecology*, 2007. 114(3): p. 325–333.

[44] O'Cathain, A., et al., Use of evidence based leaflets to promote informed choice in maternity care: randomised controlled trial in everyday practice. *British Medical Journal,* 2002. 324(7338): p. 643-647.

[45] Montgomery, A.A., et al., Two decision aids for mode of delivery among women with previous caesarean section: randomsied controlled trial. *BMJ,* 2007. 334 (7607): p. 1305-1312.

[46] Brown, S. and J. Lumley, Satisfaction with care in labor and birth: a survey of 790 Australian women. *Birth,* 1994. 21(1): p. 4-13.

[47] Drew, N., P. Salmon, and L. Webb, Mothers', midwives' and obstetricians' views on the features of obstetric care which influence satisfaction with childbirth. *Br J Obstet Gynaecol,* 1989. 96(9): p. 1084-8.

[48] Association, M.C., Recommendations from Listening to Mothers: The First U.S Survey of Women's Childbearing Experiences. . *Birth,* 2004. 31: p. 61-65.

[49] Bekker, H., et al., Informed decision making: an annotated bibliography and systematic review. *Health Technology Assessment,* 1999. 3(1): p. 1-156.

[50] Edwards, A., et al., The effectiveness of one-to-one risk communication interventions in health care: a systematic review. *Medical Decision Making,* 2000. 20(3): p. 290-7.

[51] Royal College of Obstetricians and Gynaecologists. Recommendations arising from the 41st Study Group on Pain in Obstetrics and Gynaecology. 2002 [cited 2nd of Jan]; Available from: http://www.rcog.org.uk/study/rec_41st.htm.

[52] American College of Obstetricians and Gynecologists, ACOG committee opinion. Mode of term singleton breech delivery. Number 265, December 2001. American College of Obstetricians and Gynecologists. *International Journal of Gynaecology and Obstetrics,* 2002. 77(1): p. 65-6.

[53] Smith, C.A., et al., Complementary and alternative therapies for pain management in labour. Cochrane Database of Systematic Reviews 2006, Issue 4.

[54] Eddy, D.M., A manual for assessing health practices and designing practice policies: the explicit approach. 1992, Philadelphia: American College of Physicians.

[55] Shorten, A., et al., Making choices for childbirth: development and testing of a decision-aid for women who have experienced previous caesarean. *Patient Education and Counseling,* 2004. 52(3): p. 307-313.

[56] Personal communication via email. Between Dr. W .Otten and Dr. C. Raynes-Greenow, (Author). Sydney December 2007.

In: Pain Management: New Research   ISBN: 978-1-60456-767-0
Editors: P. S. Greco, F. M. Conti   © 2008 Nova Science Publishers, Inc.

Chapter XII

Maternal Non-Pharmacological Interventions for Neonatal Pain Relief: What Do We Need to Transform them into Action?

*Thaila C. Castral[*1], Fay Warnock[2], Carmen G.S. Scochi[3], and Adriana M. Leite[3]*

1. University of São Paulo at Ribeirão Preto College of Nursing, WHO Collaborating Centre for Nursing Research Development, Ribeirão Preto-SP, Brazil.
2. University of British Columbia – School of Nursing, Vancouver-BC, Canada
3. University of São Paulo at Ribeirão Preto College of Nursing – Department of Maternal-Child and Public Health, WHO Collaborating Centre for Nursing Research Development, Ribeirão Preto-SP, Brazil

Abstract

Over the past 27 years, investigations have benefited our understanding of pain in the rapidly developing newborn. We now understand that the infant's gestational age, gender, pain history and the quality of care provided by the infant's parents and healthcare professionals greatly influence the infant's pain response. Of the many factors investigated, maternal caregiving, long considered important to promoting infant development, is now beginning to emerge as an important study variable within the infant pain field. The purposes of this paper are to summarize findings of two maternal pain caregiving interventions (breastfeeding and maternal skin-to-skin contact) during infancy and to comment on issues related to their clinical implementation. We also discuss the benefits of enhanced inclusion of maternal caregiving as a direct study variable to further the comprehensive assessment and treatment of newborn (NB) pain. Currently, few newborn pain studies examine maternal caregiving effects during the NB

[*] Corresponding author: Thaila C Castral, University of Sao Paulo at Ribeirao Preto College of Nursing, Av. Bandeirantes 3900 Ribeirão Preto – SP, Brazil CEP: 14040-902. Phone: 55 – 16 – 36023411 (office) Fax number: 55 – 16 – 36333271 e-mail: thailacastral@usp.br.

period. There is some evidence that maternal behavior before and after a painful event results in less cry intensity and duration, easy recovery and self-regulation in full term infants. Most of those studies focused on older infants, they measured the infant's global rather than individual responses to intramuscular injection pain and only one examined pain recovery. Also evident, is the lack of investigation on maternal behavior on the behavioral and physiological response of the premature infant during the first month of life although studies have been conducted that include maternal skin-to-skin contact and breastfeeding to promote neonatal acute pain relieve during minor acute pain events. These particular forms of maternal caregiving have been recommended by international groups and associations to reduce infant pain reactivity and to facilitate recovery after pain event. However, no published data exists on the efficacy of both interventions with longer or repeated painful procedures. There is also a dearth of study on the effectiveness of combining maternal skin-to-skin with other pain treatments in the clinical setting. Moreover, there is a dearth of investigation that considers the perceptions of health professionals, the experiences and the mental health status of mothers for both interventions. While knowledge gaps exist in this still evolving field, clinicians must have access to existing research for judicious clinical application. Conceptual frameworks from knowledge transfer theory and collaborative interdisciplinary research may help facilitate the clinical use of these maternal non-pharmacological interventions for adequate neonatal pain relieve in many countries.

Introduction

Over the past 27 years, investigations have benefited our understanding of pain in the rapidly developing newborn. We now understand that the infant's gestational age [1], gender [2], pain history [1] and the quality of care provided by the infant's parents [3] and healthcare professionals [4] greatly influence infant pain reactivity. Of the many factors investigated, surprising little is known about maternal caregiving; a concept considered core to understanding infant stress regulation and neurodevelopment. The small collection of infant pain studies that have included the infant's mother have primarily been interventions focused on testing the pain relieving benefits of a variety of naturalistic forms of maternal care. Most of those studies have involved the preterm infant. To help determine the potential of maternal caregiving for furthering understanding and treatment of newborn pain, especially for preterm and fullterm newborns born at-risk, it is important to examine how this factor has been viewed within the associated fields of infant study and to examine findings associated with its current use within the infant pain setting. The purposes of this chapter are to (i) summarize findings of two maternal pain caregiving interventions (breastfeeding and skin-to-skin contact) during infancy, (ii) provide direction for the inclusion of maternal caregiving as a direct study variable to further the comprehensive assessment and treatment of newborn (NB) pain and, (iii) to comment on issues related to the clinical application of maternal breast feeding and skin-to-skin contact. The chapter concludes with a discussion of translational research as a useful framework to incorporate these interventions in the clinical setting to improve neonatal clinical pain management.

Maternal Caregiving and Newborn Stress Regulation

Early experiences and the quality of early care that infants receive can profoundly impact their later adaptive abilities and health. As the primary caregiver, the infant's mother plays a crucial role in mediating environmental and biological infant risk factors. While maternal caregiving is variable and multiply determined, the repertoire of behaviors and the relationship that the mother establishes with her infant is considered the single most powerful regulator of early infant stress, serving to strengthen and shape neuronal connections throughout the child's life [5]. This view stems from works of Bowlby [6] and is based on the belief that maternal care functions to promote infant survival where maternal touch or talk is stimulated through synchronous interaction between the mother and her baby rather than through the intentions or actions of the mother alone [7]. Through reciprocal mutual influence, the sensitivity and contingent responses of the mother serves as an external organizer for the infant thus providing the basis for secure attachment [5] and later ability to cope with everyday stressful events [8].

Maternal behavior thus stands as an important factor that influences neonatal biobehavioral regulation and is the key to enhance NB self-regulation skills. Infant ability to self regulate is a marker of an effective mother-baby bond and an indicator of good infant and maternal mental health. However, it seems that the mother must first regulate herself to successfully soothe her baby [9]. Presumably, maternal inability to regulate to stress may interfere with a mother's capacity to care for her infant and this may, in turn, hamper the function and development of the early maternal infant caregiving unit. If so, further research is required on the topic of maternal stress regulation so that maternal and infant health outcomes are optimized in this setting.

Neurobehavioral Capabilities of the Young Infant

During their first days of life, most NB show a variety of primitive behaviors (e.g. to take hand to mouth, to suck hand) that indicate self stress-regulatory soothing to stressful situations [10]. Ability to self-regulate, however, varies between infants. Babies who show lower threshold to aversive stimulus tend to exhibit irritability and difficulty in regulating to incoming sensory inputs. It is particularly these infants, who may benefit from the regulating properties of the maternal-infant caregiving relationship [11].

The Synactive Theory of Development provides the framework to conceptualize the organization of the neurobehavioral capabilities of the young infant. This model is based on the assumption that the infant actively communicates through his/her behavior thresholds for sensitivity and competence. Infant ability to regulate and control behavior emerges through an interdependent and interrelated process with the environment and is expressed through five systems (autonomic/physiology, motor, state, attention/interaction and self-regulation) [11-12].

The Newborn Individualized Developmental Care and Intervention Program - NIDCAP [11] is the most well know clinical assessment tool based on the synactive theory. The goal of the NIDCAP is to protect the fragile infant from sensory overload by systematically observing how the infant responds physiologically and behaviorally to their immediate environment. Clinicians use this knowledge to structure the environment and to deliver care in a manner that enhances infant stress regulation capacity [13]. The program integrates a neurodevelopmentally supportive, individualized, and family-centered framework resulting in a relationship-based care [14]. It helps to structure care provided to the infant in clusters and it provides the framework for developing strategies aimed to promote collaborative support between healthcare providers and parents and management of the neonatal unit environment (reduced noise and light). Of particular interest, NIDCAP capitalizes on the use of infant-parent bonding, non-nutritive suckling, breastfeeding and skin-to-skin care as an adjunct to pain management and to support clinical initiatives to promote infant self-regulation [15]. By regulation, we mean infant ability to not only respond effectively to pain/stress but also ability to achieve physiological and behavioral recovery after those exposures. This is important given the frequency of infant exposure to painful and stress inducing clinical procedures and the need to determine if and how the infant has recovered from them.

While clinically significant, the complex and multifaceted nature of the NIDCAP and issues related to data collection and analysis across studies has made it difficult to demonstrate its effectiveness statistically. For instance, in a systematic review on developmental care [16], inconsistency in the reporting of the benefits and costs plus short and long term outcomes associated with NIDCAP were reported. In some of the studies reviewed, positive associations were reported between NIDCAP and moderate-severe chronic lung disease and necrotizing enterocolitis, family stress and child perception. Conversely, other studies reported an increase in mild lung disease and in the length of stay in infants who received NIDCAP compared to controls. There was also very limited evidence of the long-term positive effects of NIDCAP on behavior and movement at 5 years corrected age. Discrepancy in findings across the studies was thought to be due to differences in the collection and measurement of data associated with the NIDCAP intervention. In their conclusion, the authors recommended improved methodology to strengthen evidence on the effectiveness of clinical interventions such as NIDCAP [16].

Maternal Caregiving and Infant Pain

The foregoing discussion makes it clear that maternal caregiving has a role to play in optimizing the neurodevelopment of fragile born infants. Currently, few infant pain studies include maternal caregiving as a direct study variable during the neonatal period, either in terms of its regulative or influencing properties. There is some evidence that maternal behavior before and after a painful event results in less cry intensity and duration, easy recovery and self-regulation in full term infants. A descriptive study, for example, found maternal touch was related to less cry intensity in infants at two and six months, whereas maternal distraction and/or caretaking (e.g. change diaper) increased cry duration. Another relevant outcome of this study was reduction in infant pain reactivity when mothers held /rocked and talked to their infants [17]. Other study reported maternal holding, touching and kissing of infant after intra-muscular injection resulted in faster quieting at three months and predicted increased behavioral quieting at five months [18]. Parent vocalization 30 seconds before a painful event, had a significant impact on their child pain scores (NFCS) during intra-muscular injection after controlling for gender, gestational age and previous pain experiences in infants aged four and six months [3]. Conversely, other study did not find correlation between maternal behavior and their infant's response and recovery from vaccination in two and six month's babies as measured by infant salivary cortisol [19]. A limitation of that study was the lack of concurrent analysis of maternal behavior.

In a very interesting approach of the Sociocommunication Model of the Infant Pain, the relative contribution of maternal factors on infant behavioral pain reactivity to routine immunization was examined [20]. Maternal judgment of their child pain was determined by the combination of infant's general display of negative behaviors (face, body and cry). Mothers who evaluated themselves as dismissive had infants who showed less significantly facial expressions in response to a painful event. Higher general psychological and lower identification levels with North American culture were identified as significant stressors on day after immunization procedure when mothers were asked to recall infants pain levels on the following day after procedure by telephone interview [20].

Notably, most of the foregoing studies focused on older infants (two up to six months), they measured the infant's global rather than individual pain response to intramuscular injection pain and only two studies measured pain scores throughout and after the procedure. Also obvious, is the lack of investigation on maternal behavior on the behavioral and physiological response of the premature infant during the first month of life.

Maternal Pain Care Interventions

Breastfeeding

The effectiveness of breastfeeding has been investigated as a naturalistic maternal infant pain caregiving intervention. A Cochrane systematic review [21], analyzed five randomized clinical trials that investigated the analgesic benefit of breastfeeding during heel prick [22-24] or venipuncture [25-26] in term newborns. Five other studies have also reported on the effects of breast-milk during heel lance [27-30] or venipuncture [31] in term newborns. It is interesting to note that only one of those studies also involved preterm newborns [27]. Main findings of the systematic review were that infants who were breastfed before and after undergoing heel lance or venipuncture showed statistical significant less increases in heart rate, less time crying (percentage time or total time) and lower pain scores (PIPP, DAN and composite score) [21]. Methodological shortcomings highlighted in that Cochrane systematic [21] included lack in using validated infant pain scales and marked heterogeneity between studies in terms of the breastfeeding treatment period and type of control intervention [21]. In most studies, breastfeeding started two or three minutes before the puncture and continued throughout the painful event [22, 25]. However, in one study, babies were not breastfed during the procedure [35] and in other; infants were breastfed 45 minutes before heel prick [26].

In a more recent study [32], full term NB who were breastfeed five minutes before, during and after PKU heel prick were also reported to recover faster than a non-breastfed NB control group. In that sudy, the breast fed NB's showed more signs of emotion regulation (suckling his/her hand, looking to his/her mother's breast) while their mothers presented more actions aimed at comforting their babies (rocking their babies, pronouncing phrases to comfort and stimulating their baby to suck her nipple) [33].

Another study also examined the analgesic effects of breastfeeding in combination with skin-to-skin during infant intramuscular injection. In that study, the sixty-six infants aged two to four months who were breastfed while in full skin-to-skin contact with their mother three minutes before, during and after their immunization exhibited significantly less pain cry compared to the control group. There was no statistical significance in heart rate or oxygen saturation changes during or after the injection [34]. It is important to note that this study did not include a specific pain measure.

Many studies have compared breastfeeding or breast-milk against other non-pharmacological interventions (sucrose/glucose, non-nutritive suckling and holding). In those studies, breastfeeding was found to be less effective [35] or as effective as sucrose/glucose [25] whereas it was found to be more effective than non-nutritive suckling and holding [23].

However, while sucrose and glucose may be interpreted as being more effective than breastfeeding in terms of statistical significance, breastfeeding may have stronger clinical utility and relevance. This is because breastfeeding is a naturalistic form of maternal pain care that provides the baby four maternal stress regulative properties: maternal odor [36], antinociceptive mechanism of milk, non-nutritive suckling [37] and mother-child contact [38]. Unlike sucrose and glucose delivered via oral (syringe or pipette), with breastfeeding the baby would be simulated to suck because of smelling maternal milk on their mother's breast. During breastfeeding, these infants would also be provided with the nociceptive benefits of breast milk as they receive nurturing care and experience pleasant tactile and sensory stimulation through the physical proximity, touch, holding and talk that their mother would provide them.

The clinical implementation of breastfeeding or breast-milk for minor pain procedures may also directly benefit the infant's mother contributing to overall cost benefits to the health care system [39]. Clinical programs supportive of breastfeeding may help encourage mothers to breastfeed their infants. This in turn may help facilitate bonding and allow the mother to spend more time with her infant and enable the mother to directly participate in the care of her infant. This may be important since complex care environments can easily dismiss or ignore the mother after the birth of the infant; a perinatal time period which is critically important to both maternal and infant health.

Better understanding of the complex mechanisms underlying breastfeeding and its analgesic and comfort properties could help to clarify the most appropriated procedure to implement into clinical practice. For example, in most of the reported comparative studies, breastfeeding or breast-milk was less than or as effective as sucrose for neonatal pain relief. However, taste receptors for sucrose and breast-milk may not all work at the same rate, leading to a delay in response for some solutions [35]. Animal studies have provided evidence that breast-milk release cholecystokinin and β-casomorphine implicating in a postabsorptive analgesic mechanism [40]. Results from the foregoing comparative animal study may suggest that breastfeeding should commence before and continue during and following the entire painful procedure so that it provides its full analgesic benefit.

The effectiveness of breastfeeding requires that it be tested in different infant populations and improvements in methodology are required in order to determine its potential as an effective adjunct to infant pain management. Breastfeeding has not been systematically studied in premature infants, nor has it been evaluated when infants undergo repeated painful procedures. There is marked heterogeneity of the current studies about breastfeeding which makes difficult establish its evidence level for pain relief and to draw a protocol from systematic reviews studies for standard clinical implementation.

Maternal Skin-to-Skin

Maternal skin-to-skin contact is another naturalistic form of maternal caregiving that has been reported to effectively reduce pain in the preterm NB [41-44] and the full term NB [45]. Effectiveness in those studies has been demonstrated on the basis of statistically significant decrease in facial action (NFCS and PIPP), sleep/awake state and cry, during and after heel prick. Only one of those studies found that pre-terms in the skin-to-skin condition had a statistically significant less increase in heart rate after heel prick [42]. Conversely, higher heart rate in the skin-to-skin condition was reported [44] and other studies did not find statistically significance differences between groups [41, 43, 45]. The finding of statistical significance on heart rate that was reported in only one study [42] could be explained on the basis of the longer time that babies spent in skin-to-skin (three hours before blood collection against 15 to 30 minutes in others). The extended period of time that infants in that study [42] spent with their mothers may have enabled the infants to regain stability in heart rate. However, for the most part, researchers agree that dissociation between behavioral and physiological measures is a common challenge. Progression in this area may require improvements in technology and protocols for collecting and measuring heart-rate especially for preterm infant populations [43]. The complex issue of dissociation is discussed in another paper which suggests that dissociations between these systems may be related to individual characteristics [46].

Prolonged analgesic effects of maternal skin-to-skin care were also found in thirty preterm infants [44]. Infants in the skin-to-skin condition showed less motor disorganized activity and extension movements during blood test and more organized sleep states after heel prick even though they were already resting in the crib during the twenty minutes follow-up. The findings reported in that study [44] are similar to those reported in a comparative animal study that investigated complex mechanisms involving analgesic effect and the putative contributions of maternal caregiving [47]. In that comparative study, authors found that rats placed in contact with their anesthethized dams, remained hypoalgesic longer than rats that continued to suckle, even when they were both receiving milk infusion through the posterior tongue cannula. Escape latencies in suckling rats had returned to baseline levels within one minute after milk letdown whereas contact escape latencies were endured at least five minutes [47]. On the basis of these findings, we suggest that skin-to-skin contact may have a residual quieting effect that provides better neurobehavioral state in follow-up period as showed in a previously mentioned study [44].

There is also evidence that maternal touch-based interventions (massage-like stroking) may induce oxytocinergic mechanisms resulting in acute antinoceptive effects in rats [48]. Further research is needed to investigate the involvement of inhibitory mechanisms and endorphins and if and how they relate to maternal pain caregiving interventions.

In addition to demonstrating nociceptive benefits, maternal infant skin-to-skin contact is natural, economical and simple to implement. Moreover, skin-to-skin contact has been shown to promote breastfeeding and the combinations of these two interventions in promoting maternal infant interaction and infant development are well documented. For example, in a Cochrane systematic review [49], seventeen studies were analyzed, involving 806 participants (mothers and babies). They found positive statistically significant association between early skin-to-skin contact and breastfeeding at one to three months post-birth. Breastfeeding duration was associated with increases in maternal affectionate love/touch. Maternal attachment behavior was associated with early skin-to-skin contact during breastfeeding within the first few days post-birth [49].

Additional infant benefits of skin-to-skin care are improved self-organization behavior through more quite sleep states and flexor movements [50], prevention of neonatal hypothermia [51] and stability of heart and respiratory function [52].

On the basis of the foregoing evidence, maternal skin-to-skin contact is now recommended as a non-pharmacological intervention to promote infant pain relief during minor acute pain procedures [53-54]. It is interesting to note, however, that no published data exists on the efficacy of maternal skin-to-skin with other types of painful procedures (intra-muscular injection, venipuncture, post-operative pain, suctioning) or with other individuals who may also serve as primary caregivers or that play a significant parenting or caregiving role (eg., fathers, siblings and healthcare provider). Maternal skin-to-skin care is a very proximal intervention between child-mother. Conducting more clinical studies to determine if skin-to-skin provided by caregivers other than the mother is essential as it may help broaden the use of the intervention. This is important given that the infant's mother may not be available and given the frequency of pain and stress inducing procedures that the ill full-term and preterm infant often undergo and their potential implications.

There is also a dearth of study on the effectiveness of combining maternal skin-to-skin with other pain treatments in the clinical setting. Combing maternal skin-to-skin with other non-pharmacological interventions (sucrose, glucose, maternal touch, breast-milk and music) may increase analgesic benefits for the baby. For example, maternal gentle touch may have additive effects that have not been investigated in skin-to-skin studies. It is possible that maternal gentle touch buffers and helps regulate the infant's response to the stressor of the pain stimulation. Enhancing our understanding of these potential effects may enable a more clear understanding of why the skin-to-skin is effective and may help guide the clinical development of comprehensive maternal infant pain treatment protocols.

Requirements for Further Research

While the evidence favors the use of breastfeeding and skin-to-skin for infant pain relief, the science remains incomplete. In addition to those already mentioned, there appears to be no studies that have examined the perceptions of health professionals or the experiences of mothers for either the breastfeeding or skin-to-skin intervention. For example, it is well known that maternal mental mood (depression and anxiety) diminishes maternal caregiving capacity and interferes with the functional regulatory role of maternal caregiving on NB stress regulation [55]. In a recent systematic observation study, mothers with history of depression (either treated or not treated with antidepressant medications) exhibited less responsiveness to their infant's pain cry than did a control group of non-depressed mothers [56]. Given the prevalence of perinatal depression, it is possible that alterations in maternal mental mood could serve as a potential confounder that may interfere with a mother's ability to engage in skin-to-skin. It is also possible that this may in turn reduce the effectiveness of the maternal pain caregiving intervention. We found no breastfeeding or skin-to-skin infant pain study that reported excluding mothers with history of mood alterations (eg., depression, anxiety) or if such maternal factors were controlled for during data analysis. Given their potential confounding effects, this information will need to be collected and clarified in future maternal pain caregiving intervention studies.

Transforming Current Evidence of Maternal Pain Care Interventions into Action

This paper has provided a brief overview of the effectiveness of two maternal caregiving interventions for NB pain relief. Despite best available evidence, improved options, and regulatory mandates, the pain management of neonates remains inadequate. One reason may be due to the ineffective translation of research data into clinical practice [57].

While knowledge gaps exist in this still evolving field, clinicians must have access to existing research for judicious clinical application. The act of linking research to action in clinical environments has raised many issues to be discussed among academics and clinicians.

A multidisciplinary approach to pain management in a neonatal unit [58] is now recommended. This would encompass a collaborative multi-center effort which is considered essential for translating and integrating research into best practice guidelines and clinical practice [58].

Several essential components have been identified as important for creating an effective collaborative group for changing practices. Change concepts can be based on the literature and empirical evidence; however, for sustained positive results to be achieved in clinical settings, it is important to demonstrate measurable improvement [57].

The knowledge creation model (Figure 1) proposed by Graham and colleagues [59] is a useful evidence-based practice framework to support changing practices initiatives. The knowledge creation process (knowledge tools, synthesis and inquiry) incorporates the major types of research that can be used in health care and the action cycle represents the steps that may be followed for knowledge application.

Currently, there are eleven systematic reviews of the literature on the Cochrane Library about neonatal pain management. Two of the reviews were already updated and give recommendations about the use of sucrose [60-62] for pain relieve and for venipuncture versus heel lance [63-65]. There is also one Cochrane review about breastfeeding and breast milk that has not been updated yet [21].

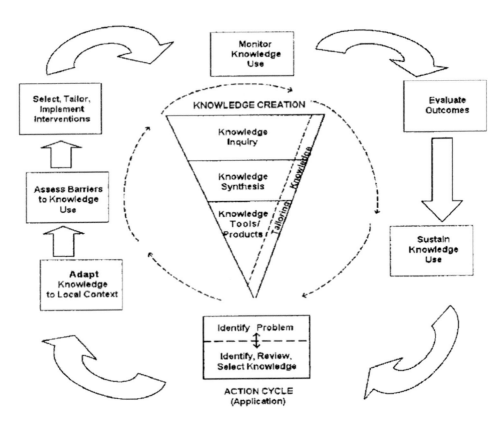

Figure 1- Knowledge to action process. In: Graham et al. Lost in knowledge translation: time for a map? *The Journal of Continuing Education in the Health Professions*, 2006 16, 13-24.

Systematic reviews about neonatal pain management published in paper-based journals [66-67], evidence-based guidelines [53-54, 68- 69] and policies [68, 70] are also already available in the literature. Workshops and web-sites that provide information about neonatal pain management have also been developed.

Notably, however, most of these knowledge sources are only accessible in high income countries. The lack of resources and infrastructure in low-income or developing countries raises the need for collaborative research within the developed world and direct attention to specific cultural, disease-related conditions and economical issues in these countries [71].

There is still a need to better understand how best to transfer knowledge on infant pain interventions to health professionals in the form of high quality systematic reviews, guidelines and policies of pain-relieving interventions for neonates, and the use of translational research to support evidence-based practice in clinical pain management. Conceptual frameworks from knowledge transfer theory and collaborative interdisciplinary research may help facilitate the clinical use of these maternal non-pharmacological interventions for adequate neonatal pain relieve in many countries. Free international electronic libraries access, inclusion of policy-makers, managers and health care professionals in the research planning and dissemination process, and developing practice guidelines considering local adaptations are some initiatives that should be encouraged.

Conclusion

In conclusion, maternal caregiving is an early form of experience and is crucial to infant development. There is evidence to support the use of maternal caregiving interventions for neonatal pain relief although there are many issues to be addressed in future studies. Breastfeeding and skin-to-skin contact, in particular, may have an advantage over current approaches to provide analgesia in the neonatal clinical setting. These naturalistic forms of maternal pain care may help promote the function and development of the maternal-infant caregiving relationship and facilitate infant-maternal and family attachment and care by professional caregivers working in complex care environments. Translational research is a promising area to support the use of these interventions on neonatal pain management.

Acknowledgments

The authors gratefully acknowledge the editor of Nova Science Publishers for the invitation for this chapter. TC Castral is supported by The State of São Paulo Research Foundation, F Warnock is granted by Michael Smith Scholar Award and CGS Scochi by The National Council for Scientific and Technological Development.

References

[1]   Grunau, RE; Oberlander, TF; Whitfield, MF; Fitzgerald, C; Lee, SK. Demographic and therapeutic determinants of pain reactivity in very low birth weight neonates at 32 weeks'postconceptional age. *Pediatrics*, 2001 107, 105-112.

[2]   Guinsburg, R; Peres, CA; Almeida, MFB; Balda, RCX; Bereguel, RC; Tonelotto, J. et al. Differences in pain expression between male and female newborn infants. *Pain*, 2000 85, 127-133.

[3]   Piira, T; Champion, GD; Bustos, T; Donnelly, N; Lui, K. Factors associated with infant pain response following an immunization injection. *Early Human Development*, 2007 83, 319-26.

[4]   Sweet, SD; McGrath, PJ; Symons, D. The roles of child reactivity and parenting in infant pain response. *Pain*, 1999 80, 655-661.

[5]   Schore, AN. Attachment and the regulation of the right brain. *Attachment and Human Development*, 2000 2, 23–47.

[6]   Bowlby, J. *Attachment and loss,* 2nd ed. New York: Basic Books; 1987.

[7]   Kopp CB. Antecedents of self-regulation: a developmental perspective. *Developmental Psychology*, 1982 18, 199-214.

[8]   Levine, S. The ontogeny of the hypothalamic-pituitary-adrenal axis: the influence of maternal factors. *Annals of the New York Academy of Sciences* 1994 746, 275–288.

[9]   Schore, AN. Attachment, affect regulation, and the developing right brain: linking developmental neuroscience to pediatrics. *Pediatrics in Review*, 2005 26, 204-13.

[10]   Brazelton, TB Early Intervention. What does it means? In: Fitzgerald, HE; Lester, BM; Yogman, MW. *Theory and research in behavioral pediatrics*. New York: Plenum Press, 1982.

[11]   Als, H; Lester, BM; Tronick, EZ; Brazelton, B. Toward a research instrument for the assessment of preterm infant's behavior (APIB). In: Fitzgerald, HE; Lester, BM; Yogman, MW. *Theory and research in behavioral pediatrics*. New York: Plenum Press; 1982.

[12]   Vanderberg, k. Individualized developmental care for high risk newborns in the NICU: a practice guideline. *Early Human Development*, 2007 83, 433-442.

[13]   Aita, M; Snider, L. The art of developmental care in the NICU: a concept analysis. *Journal of Advanced Nursing*, 2003 41, 223-232.

[14]   Als, H. NIDCAP Program Guide. Boston: NICAP Federation International; 2006.

[15]   Byers IF. Care and the evidence for their use in the NICU. Components of developmental. *MCN American Journal of Maternal and Child Nurse*, 2003 28, 175-80.

[16]   Symington, A; Pinelli, J. Developmental care for promoting development and preventing morbidity in preterm infants. *Cochrane Database of Systematic Reviews*, 2003 4, 1-55.

[17]   Jahromi, LB; Putmam, SP; Stifter, CA. Maternal regulation of infant reactivity from 2 to 6 months. *Developmental Psychology*, 2004 40, 477-487.

[18]   Axia, G; Bonichini, S. Are babies sensitive to the context of acute pain episodes? Infant distress and maternal soothing during immunization routines at 3 and 5 months of age. *Infant and Child Development*, 2005 14, 51-62.

[19]   Lewis, M; Ramsay, D. Effect of maternal soothing on infant stress response. *Child Development*, 1999 70, 11-20.

[20]   Pillai Riddell, RR; Stevens, BJ; Cohen, LL; Flora, BD; Greenberg, S. Predicting maternal and behavioral measures of infant pain: the relative contribution of maternal factors. *Pain,* 2007 133, 138-149.

[21]   Shah, PS; Aliwalas, LI; Shah, V. Breastfeeding or breast milk for procedural pain in neonates. *Cochrane Database Systematic Review*, 2006 19, 1-32. CD004950.

[22]   Gray, L; Miller, LW; Philipp, BL; Blass, E.M. Breastfeeding is analgesic in healthy newborns. *Pediatrics*, 109:590-593, 2002.

[23]   Phillips, RM; Chantry, CJ; Gallagher, MP. Analgesic effects of breast-feeding or pacifier use with maternal holding in term infants. *Ambul Pediatr*, 2005 5, 359-64.

[24] Shendurnikar, N; Gandhi, K. Analgesic effects of breastfeeding on heel lancing. *Indian Pediatrics*, 2005 42, 730-732.

[25] Carbajal, R; Veerapen, S; Couderc, S; Jugie, M; Ville, Y. Analgesic effect of breast feeding in term neonates: randomized controlled trial. *British Medical Journal*, 2003 320, 1-5.

[26] Gradin, M; Finnström, O; Schollin, J. Feeding and oral glucose-additive effects on pain reduction in newborns. *Early Human Development*, 2004 77, 57-65.

[27] Skogsdal, Y; Eriksson, M; Schollin, J. Analgesia in newborns given oral glucose. *Acta Paediatrica* 1997 86, 217-220.

[28] Bucher, HU; Baumgartner, R; Bucher, N; Seiler, M; Fauchere, JC. Artificial sweetener reduces nociceptive reaction in term newborn infants. *Early Human Development* 2000 59, 51-60.

[29] Blass EM, Miller LW. Effects of colostrum in newborn humans: dissociation between analgesic and cardiac effects. *Journal of Developmental and Behavioral Pediatrics* 2001 22, 385-390.

[30] Uyan, ZS; Ozek, E; Bilgen, H; Cebeci,D; Akman, I. Effect of foremilk and hindmilk on simple procedural pain in newborns. *Pediatrics International* 2005 47, 252-257.

[31] Upadhyay, A; Aggarwal, R; Narayan, S; Joshi, M; Paul, VK; Deorari, AK. Analgesic effect of expressed breast milk in procedural pain in term neonates: a randomized, placebo-controlled, double-blind trial. *Acta Paediatrica* 2004 93, 518-522.

[32] Leite, AM; Linhares, MBM; Lander, J; Castral, TC; Santos, CB; Scochi, CGS. Effects of breastfeeding on pain relief in full-term newborns [*under review*].

[33] Leite, AM; Linhares, MBM; Castral, TC; Scochi, CGS; Fonseca, LMM; Góes, FSN. [*abstract*] Effects of breastfeeding on maternal and neonatal behavioral during PKU test. *Pain Research and Management*, 2006 11(suppl B), 44B.

[34] Efe, E; Ozer, ZC. The use of breast-feeding for pain relief during neonatal immunization injections. *Applied Nursing Research*, 2007 20, 10–16.

[35] Bilgen, H; Ozek, E; Cebeci, D; Ors, R. Comparison of sucrose, expressed breast milk, and breast-feeding on the neonatal response to heel prick. *Journal of Pain* 2001 2, 301-305.

[36] Varendi, H; Ghistensson, K; Porter, R; Windberg, J. Soothing effect of amniotic fluid smell in newborn infants. *Early Human Development*, 1998 51, 47-55.

[37] Blass, EM; Shide, DJ. Endogenous cholescystokinin reduces vocalization in isolated 10-day-old rats. *Behavior Neuroscience*, 1993 107, 488-92.

[38] Blass, EM; Fillion, TJ; Weller, A; Brunson, L. Separation of opiod from nonopiod mediation of affect in neonatal rats: nonopioid mechanisms mediate maternal contact influences. *Behavior Neuroscience*, 1990 104, 625-36.

[39] Shah, PS; Aliwallas, LI; Shah, V. Breastfeeding or breast milk to alleviate procedural pain in neonates: a systematic review. *Breastfeeding Medicine, 2007* 2, 74-82.

[40] Blass, EM. Mothers and their infants: peptide-mediated physiological, behavioral and affective changes during suckling. *Regulatory Peptides*, 1996 66,109-112.

[41] Johnston, CC; Stevens, B; Pinelli, J; Gibbins, S; Fillion, F; Jack, A. et al. A. Kangaroo care is effective in diminishing pain response in preterm neonates. *Archives of Pediatrics and Adolescent Medicine*, 2003 157, 1084-088.

[42] Ludington-Hoe, SM; Hosseini, R; Torowiez, DL. Skin-to-skin contact (kangaroo Care) analgesia for preterm infant heel stick. *AACN Clinical Issues*, 2005 16, 373-87.

[43] Castral, TC; Warnock, F; Leite, AM; Haas, V; Scochi, CGS. The effects of skin-to-skin contact during acute pain in pre-term newborns. *European Journal of Pain* 2007 [*in press*].

[44] Ferber, SG; Makhoul, IR. Neurobehavioural assessment of skin-to-skin effects on reaction to pain in preterm infants: a randomized, controlled within-subject trial. *Acta Paediatrica*, 2008 97, 171-176.

[45] Gray, L; Watt, L; Blass, EM. Skin-to-skin contact is analgesic in healthy newborns. *Pediatrics*, 2000 105, 1-6.

[46] Barr, RG. Reflections on measuring pain in infants: dissociation in responsive systems and "honest signaling". *Archives of Disease inCchildhood. Fetal and Neonatal Edition* 1998 79, 152-156.

[47] Blass, EM. Interactions between contact and chemosensory mechanisms in pain modulation in 10-day-old rats. *Behavioral Neuroscience*, 1997 111, 147-154.

[48] Lund, I; Yu, L; Uvnas-Moberg, K; Wang, J; Yu, C; Kurosawa, M; Agren, G; Rose, A; Lekman, M; Lundeberg, T. Repeated massage-like stimulation induces long-term effects on nociception: contribution of oxytocinergic mechanisms. *European Journal of Neuroscience*, 2002 16, 330-338.

[49] Anderson, GC; Moore, E; Hepworth, J; Bergman, N. Early skin-to-skin contact for mothers and their healthy newborn infants. *Cochrane Database of Systematic Reviews*, 2005 3, 1-53.

[50] Ferber, SG; Makhoul, IR. The effect of skin-to-skin contact (Kangaroo Care) shortly after birth on the neurobehavioral responses of the term newborn: a randomized, controlled trial. *Pediatrics*, 2004 113, 858-865.

[51] Galligan, M. Skin-to-skin treatment of neonatal hypothermia. *MCN American Journal of Maternal and Child Nurse*, 2006 31, 298-304.

[52] Lundington-Hoe, SM; Sminth, J. Developmental aspects of kangaroo care. *Journal of Obstetric, Gynecologic, and Neonatal Nursing*, 1996 25, 671-703.

[53] Anand, KJS; Dphil, MBBS; The International Evidenced-Based Group for Neonatal Pain. Consensus statement for prevention and management of pain in the newborn. *Archives of Pediatric and Adolescent Medicine*, 2001 155, 173-181.

[54] Anand, KJS; Aranda, JV; Berde, CB; Buckman, S; Capparelli, EV; Carlo, W. et al. Summary proceedings from the Neonatal Pain-Control Group. *Pediatrics*, 2006 117, 9-22.

[55] Gunnar, MR; Vazquez, DM. Stress neurobiology and developmental psychopathology. In: Cicchetti, D; Cohen, D. *Developmental psychopathology: Developmental neuroscience*. 2nd ed., New York: Wiley; 2006.

[56] Warnock, F; Bakeman, R; Oberlander, TF; Shearer, K; Misri, S. Caregiving behavior and interactions of depressed mothers (antidepressant treated and non-antidepressant treated) during newborn acute pain [*under review*].

[57] Sharek, PJ; Powers, R; Koehn, A; Anand, KJS. Evaluation and development of potentially better practices to improve pain management of neonates. *Pediatrics*, 2006 118, S78-S86.

[58] Golianu, B; Krane, E; Seybold, J; Almgren, C; Anand, KJS; DPhil, MBBS. Non-pharmacological techniques for pain management in neonates. *Seminars in Perinatology*, 2007 31, 318-322.

[59] Graham, ID; Logan, J; Harrison, MB; Straus, SE; Tetroe, J; Caswell, W. et al. Lost in knowledge translation: time for a map? *The Journal of Continuing Education in the Health Professions*, 2006 16, 13-24.

[60] Stevens B, Ohlsson A Sucrose for analgesia in newborn infants undergoing painful procedures. *Cochrane Database of Systematic Reviews*, 2:CD001069, 2000.

[61] Stevens, B; Yamada, J; Ohlsson, A. Sucrose for analgesia in newborn infants undergoing painful procedures. *Cochrane Database of Systematic Reviews*, 2001 4, CD001069.

[62] Stevens, B; Yamada, J; Ohlsson, A. Sucrose for analgesia in newborn infants undergoing painful procedures (Review), *Cochrane Database of Systematic Reviews*, 2004 3, CD001069.

[63] Shah, V; Ohlsson, A. Venepuncture versus heel lance for blood sampling in term neonates. *Cochrane Database Systematic Review*, 2001 2, CD001069.

[64] Shah, V; Ohlsson, A. Venepuncture versus heel lance for blood sampling in term neonates. *Cochrane Database Systematic Review*, 2004 2, CD001452.

[65] Shah, V; Ohlsson, A. Venepuncture versus heel lance for blood sampling in term neonates. *Cochrane Database Systematic Review*, 2007 17, CD001452.

[66] Gaspardo, CM; Linhares, MBM; Martinez, FE. The efficacy of sucrose for the relief of pain in neonates: a systematic review of the literature. *Jornal de Pediatria*, 2005 8, 435-42.

[67] Cignacco, E; Hamers, JPH; Stoffel, L; van Lingen, RA; Gessler, P; Mcdougall, J. et al. The efficacy of non-pharmacological interventions in the management of procedural pain in the preterm and term neonates. A systematic literature review. *European Journal of Pain*, 2007 11, 139-52.

[68] American Academy of Pediatrics, Canadian Pain Society. Prevention and Management of Pain in the neonate: an update. *Pediatrics*, 2006 118, 2231-2241.

[69] Lefrak, L; Rheta, C; Knoerlein, K; DeNolf, N; Duncan, J; Hampton, F. et al. Sucrose analgesia: identifying potential better practices. *Pediatrics*, 2006 118, S197-S202.

[70] Morash, D; Fowler, K. An evidence-based approach to changing practice: using sucrose for infant analgesia. *Journal of Pediatric Nursing*, 2004 19, 366-370.

[71] Abertyn, R; van Dijk, M; Tibboel, D; Liefde, I; Bosenberg, AT; Rode, H et al. Infant pain in developing countries: a South African perspective. In: Anand, KJS; Stevens, BJ; McGrath, PJ. *Pain in neonates and infants*. 3rd ed. Philadelphia: Elsevier; 2007.

In: Pain Management: New Research   ISBN: 978-1-60456-767-0
Editors: P. S. Greco, F. M. Conti   © 2008 Nova Science Publishers, Inc.

Chapter XIII

Clinical Staff Perceptions of the Treatment of Procedural Pain in Neonates: Exploring a Change Process

Randi Dovland Andersen [1], Alf Meberg [2], Lars Wallin [3,4], and Leena Jylli [3,5]

[1]Department of Pediatrics, Telemark Hospital, Skien, Norway
[2]Department of Pediatrics, Vestfold Hospital, Tonsberg, Norway
[3]Department of Neurobiology, Care Sciences and Society, Division of Nursing, Karolinska Institutet, Stockholm, Sweden
[4]Clinical Research Utilization (CRU), Karolinska University Hospital, Stockholm, Sweden
[5]Acute Pain Treatment Service, Astrid Lindgren Children's Hospital, Karolinska University Hospital, Stockholm, Sweden

Abstract

Background

The gap between scientific knowledge and clinical practice is a major challenge in neonatal pain management. The aim of this study was to describe the perceptions of physicians and nurses regarding the treatment of procedural pain in neonates two years after they had been exposed to new pain-management strategies, and how their perceptions changed over the period.

Materials and methods

The study population consisted of physicians and nurses in two neonatal intensive care units in southern Norway. A multifaceted approach to changing practice was evaluated. It comprised the establishment of multiprofessional groups, the active support of leaders and the senior neonatologists at both study-sites, facilitation, education, and the introduction of evidence-based guidelines and procedures for blood collection. Data were collected before (2003) and after (2005) the intervention, with a questionnaire. Ten commonly performed procedures were assessed. The response rates were 79% and 73%, respectively.

Results

Although the answers of both the nurses and physicians indicated a slight increase in the use of pharmacological agents, they also displayed a persisting significant difference between what clinicians believe to be the current and optimal treatment for procedural pain. Only the nurses' answers indicated a change in their views about procedure painfulness, the current use of comfort measures, and the optimal treatment of pain. These changes have not diminished the differences between the views of nurses and physicians concerning procedure painfulness and the treatment of procedural pain.

Conclusions

Despite the use of a multifaceted intervention to support evidence-based practice, pharmacological agents and comfort measures appear to be underutilized in the treatment of procedural pain in neonates. Pharmacological treatments for procedural pain might have improved, but the overall results point clearly to difficulties in applying evidence to practice.

Background

One of the major challenges in neonatal pain management is the persistent gap between scientific knowledge and clinical practice [1]. The dissemination of scientific knowledge into clinical practice takes time, but a lack of knowledge alone cannot explain the discrepancy between available evidence and practice. Studies have shown that although knowledge can be well developed and appropriate, clinical practice does not change accordingly [2-4]. Therefore, it is necessary to explore how scientific knowledge about neonatal pain management can be implemented in clinical practice.

Social Context of Neonatal Pain

In the past, most clinicians have believed that neonates are unable to feel or respond to pain [5]. The scientific work of Anand and changes in public opinion caused by parental lobbying contributed to a new perspective on infant pain in the late 1980s [6]. At that time, the standard procedures for infant surgery involved minimal (muscle relaxants and nitrous oxide) or no (muscle relaxants and oxygen) anesthesia. In a series of studies, Anand and colleagues demonstrated that this practice lead to an increase in mortality and morbidity compared with cases where infants also received fentanyl during surgery [7-11]. This groundbreaking work was followed by a significant increase in the scientific knowledge regarding pain in neonates [12]. During the same period, continuous advances in perinatal care resulted in not only increased survival rates for prematurely born infants but also an increased use of invasive and often painful procedures [13-16]. The procedure performed most often in neonates is the heel stick for blood sampling [13-15]. Other common procedures are tracheal suctioning, the insertion of a gavage tube, the insertion of a peripheral intravenous line, endotracheal intubation, and intramuscular injection [16-18]. Different procedures cause varying levels of pain, related to their invasiveness [19, 20].

In 2001, the first international guidelines for the assessment and management of neonatal pain were published [17]. They served as a starting point for the development of locally adapted guidelines. Two different studies have shown the more frequent use of pharmacologic agents in neonatal intensive care units (NICUs) with the use of guidelines [21, 22]. However, despite the scientific advances over the past decades, pain in neonates is still poorly treated. Several studies have demonstrated a failure to treat pain in neonates efficiently, even for the most painful procedures [3, 14, 16, 21, 23-25].

Consequences of Untreated Pain in the Neonatal Period

All neonates have the functional capacity to experience pain at birth, but their nervous systems are still immature. This causes a prolonged and enhanced pain experience compared with that of older children or adults and makes neonates more vulnerable to the deleterious effects of pain [26, 27]. Their pain modulation systems are not fully developed and functional [26]. Pain consumes energy needed for growth and development, and disturbs infant homeostasis, which can result in instability in their blood pressure and heart rate, increases in oxygen consumption and stress hormones, and changes in sleep-wake-cycles, nutrition and their ability to be comforted [28]. Rapid changes in blood pressure are followed by changes in intracranial pressure, which increase the risk of intracranial bleeding and neurological damage [29]. Pain in the neonatal period may alter pain perception later in life [30, 31]. Reviewing the available evidence, Grunau concluded that early pain may have a substantial effect on later cognitive, social, and emotional functioning [32]. The need to narrow the knowledge-practice gap is obvious because unrelieved pain results in unnecessary and potentially persistent suffering for individual children.

Pain Assessment in Neonates

The assessment of pain is the cornerstone of efficient pain management [28]. The subjective nature of pain makes it impossible to understand fully the suffering of another person. Assessing pain in neonates remains a great challenge because this group of patients cannot express their pain verbally [33]. Behavioral changes can be viewed as an infantile form of self-report [34]. The implementation and sustained use of structured pain-assessment tools can improve infant pain assessment and management [35]. Studies have shown a deficiency in the use of structured pain-assessment measures in NICUs [21, 24, 25]. Instead, clinicians observe infant behavior and physiological parameters, identify signs of pain, and use these observations and their knowledge to determine whether infants are in pain and whether they require pain treatment [34]. Studies have shown that clinicians underestimate the magnitude and severity of pain in children [36, 37]. There is no reason to believe that this phenomenon is different in the assessment of neonatal pain.

Neonatal Pain Management

Shielding the neonate from light, sounds and unnecessary handling and procedures can efficiently prevent pain and/or stress. If a procedure, such as blood sampling, is necessary, pain can be lessened by choosing the least painful method. The recently updated Cochrane review documented that venous punctures are less painful than heel sticks [38]. Comfort measures are the foundation for all pain management [39] and include, among others, sweet tasting solutions [40], nonnutritive sucking [41], and facilitated tucking [42, 43]. Although each measure can relieve pain and discomfort in neonates to a certain degree, a combination of several measures is more effective [44]. Comfort measures have little effect without a person reassuring the baby during the procedure [45]. To achieve optimal pain relief, it is recommended that comfort measures be combined with analgesics because a multifaceted intervention is thought to have additive or synergistic effects [39]. Opioids, paracetamol (acetaminophen), and local anesthetics are the most commonly used analgesics in the treatment of neonatal pain [18].

Current Knowledge on the Implementation of Change and Knowledge Translation

Implementation research, or knowledge translation (i.e., research into how to apply evidence to practice), is an emerging field in health care science [46, 47]. It is certainly not a new idea. The use of research has been on the health care agenda for a long time but has received greater prominence only in the last two decades. It is a research field with significance for all health care professionals and has immense global implications [48]. In a widely cited report based on data from the USA and the Netherlands, Grol and Grimshaw [49] reported that 30%-40% of all patients do not receive health care based on current relevant knowledge and that as many as 20%-25% of all patients receive harmful or unnecessary care. The World Health Organization (WHO) has realized the serious nature of this situation, stating "stronger emphasis should be placed on translating knowledge into action to improve public health by bridging the gap of what is known and what is actually done" [50, p. V]. Neonatal pain management is a clinical area with great potential for improvement if available knowledge is put into action.

Several systematic reviews have been published on interventions intended to change practitioners' behaviour [49, 51-53]. A range of implementation interventions appear to be useful, although at present, it is not feasible to recommend a particular intervention to support implementation in a specific setting [52]. A limitation of these reviews is their focus on studies on medical practice and outcomes linked to physician performance. Evidence of the effectiveness of strategies that change nursing practice is largely lacking [54]. Two issues currently receiving much attention in the knowledge translation field are the need for theory to guide implementation research [55, 56] and the influence of individual and contextual factors on the implementation of change [57]. A principal argument for the use of theory is the need to gain a fuller understanding of a range of factors at different levels, which interact to determine whether and to what extent an implementation intervention results in change

[58]. According to social learning theory, human behavior can be changed by changing the context in which the behavior occurs. The experience of rewards or unfavorable results plays an important role in shaping behavior, together with cognitive processes. Learning often occurs by observation or imitation [59]. Social influence may be normative or informal. It is normative when the group provides a frame of reference in which its members can evaluate their own behavior against the norms of the group, and informal when the group is a source of new knowledge and information [59]. The influence of individual factors has been investigated extensively [60], and it appears that the difficulties in implementing evidence might be explained largely in terms of contextual influences. Proving that an intervention works in one setting does not necessarily mean it will work in a different context [61, 62]. Factors frequently described as influencing the success or failure of a process of change include leadership, resources, time, support functions, staff development, interpersonal relationships, job pressures, and organizational culture and climate [63, 64].

Rationale of this Study

When this study was planned, little systematic work had been done on the implementation of change in the field of neonatal pain management. In 1993 and again in 2002, McGrath and Unruh [6, 65] described change as a social process, stating that social influence is a necessary prerequisite for change, together with scientific and technical knowledge. Based on their ideas and social learning theory [59], the following premises underlying the change of practice in this study were outlined. Knowledge is a necessary but not sufficient prerequisite for change and must be disseminated and made available to all members of the group. Clinical practice is influenced by both individual and social/contextual factors, and a strategy to change clinical practice must target both. Multiprofessional interventions are necessary; no health profession can adequately manage pain alone.

Clinicians' perceptions of the treatment of procedural pain in neonates have been described previously [3]. Those findings indicated that clinical practice was not in accordance with international [17] and Swedish national guidelines [66]. An intervention was planned and implemented based on the premises described above. The aim of this chapter is to describe the perceptions of physicians and nurses in two NICUs of the treatment of procedural pain in neonates, two years after the implementation of new pain management strategies, and how perceptions changed over the study period.

We hypothesized that the respondents' answers would indicate:

- an increase in the use of both pharmacological agents and comfort measures,
- a diminished gap between their perceptions regarding current and optimal treatments of neonatal pain, and
- increased homogeneity in the perceptions of nurses and physicians.

The results will be discussed in relation to recent research and knowledge concerning the implementation of change. Some of the areas requiring further research will be outlined.

Materials and Methods

Subjects and Setting

Physicians and nurses working in two NICUs in southern Norway was eligible for the study (N=92). Table 1 shows the characteristics of the sample.

In 2003, 73 questionnaires were completed. The response rate was 79%. Seven persons (members of the project groups, including the project manager) were excluded because of previous knowledge of the questionnaire, and 12 were not present when the survey was conducted. In 2005, 67 questionnaires were completed, a response rate of 73%. The project manager was excluded from the sample, and 24 members of staff were not present when the survey was conducted.

Instrument

The data collection was based on a questionnaire [23], which consisted of a series of questions on pain and pain management with reference to 12 procedures frequently performed in neonates. In our study, 10 of the procedures were included (table 2). Circumcision and arterial or venous cutdown were excluded because these procedures were not performed in the units being studied. The responses were in a Likert-scale format, ranging from 0 to 4, and the participants were asked to grade the painfulness of the 10 procedures, the frequencies of the current use of pharmacological agents and comfort measures, and the optimal use of such measures (table 2).

Definitions

- Procedure: A therapeutic or diagnostic intervention carried out in neonates by health personnel.
- Pharmacological agents: Paracetamol (acetaminophen), opioids and/or local anesthetics.
- Comfort measures: Containment and support during a procedure, reduction of stimuli, nonnutritive sucking, sweet-tasting solutions, warming of heel before a heel stick, and others.
- Procedure painfulness: The painfulness of each procedure, rated by the respondent on a five-item ordinal scale from "not painful" to "very painful".
- Current use of pharmacological agents/comfort measures: How often the respondent believed that each procedure was performed with pharmacological agents/comfort measures, rated on a five-item ordinal scale from "never" to "always".
- Optimal use of pharmacological agents/comfort measures: How often the respondent believed that each procedure should be performed with pharmacological agents/comfort measures, on a five-item ordinal scale from "never" to "always".

Table 1. Demographic Characteristics of the sample

	2003	2005	*P* value
Number of respondents and percentage of total population (N=92)	73 (79)	67 (73)	
Hospital I, n (%)	38 (52)	33 (49)	
Hospital II, n (%)	35 (48)	34 (51)	0.866
Physicians, n (%)	20 (27)	17 (25)	
Nurses, n (%)	53 (73)	50 (75)	0.849
Senior pediatricians (n) and % of total number of pediatricians	11 (55)	8 (47)	0.746
Specialist nurses (n) and % of total number of nurses	13 (25)	16 (32)	0.511
Nurses participated in the external competence program (n) and % of total number of nurses	21 (40)	39 (78)	0.001*
Age (mean ±SD) in years	39,6 ± 8,2	42,1 ± 10,4	0.116
Female, n (%)	59 (81)	52 (78)	0.680
Experience > 12 years, n (%)	29 (40)	30 (45)	0.699

Procedures

The respondents received information about the study before the completion of the questionnaire. Data were collected during staff meetings before (2003) and after (2005) the intervention. A multifaceted intervention was designed, based on the premises described above. The intervention included the establishment of multiprofessional groups, active support from leaders and the senior neonatologists at both study sites, facilitation, education, and the implementation of evidence-based guidelines and procedures for blood collection. A multi professional project group (physician, nurse and nurse assistant) was established at each hospital. These groups worked with the implementation of the guidelines and the new procedure for blood collection at each work place but met regularly during the intervention period to discuss progress and problems. The management of both pediatric departments supported their participation in the project and provided the initial funding. The leaders encouraged the staff to support and participate in the change process. The senior neonatologist at both NICUs approved the medical content of the intervention. The project manager and the members of the project groups performed their daily work in the units, acted as role models regarding pain management, and supported colleagues when various pain management issues arose. Members of the project groups were given time during working hours for meetings and to work on project issues.

Education included one-day neonatal pain-management seminars and half-day seminars on implementing change, personal and organizational reactions to change, and the change process. The content of the pain-management seminars was based on the new guidelines, including the development, anatomy and physiology of the pain system, the consequences of pain, pain assessment, pharmacological treatments, and environmental and behavioral pain-management strategies.

Table 2. Infant Pain Questionnaire

The following procedures were evaluated.

INTU	Endotracheal intubation
TUBE	Insertion of chest tube
GAV	Insertion of gavage tube
SUCT	Tracheal suctioning
LP	Lumbar puncture
SHOT	Intramuscular injection
UAC	Insertion of umbilical catheter
PIV	Insertion of peripheral intravenous line
STK	Heel stick
RAC	Insertion of radial or tibial arterial catheter

Questions
1) Rate the painfulness of each procedure.
2) Rate how often you believe each procedure is performed with pharmacological agents (e.g., paracetamol, opioids and/or local anesthetics).
3) Rate how often you believe each procedure is performed with comfort measures (e.g., containment and support during the procedure, reduction of stimuli, nonnutritive sucking, sweet-tasting solutions, warming of the heel before a heel stick, or others).
4) Rate how often you believe each procedure should be performed with pharmacological agents.
5) Rate how often you believe each procedure should be performed with comfort measures.

Questions were answered by the clinical staff according to the following scales.

Question 1	Questions 2-5
0 = not painful	0 = never
1 = somewhat painful	1 = rarely
2 = moderately painful	2 = often
3 = quite painful	3 = usually
4 = very painful	4 = always

Members of the project group conducted *ad hoc* bedside teaching concerning pain assessment, pain management, and venous blood sampling, as needed during the intervention period.

Local, evidence-based guidelines were developed, containing information on pain in neonates, pain assessment, and pain management with pharmacological agents and comfort measures, was developed. The guidelines were based on international [17] and Swedish national guidelines [66] and were implemented in both units after the completion of the neonatal pain seminars.

A new procedure for blood collection replaced heel-stick with venous blood sampling. All nursing staff were taught to perform venous blood sampling. By the end of the intervention period, almost all members of the nursing staff had mastered the new procedure. Ethical approval was obtained from the Regional Ethics Committee in southern Norway.

Statistical Analyses

Background variables for the two time points were compared using the χ^2 test, except for variable age (t test). The respondents were sorted into groups based on profession, and data for the two time points analyzed separately using the Mann-Whitney U test. The scores for current and optimal treatments of procedural pain were compared using the Wilcoxon paired-groups test. The results for the two time points were then compared for each question and procedure, with the Mann-Whitney U test. When a significant difference was detected, respondents were divided into subgroups based on profession and a *post hoc* test was performed. For each respondent, a mean score for each series of questions was calculated and the effects of time (before and after the intervention) and profession (nurse *vs* physician) were assessed using the Mann-Whitney U test. P ≤ 0.05 was considered statistically significant.

Results

The only significant change in the demographic variables was the number of nurses who participated in an external competence program (table 1).

Procedure Painfulness

A significant change in the respondents' perception of procedure painfulness was observed for 4/10 procedures (Figure 1). Only the nurses changed their views, considering the insertion of a chest tube ($P = 0.006$) and the heel stick ($P = 0.039$) more painful, and the insertion of a peripheral intravenous line ($P = 0.015$) and the insertion of an umbilical catheter ($P = 0.001$) less painful. There were no significant changes in physicians' answers between the two measurement events. In general, the physicians ascribed lower pain scores (mean 2.46 ± 0.43) to the different procedures than those ascribed by the nurses (mean 2.75 ± 0.39; $P = 0.030$).

Current Use of Pharmacological Agents

Although the respondents described an infrequent use of pharmacological agents for most procedures on both measurement occasions, a tendency to the increased use for several procedures was observed. The increase was significant for several procedures: the insertion of a chest tube, insertion of lumbar puncture, insertion of a peripheral intravenous line, insertion of radial or tibial arterial catheter, and tracheal suctioning (Figure 2).

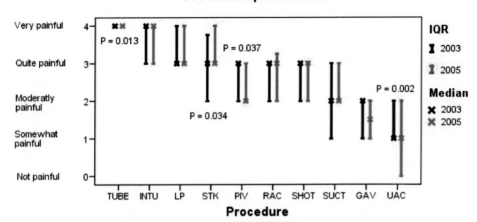

TUBE=insertion of chest tube, INTU=endotracheal intubation, LP=lumbar puncture, STK=heel stick, PIV=insertion of peripheral intravenous line, RAC=insertion of radial or tibial arterial catheter, SHOT=intramuscular injection, SUCT=tracheal suctioning, GAV=insertion of gavage tube and UAC=insertion of umbilical catheter.

Medians and interquartile ranges (IQR) of physicians' and nurses' answers in 2003 (N=73) and 2005 (N=67)

Figure 1.

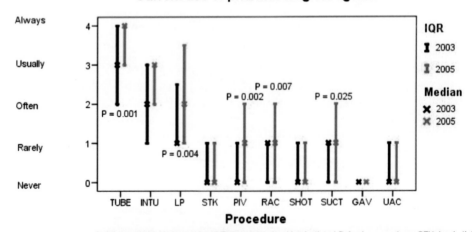

TUBE=insertion of chest tube, INTU=endotracheal intubation, LP=lumbar puncture, STK=heel stick, PIV=insertion of peripheral intravenous line, RAC=insertion of radial or tibial arterial catheter, SHOT=intramuscular injection, SUCT=tracheal suctioning, GAV=insertion of gavage tube and UAC=insertion of umbilical catheter.

Medians and interquartile ranges (IQR) of physicians' and nurses' answers in 2003 (N=73) and 2005 (N=67).

Figure 2.

Table 3. Current use of pharmacological agents. Results for subgroups (physicians and nurses). Presented as medians and interquartile ranges (IQR). Statistical comparisons made with Mann-Whitney U test. Only procedures where a significant difference for the whole group was found are presented.

| Procedure | Physicians | | | | Nurses | | | | P values | |
| | 2003 | | 2005 | | 2003 | | 2005 | | Subgroups | |
	Median	IQR	Median	IQR	Median	IQR	Median	IQR	Physicians	Nurses
TUBE	3	2-4	4	3-4	3	2-4	4	3-4	0.056	0.005*
LP	1	0-2	2	2-3	1	1-3	2,5	1-4	0.004*	0.075
PIV	0,5	0-1	1	1-2	0	0-1	1	0-1	0.052	0.013*
RAC	1	0-1	2	1-3	1	0-1	1	0-2	0.008*	0.076
SUCT	0	0-1	1	0-2	1	0-1	1	0-3	0.081	0.118

* significant difference, IQR=Interquartile range
TUBE=insertion of chest tube, LP=Lumbar puncture, PIV=insertion of peripheral intravenous line, RAC=insertion of radial or tibial arterial catheter, SUCT=tracheal suctioning

Nurses' and physicians' scores tended to change in the same direction, although the changes were significant for only one of the subgroups for each procedure (table 3).

Optimal Use of Pharmacological Agents

The answers regarding the optimal use of pharmacological agents were in accordance with the respondents' ratings of procedure painfulness. The respondents would use pharmacological agents most frequent for those procedures with the highest ratings for pain, except the heel stick (Figure 3). The nurses' answers pointed to a less frequent optimal use of pharmacological agents than had been previously indicated for several procedures: heel stick ($P = 0.001$), insertion of a gavage tube ($P = 0.002$), and insertion of an umbilical catheter ($P = 0.001$). Physicians' perceptions did not change between the two time points.

Current Use of Comfort Measures

The respondents' scores concerning the current use of comfort measures exceeded "often" (median ≥ 2) for all procedures, except intubation (Figure 4). In general, there was a significant difference between the perceptions of the nurses and those of the physicians ($P = 0.020$). Whereas the nurses' answers indicated an increased use of comfort measures during the heel stick ($P = 0.034$), and the insertion of a gavage tube ($P = 0.001$), there were no significant changes in physicians' answers. The nurses rated the current use of comfort measures (mean 2.44 ± 0.74) significantly higher than did the physicians (mean 1.95 ± 0.76; $P = 0.012$).

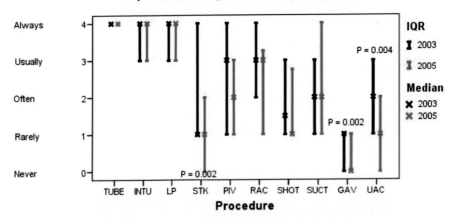

TUBE=insertion of chest tube, INTU=endotracheal intubation, LP=lumbar puncture, STK=heel stick,
PIV=insertion of peripheral intravenous line, RAC=insertion of radial or tibial arterial catheter,
SHOT=intramuscular injection, SUCT=tracheal suctioning, GAV=insertion of gavage tube and
UAC=insertion of umbilical catheter.

Medians and interquartile ranges (IQR) of physicians' and nurses' answers in 2003 (N=73) and 2005
(N=67).

Figure 3.

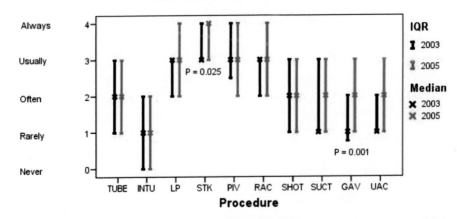

TUBE=insertion of chest tube, INTU=endotracheal intubation, LP=lumbar puncture, STK=heel stick,
PIV=insertion of peripheral intravenous line, RAC=insertion of radial or tibial arterial catheter,
SHOT=intramuscular injection, SUCT=tracheal suctioning, GAV=insertion of gavage tube and
UAC=insertion of umbilical catheter.

Medians and interquartile ranges (IQR) of physicians' and nurses' answers in 2003 (N=73) and 2005
(N=67).

Figure 4.

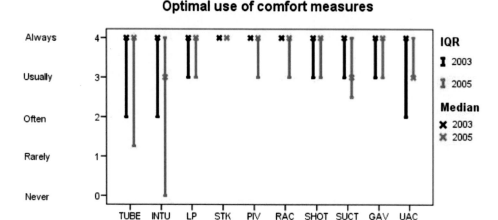

Optimal use of comfort measures

TUBE=insertion of chest tube, INTU=endotracheal intubation, LP=lumbar puncture, STK=heel stick, PIV=insertion of peripheral intravenous line, RAC=insertion of radial or tibial arterial catheter, SHOT=intramuscular injection, SUCT=tracheal suctioning, GAV=insertion of gavage tube and UAC=insertion of umbilical catheter.

Medians and interquartile ranges (IQR) of physicians' and nurses' answers in 2003 (N=73) and 2005 (N=67).

Figure 5.

Optimal Use of Comfort Measures

Both physicians and nurses expressed the perception that comfort measures should be used more frequently than they are currently used, but the nurses rated the optimal use of comfort (mean 3.34 ± 0.85) significantly higher ($P = 0.007$) than did the physicians (mean 2.75 ± 0.82). No significant changes in single procedures were observed (figure 5).

Comparing the Two Time Points

Both before and after the intervention, the respondents considered the current use of comfort measures to be more frequent than the current use of pharmacological agents ($P = 0.001$). The differences in their perceptions regarding the current and optimal use of pharmacological agents and comfort measures were significant at both time points (all P-values < 0.05).

Discussion

This chapter describes how the perceptions of clinical staff concerning procedural pain in neonates changed after the implementation of new pain-management strategies in two NICUs. Although both the nurses' and physicians' answers indicated a slight increase in the current use of pharmacological agents, there was also a persisting significant difference between what the clinicians perceived to be the current and optimal treatments of procedural pain. Only the nurses reported changes in their views of procedure painfulness, the current use of comfort measures, and the perceived optimal treatment for procedural pain. These changes did not diminish the differences between the views of the nurses and those of the physicians on procedure painfulness or the treatment of procedural pain.

The study has several weaknesses. Most important is the lack of a control group and controls for confounding factors. The observed changes may have been influenced by factors other than the intervention. During the period, nurses from both units participated in a 60 h external competence program for nurses, which included a 3 h session on neonatal pain and pain management. However, its content was mainly in line with the first education program provided as part of the intervention. In 2004, the Norwegian Pediatric Pain Society was founded during a meeting initiated by the pediatric department at one of the study sites. In general, there was a growing attention to pediatric pain issues among Norwegian health personnel during this period.

The sample sizes were small, especially the numbers of physicians. Some of the findings should be evaluated with caution, because the statistical power is probably low. The strength of the study is the small turnover in the clinical staff at both hospitals during the project period, so that the same respondents generally replied at both time points.

The results are the respondents' perceptions only and may differ from the actual pain-management practices in the units. Various studies have found significant differences between clinicians' self-reported actions and objective observational data. Respondents systematically overestimate their own performance [67-69] and tend to rate their own performance as better than the average performance of their peers [67]. The respondents' professional backgrounds may also influence their answers differently. The pharmacological treatment of pain is the physicians' responsibility, although it is carried out by nurses. The nurses' answers on the current use of pharmacological agents can be viewed as an evaluation of physicians' practice and not their own, whereas the physicians' answers reflect an evaluation of their own practice, and *vice versa* for the current use of comfort measures. The differences in the nurses' and physicians' answers may reflect the extent to which they were responsible for the treatment in question, rather than accurately reflecting actual pain-management practice in the two units studied. The self assessment of practice is not a good proxy measure of actual practice [67], and further studies are required to investigate the relationship between assessed and observed practice.

The differences between the nurses' and physicians' perceptions persisted over the study period. The nurses still believed the different procedures to be more painful than did the physicians, and their answers indicated a more frequent optimal use of comfort measures and pharmacological agents than did the physicians' answers. Different education, different roles and different areas of responsibility are plausible explanations.

The answers of both groups indicate an increase in the pharmacological treatment of neonatal pain, but only the nurses reported changes in the use of comfort measures. Both methods were included in the education program and in the guidelines, but it is likely that more emphasis was put on the use of pharmacological agents. Another possible explanation is that whereas pharmacological treatments are concrete, clearly defined, measurable, and documented in the infants' medical charts, comfort measures are less clearly defined, individual, and not documented in a systematic manner. Differences in the physicians' and nurses' views on the use of comfort measures may influence the extent to which comfort is given. The nurses' answers indicated a significant increase in the use of comfort measures only for procedures that were carried out independently by the nurses.

The respondents' views on procedure painfulness and the optimal treatment of procedural pain are largely consistent with international guidelines [17] and previous studies [16, 23]. Their answers showed only minor changes over two years, indicating that these are relatively stable beliefs. However, the few changes observed are noteworthy: The nurses were predominantly involved in changing the procedure of blood sampling. They rated heel stick as more painful after the intervention period, probably influenced by both their increased knowledge of blood sampling and their own observations during the change in the procedure. Venous punctures are less painful than heel sticks [38], and predominantly the nurses observed the differences in the neonates' behavioral responses. Previously, nurses had performed the heel stick or assisted phlebotomists in performing the procedure. Based on the new method, the nurses were trained to perform venous punctures for blood sampling. The procedure detailed the environmental and behavioral interventions that should be applied during blood sampling, and the nurses' answers indicated a significant increase in the use of comfort measures during heel-stick sampling. Knowledge about the available pharmacological treatments for the different procedures was disseminated throughout the intervention period. No appropriate pharmacological treatment is currently available for the heel-stick procedure. This knowledge is reflected in the nurses' answers, which indicated a significant drop in the optimal use of pharmacological agents for this procedure.

It appears that the intervention, although designed for a multi-professional group, influenced the nurses more than the physicians. Future research should investigate this difference and explore whether it is beneficial to target interventions differently according to the profession of the recipients.

When this intervention was designed, we were unavare of useful models for the implementation of knowledge in practice, and social learning theory was used as a guide for the elements that were included in the intervention. During the implementation period, we discovered other and maybe more sophisticated models, developed for the implementation of evidence in practice, like the Promoting Action on Research Implementation in Health Services (PARIHS) framework [70-72] and the Pettigrew and Whipp model of strategic change [73].

The PARIHS framework is based on the assumption that the successful implementation of evidence in practice is the result of the interplay between three factors: evidence, context, and facilitation [70, 72].

Evidence is understood to include research, clinical experience, and patient preferences [71]. One of the premises for this intervention was that knowledge or evidence is a prerequisite for change. Both the guidelines and the change in the procedure for blood sampling were based on research evidence. The international guidelines, which were the basis for the local guidelines, were also based on the collective clinical experience of the leading experts in the field of neonatal pain management in areas where research evidence is sparse. Both the NICUs included in the study had relatively little practical experience with systematic pain management before the intervention. Although the project group members possessed sufficient theoretical skills at the beginning of the intervention period, this knowledge had only been applied to clinical practice to a limited extent. The challenge was to acquire sufficient clinical skills and at the same time guide colleagues. The influence of clinical experience was most evident during the implementation of venous blood sampling, where members of the project group first helped each other to master the new procedure, with some help from another hospital, then used their newly acquired clinical expertise to help colleagues master the procedure. Patient preferences are difficult to measure when the patients are preverbal infants, but the differences in their behavioral responses to heel stick *vs* venous puncture motivated the nurses to change their perceptions. The mothers' responses also contributed to that change.

The PARIHS framework emphasizes the context, understood as including supportive leadership, a learning organization, and evaluation [70]. One of the premises for this intervention was that social or contextual factors influence change. Desired changes in practice are introduced to a complete social setting, not to single groups or individuals within this setting. Based on social learning theory, we believed that this would create a social pressure that would positively enhance the implementation of change. We did not formally evaluate the support provided by the local leadership, but it was important that the intervention was approved and supported by leaders at different levels of the pediatric departments before the intervention was performed. Neither did we focus on the characteristics of the learning organization. The approval of the senior neonatologists at both NICUs was essential for the credibility of the intervention and for the cooperation of the medical staff.

We carried out an evaluation as described in the PARIHS framework. A questionnaire that aimed to evaluate their knowledge, values, and beliefs regarding neonatal pain management, and the perceived barriers to sufficient pain-management practice, was distributed to each member of staff before the intervention was started. The results were fed back to the staff and have since been presented in two separate articles [3, 74].

The third pillar of the PARIHS framework is facilitation. Facilitation is a process in which an external or internal facilitator acts to support and enable the implementation of evidence in practice [70]. Facilitation was not considered an independent factor in the outlined premises. However, reviewing the intervention, the project manager had some facilitating role during the intervention period, together with the other members of the project groups. The project manager compiled the guidelines, supplied the staff and parents with oral and written information, organized the materials for the implementation of systematic pain assessment, and provided educational sessions. Both the project manager and members of the project groups engaged in bedside teaching, and members of the project groups underwent practical training of the nursing staff in venous blood sampling. Although the PARIHS framework was not known to us when the intervention was designed, it provides a useful framework with which to understand and evaluate elements of the intervention and the intervention process. All three elements in the framework were included in the intervention to some extent.

Conclusions

Despite the performance of a multifaceted intervention to support evidence-based practice, pharmacological agents and comfort measures appear to be underutilized in the treatment of procedural pain in neonates. The pharmacological treatment of procedural pain might have improved, but the overall results point clearly to the difficulties in applying evidence to practice.

Change is not easy or a straightforward process. It is necessary to gain a better understanding of the factors that influence the change process. Clinical research is of little value if the results cannot be disseminated and implemented in clinical practice, to benefit patients and practitioners.

Acknowledgements

The authors would like to express their gratitude to the physicians and nurses who participated in this study and to Fran Lang Porter for permission to use the questions from her survey. The study has been financed with the aid of EXTRA funds from the Norwegian Foundation for Health and Rehabilitation and financial support from Telemark Hospital and Vestfold Hospital.

References

[1]   Stevens BJ, Anand KJS, McGrath PJ: An overview of pain in neonates and infants. In: *Pain in neonates and infants*. Third edition. Edited by Anand KJS, Stevens BJ, McGrath PJ. Philadelphia: Elsevier; 2007: 1-7.

[2]   Salantera S: Finnish nurses' attitudes to pain in children. *J Adv Nurs* 1999, 29(3):727-736.

[3]   Andersen RD, Greve-Isdahl M, Jylli L: The opinions of clinical staff regarding neonatal procedural pain in two Norwegian neonatal intensive care units. *Acta Paediatr* 2007, 96(7):1000-1003.

[4]   Wallin L: Knowledge Utilization in Swedish Neonatal Nursing. Studies on Guideline Implementation, Change Processes and Contextual Factors. Doctoral dissertation. Uppsala: Uppsala University; 2003.

[5]   Rouzan IA: An analysis of research and clinical practice in neonatal pain management. *J Am Acad Nurse Pract* 2001, 13(2):57-60.

[6]   McGrath PJ, Unruh AM: The social context of neonatal pain. *Clin Perinatol* 2002, 29(3):555-572.

[7]   Anand KJ, Hickey PR: Pain and its effects in the human neonate and fetus. *N Engl J Med* 1987, 317(21):1321-1329.

[8]   Anand KJ, Sippell WG, Aynsley-Green A: Pain, anaesthesia, and babies. *Lancet* 1987, 2(8569):1210.

[9] Anand KJ, Sippell WG, Aynsley-Green A: Randomised trial of fentanyl anaesthesia in preterm babies undergoing surgery: effects on the stress response. *Lancet* 1987, 1(8524):62-66.

[10] Anand KJ, Sippell WG, Schofield NM, Aynsley-Green A: Does halothane anaesthesia decrease the metabolic and endocrine stress responses of newborn infants undergoing operation? *Br Med J (Clin Res Ed)* 1988, 296(6623):668-672.

[11] Anand KJ, Ward-Platt MP: Neonatal and pediatric stress responses to anesthesia and operation. *Int Anesthesiol Clin* 1988, 26(3):218-225.

[12] Banos JE, Ruiz G, Guardiola E: An analysis of articles on neonatal pain published from 1965 to 1999. *Pain Res Manag* 2001, 6(1):45-50.

[13] Barker DP, Rutter N: Exposure to invasive procedures in neonatal intensive care unit admissions. *Arch Dis Child Fetal Neonatal Ed* 1995, 72(1):F47-48.

[14] Johnston CC, Collinge JM, Henderson SJ, Anand KJ: A cross-sectional survey of pain and pharmacological analgesia in Canadian neonatal intensive care units. *Clin J Pain* 1997, 13(4):308-312.

[15] Porter FL, Anand KJ: Epidemiology of pain in neonates. *Res Clin Forums* 1998, 20(4):9-18.

[16] Simons SH, van Dijk M, Anand KS, Roofthooft D, van Lingen RA, Tibboel D: Do we still hurt newborn babies? A prospective study of procedural pain and analgesia in neonates. *Arch Pediatr Adolesc Med* 2003, 157(11):1058-1064.

[17] Anand KJ: Consensus statement for the prevention and management of pain in the newborn. *Arch Pediatr Adolesc Med* 2001, 155(2):173-180.

[18] Anand KJ, Johnston CC, Oberlander TF, Taddio A, Lehr VT, Walco GA: Analgesia and local anesthesia during invasive procedures in the neonate. *Clin Ther* 2005, 27(6):844-876.

[19] Porter FL, Wolf CM, Miller JP: Procedural pain in newborn infants: the influence of intensity and development. *Pediatrics* 1999, 104(1):e13.

[20] Anand KJ, Aranda JV, Berde CB, Buckman S, Capparelli EV, Carlo W, Hummel P, Johnston CC, Lantos J, Tutag-Lehr V *et al*: Summary proceedings from the neonatal pain-control group. *Pediatrics* 2006, 117(3 Pt 2):S9-S22.

[21] Lago P, Guadagni A, Merazzi D, Ancora G, Bellieni CV, Cavazza A: Pain management in the neonatal intensive care unit: a national survey in Italy. *Paediatr Anaesth* 2005, 15(11):925-931.

[22] Gharavi B, Schott C, Nelle M, Reiter G, Linderkamp O: Pain management and the effect of guidelines in neonatal units in Austria, Germany and Switzerland. *Pediatr Int* 2007, 49(5):652-658.

[23] Porter FL, Wolf CM, Gold J, Lotsoff D, Miller JP: Pain and pain management in newborn infants: a survey of physicians and nurses. *Pediatrics* 1997, 100(4):626-632.

[24] Rohrmeister K, Kretzer V, Berger A, Haiden N, Kohlhauser C, Pollak A: Pain and stress management in the Neonatal Intensive Care Unit--a national survey in Austria. *Wien Klin Wochenschr* 2003, 115(19-20):715-719.

[25] Harrison D, Loughnan P, Johnston L: Pain assessment and procedural pain management practices in neonatal units in Australia. *J Paediatr Child Health* 2006, 42(1-2):6-9.

[26] Coskun V, Anand KJS: Development of supraspinal pain processing. In: *Pain in Neonates,* vol. 10. Second Revised and Enlarged Edition. Edited by Anand KJS, Stevens BJ, McGrath PJ. Amsterdam: Elsevier; 2000: 23-54.

[27] Fitzgerald M: Development of the peripheral and spinal pain system. In: *Pain in Neonates,* vol. 10. Second Revised and Enlarged Edition. Edited by Anand KJS, Stevens BJ, McGrath PJ. Amsterdam: Elsevier; 2000: 9-22.

[28] Stevens B, Johnston C, Gibbins S: Pain assessment in neonates. In: *Pain in Neonates,* vol.10. Second Revised and Enlarged Edition. Edited by Anand KJS, Stevens BJ, McGrath PJ. Amsterdam: Elsevier; 2000: 101-134.

[29] Mitchell A, Boss BJ: Adverse effects of pain on the nervous systems of newborns and young children: a review of the literature. *J Neurosci Nurs* 2002, 34(5):228-236.

[30] Whitfield MF, Grunau RE: Behavior, pain perception, and the extremely low-birth weight survivor. *Clin Perinatol* 2000, 27(2):363-379.

[31] Taddio A, Katz J: The effects of early pain experience in neonates on pain responses in infancy and childhood. *Paediatr Drugs* 2005, 7(4):245-257.

[32] Grunau RE: Long-term consequences of pain in human neonates. In: *Pain in Neonates,* vol. 10. Second Revised and Enlarged Edition. Edited by Anand KJ, Stevens B, McGrath PJ. Amsterdam: Elsevier; 2000: 55-76.

[33] Stevens BJ, Riddell RRP, Oberlander TE, Gibbins S: Assessment of pain in neonates and infants. In: *Pain in neonates and infants.* Third edition. Edited by Anand KJS, Stevens BJ, McGrath PJ. Amsterdam: Elsevier; 2007: 67-90.

[34] Anand KJ, Craig KD: New perspectives on the definition of pain. *Pain* 1996, 67(1):3-6; discussion 209-211.

[35] Duhn LJ, Medves JM: A systematic integrative review of infant pain assessment tools. *Adv Neonatal Care* 2004, 4(3):126-140.

[36] Jylli L, Olsson GL: Procedural pain in a paediatric surgical emergency unit. *Acta Paediatr* 1995, 84(12):1403-1408.

[37] Knutsson J, Tibbelin A, Von Unge M: Postoperative pain after paediatric adenoidectomy and differences between the pain scores made by the recovery room staff, the parent and the child. *Acta Otolaryngol* 2006, 126(10):1079-1083.

[38] Shah V, Ohlsson A: Venepuncture versus heel lance for blood sampling in term neonates. *Cochrane Database Syst Rev* 2007(4):CD001452.

[39] Franck LS, Lawhon G: Environmental and behavioral strategies to prevent and manage neonatal pain. In: *Pain in Neonates,* vol. 10. Second Revised and Enlarged Edition. Edited by Anand KJS, Stevens BJ, McGrath PJ, vol. Amsterdam: Elsevier; 2000: 203-216.

[40] Stevens B, Taddio A, Ohlsson A, Einarson T: The efficacy of sucrose for relieving procedural pain in neonates--a systematic review and meta-analysis. *Acta Paediatr* 1997, 86(8):837-842.

[41] Pinelli J, Symington A, Ciliska D: Nonnutritive sucking in high-risk infants: benign intervention or legitimate therapy? *J Obstet Gynecol Neonatal Nurs* 2002, 31(5):582-591.

[42]   Ward-Larson C, Horn RA, Gosnell F: The efficacy of facilitated tucking for relieving procedural pain of endotracheal suctioning in very low birthweight infants. *MCN Am J Matern Child Nurs* 2004, 29(3):151-156; quiz 157-158.

[43]   Corff KE, Seideman R, Venkataraman PS, Lutes L, Yates B: Facilitated tucking: a nonpharmacologic comfort measure for pain in preterm neonates. *J Obstet Gynecol Neonatal Nurs* 1995, 24(2):143-147.

[44]   Bellieni CV, Bagnoli F, Perrone S, Nenci A, Cordelli DM, Fusi M, Ceccarelli S, Buonocore G: Effect of multisensory stimulation on analgesia in term neonates: a randomized controlled trial. *Pediatr Res* 2002, 51(4):460-463.

[45]   Bellieni CV, Bagnoli F, Buonocore G: Alone no more: pain in premature children. *Ethics Med* 2003, 19(1):5-9.

[46]   Eccles M, Mittman B: Welcome to Implementation Science. In: *Implement Sci* 2006, 1(1):1.

[47]   About Knowledge Translation. The KT Portfolio at CIHR. Accessed 2008-01-13 at http://www.cihr-irsc.gc.ca/e/29418.html#The.

[48]   Sanders D, Haines A: Implementation research is needed to achieve international health goals. *PLoS Med* 2006, 3(6):e186.

[49]   Grol R, Grimshaw J: From best evidence to best practice: effective implementation of change in patients' care. *Lancet* 2003, 362(9391):1225-1230.

[50]   WHO: World report on knowledge for better health. World Health Organisation: Geneva; 2004. Accessed 2008-01-14 at: http://www.who.int/rcp/meetings/publ/en/.

[51]   Bero LA, Grilli R, Grimshaw JM, Harvey E, Oxman AD, Thomson MA: Closing the gap between research and practice: an overview of systematic reviews of interventions to promote the implementation of research findings. The Cochrane Effective Practice and Organization of Care Review Group. *BMJ* 1998, 317(7156):465-468.

[52]   Grimshaw JM, Thomas RE, MacLennan G, Fraser C, Ramsay CR, Vale L, Whitty P, Eccles MP, Matowe L, Shirran L *et al*: Effectiveness and efficiency of guideline dissemination and implementation strategies. *Health Technol Assess* 2004, 8(6):iii-iv, 1-72.

[53]   Grimshaw JM, Shirran L, Thomas R, Mowatt G, Fraser C, Bero L, Grilli R, Harvey E, Oxman A, O'Brien MA: Changing provider behavior: an overview of systematic reviews of interventions. *Med Care* 2001, 39(8 Suppl 2):II2-45.

[54]   Thompson DS, Estabrooks CA, Scott-Findlay S, Moore K, Wallin L: Interventions aimed at increasing research use in nursing: a systematic review. *Implement Sci* 2007, 2:15.

[55]   Estabrooks CA, Thompson DS, Lovely JJ, Hofmeyer A: A guide to knowledge translation theory. *J Contin Educ Health Prof* 2006, 26(1):25-36.

[56]   Rycroft-Malone J: Theory and knowledge translation: setting some coordinates. *Nurs Res* 2007, 56(4 Suppl):S78-85.

[57]   Wallin L, Ewald U, Wikblad K, Scott-Findlay S, Arnetz BB: Understanding work contextual factors: a short-cut to evidence-based practice? *Worldviews Evid Based Nurs* 2006, 3(4):153-164.

[58] Grol RP, Bosch MC, Hulscher ME, Eccles MP, Wensing M: Planning and studying improvement in patient care: the use of theoretical perspectives. *Milbank Q* 2007, 85(1):93-138.

[59] Atkinson RL, Atkinson RC, Smith EE, Bem DJ: *Introduction to Psychology*, 11th Edition. Forth Worth: Harcourt Brace Jovanovitch College Publishers; 1993.

[60] Estabrooks CA, Floyd JA, Scott-Findlay S, O'Leary KA, Gushta M: Individual determinants of research utilization: a systematic review. *J Adv Nurs* 2003, 43(5):506-520.

[61] Greenhalgh T, Robert G, Macfarlane F, Bate P, Kyriakidou O: Diffusion of innovations in service organizations: systematic review and recommendations. *Milbank Q* 2004, 82(4):581-629.

[62] Dopson S, Fitzgerald L: The role of the middle manager in the implementation of evidence-based health care. *J Nurs Manag* 2006, 14(1):43-51.

[63] Estabrooks CA, Midodzi WK, Cummings GG, Wallin L: Predicting research use in nursing organizations: a multilevel analysis. *Nurs Res* 2007, 56(4 Suppl):S7-23.

[64] Cummings GG, Estabrooks CA, Midodzi WK, Wallin L, Hayduk L: Influence of organizational characteristics and context on research utilization. *Nurs Res* 2007, 56(4 Suppl):S24-39.

[65] McGrath PJ, Unruh AM: Social and legal issues. In: *Pain in Neonates* Vol.5. Edited by Anand KJ, McGrath PJ. Amsterdam: Elsevier Science Publishers B.V.; 1993: 295-320.

[66] Larsson BA, Gradin M, Lind V, Selander B: [Swedish guidelines for prevention and treatment of pain in newborn infants]. In Swedish. *Lakartidningen* 2002, 99(17):1946-1949.

[67] Saturno PJ, Palmer RH, Gascon JJ: Physician attitudes, self-estimated performance and actual compliance with locally peer-defined quality evaluation criteria. *Int J Qual Health Care* 1999, 11(6):487-496.

[68] Jenner EA, Fletcher BC, Watson P, Jones FA, Miller L, Scott GM: Discrepancy between self-reported and observed hand hygiene behaviour in healthcare professionals. *J Hosp Infect* 2006, 63(4):418-422.

[69] Hennes H, Kim MK, Pirrallo RG: Prehospital pain management: a comparison of providers' perceptions and practices. *Prehosp Emerg Care* 2005, 9(1):32-39.

[70] Rycroft-Malone J: The PARIHS framework--a framework for guiding the implementation of evidence-based practice. *J Nurs Care Qual* 2004, 19(4):297-304.

[71] Rycroft-Malone J, Kitson A, Harvey G, McCormack B, Seers K, Titchen A, Estabrooks C: Ingredients for change: revisiting a conceptual framework. *Qual Saf Health Care* 2002, 11(2):174-180.

[72] Rycroft-Malone J, Harvey G, Kitson A, McCormack B, Seers K, Titchen A: Getting evidence into practice: ingredients for change. *Nurs Stand* 2002, 16(37):38-43.

[73] Stetler CB, Ritchie J, Rycroft-Malone J, Schultz A, Charns M: Improving quality of care through routine, successful implementation of evidence-based practice at the bedside: an organizational case study protocol using the Pettigrew and Whipp model of strategic change. *Implement Sci* 2007, 2:3.

[74] Andersen RD, Greve-Isdahl M, Meberg A, Jylli L: [Knowledge and barriers of neonatal pain and pain management. A survey among clinical staff in two Norwegian neonatal intensive care units]. In Norwegian. *Vaard i Norden* 2007, 27(1):22-26.

In: Pain Management: New Research
Editors: P. S. Greco, F. M. Conti

ISBN: 978-1-60456-767-0
© 2008 Nova Science Publishers, Inc.

Chapter XIV

Immediate Pain Relief at Home

Jiman He[1], Wei Zhao[2] and Qiu Chen[3]
1 Rhode Island Hospital, Brown University, RI 02903, USA
2 College of Medical Sciences, Qingdao University, Qingdao, 266071, China
3 Affiliated Hospital of Luzhou, Luzhou Medical College, Sichuan, 646000, China

Abstract

Pain may afflict humans anytime, anywhere. There are usually considerable delays before relief, for example, time to find a doctor, expert, or pharmacist, or, time for the analgesic to take effect. To quickly overcome the pain is the goal sought by researchers for a very long time. We recently published a new analgesic method, acute mechanical pressure stimulation of the sciatic nerves, which resulted in relief of pain within a few minutes. The method is generally useful, and has been tested on pain from many diseases seen in emergency clinics as well as pain from various dental, renal, and tumor pathologies. The technique is simple, can be applied at home, immediately upon the onset of pain. No side effects have yet been observed in more than 600 subjects tested at 10 hospitals and universities. This chapter discusses more aspects of this new analgesic method.

Background

Pain is the most common medical problem. However, current analgesics are not satisfactory. In most cases, pain cannot be immediately relieved. The time necessary to acquire pain medications, and the time needed to reach effective levels too often are considerable. Overcoming pain in as fast and convenient a way possible is a worthwhile goal that has yet to be achieved despite considerable research into the subject.

Besides drawbacks in the relief delay, analgesic drugs have well known side effects (Fowler PD, 1987; Davis MP, 2003; Stiel D, 2000; Forman WB, 1996; Hersh EV, 2000). For example, corticosteroids lead to hypertension and psychosis; commonly prescribed NSAIDs cause ulcers and gastrointestinal bleeding, and, opioids cause constipation, nausea, respiratory depression, etc. According to the American Geriatrics Society 1998, some of the adverse effects are even more serious for the elderly.

A number of non-pharmacological analgesics have been reported in current clinical practice, for example, acupuncture, transcutaneous electrical nerve stimulation (TENS), various temperature modalities, manual therapies (e.g. massage), exercise, education, etc. (Wright A, 2001; Rakel B, 2003; Ernst E, 1994; Rusy LM, 2000; Driscoll CE,1987; Cherny NI,1994; Golianu B, 2007). Combinations of these non-pharmacological analgesics with pharmacological analgesics comprise an integral profile for pain management (Driscoll CE,1987; Ahmad M, 2002; Cherny NI, 1994). Among the non-pharmacological analgesics, however, the efficacy, advantages and limitations vary greatly. The efficacy of some non-pharmacological analgesic interventions was supported by some literature reviews (Wright A, 2001; Trescot AM, 2003; Nadler SF, 2004; Ying KN, 2007; Titler MG, 2001), but refuted by others (Ernst E, 2006; Milne S, 2001; Carroll D, 2001). Furthermore, the use of these analgesics is still limited to a small proportion of hospitals and clinics.

Acupuncture, a Traditional Chinese Medicine (TCM) has been applied in a wide variety of disease conditions for centuries (Han JS, 1985; Luu M, 1989; Golianu B, 2007). The key features for conventional acupuncture are the use of needles inserted selectively into precise points on the body surface and manipulated in various ways. However, reports on the efficacy of the method are contradictory (Cheuk DK, 2007; Golianu B, 2007; Aker PD, 1996). Also, acupuncture requires a highly trained specialist.

TENS is a relatively new procedure, which has been used on a variety of diseases for pain relief, generally the more chronic pain conditions (Herman E, 1994; Tan JC, 1998). However, several studies of clinical efficacy reported opposite results (Deyo RA, 1990; van Tulder MW, 1997). Also, studies indicated limitations on the use of TENS, such as its unsuitability for children and some heart disease patients (Chen D, 1990; Buonocore M,1992).

Temperature modalities have demonstrated effectiveness for pain relief (Feine JS,1997; Trescot AM, 2003). Their use, however, is limited to shallow depths in tissue. Also, peripheral nerve injury has been described, such that, unmonitored direct application over peripheral nerves of the skin is not suggested (Fisher S, 1965; Bassett FH,1992).

Similarly, exercise, education, psychological intervention and other adjunctive therapies may have advantages in some situations and drawbacks in others. Drawbacks may include costing a great deal, taking considerable time, requiring special settings or application experts, giving limited pain relief, or applying only to very limited special situations.

We recently reported a new physical analgesic, a 2-minute sciatic nerve press, for immediate relief of pain brought on by different pathologies, which imparted significant pain relief lasting throughout the observed period of one hour (He J, 2007; 2008a). The method was introduced in reports on tests of dental, renal, tumor and emergency patients. Pain was relieved immediately within a few minutes of pressure. Though some patients did obtain relief for several hours, the best pain relief occurred from 10 – 20 minutes after two minutes pressure stimulation of the sciatic nerves.

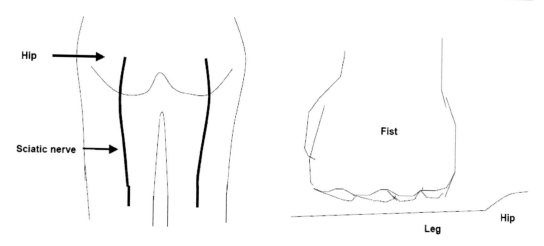

Figure 1. Sciatic nerve and fist gesture.

The method can be used repeatedly, but there was a diminishing effect if the method was repeated too frequently. However, the effectiveness returned after discontinuing use. Our further preliminary studies have shown that this simple method also worked excellently on immediate relief of non-painful discomfort (He J, 2008b). The technique is simple, can be applied anytime, anyplace, even at home, and immediately upon the onset of pain. This chapter will discuss this new method, a two-minute pressure stimulation of the sciatic nerves, in more detail.

The Procedural Points

As a simple physical analgesic method, the procedure consists of three principal actions: applying pressure directly over the sciatic nerve, achieving 11 – 20kg of mechanical pressure on each sciatic nerve, and holding the pressure for 2 minutes.

Figure 1 shows the fist pressing on the sciatic nerve with the patient lying on his stomach. Pressure is applied with the dorsal, proximal phalangeal surface of the fists, or the heel of palm but not the knuckles, or the finger tips. The easiest way to apply the method is to have a third person pressing on the sciatic nerves simultaneously with the patient lying prone. The pressure force applied is not a rigid parameter. The amount of force we use is within the range of 11 - 20 kg, and, depends on the patient's body type, with heavily muscled, or large-bodied patients receiving higher pressures than thin patients. Usually, 11 - 13 kg per hand is reserved for weak and thin patients. Greater pressure than 14 kg per hand will produce better relief. Time is also not a rigid parameter, and can be a little shorter or longer than two minutes. If two minutes of pressure does not result in immediate pain relief, one or two more minutes pressure may achieve relief. The two-minute period was optimal in our pilot studies, and is used in our clinical studies. However, pressure for a much longer time period does not result in better or longer relief of pain. Some patients will feel pain relief even after a one minute press, but pressing for too short a time will result in failure to achieve relief.

Discussion

It is well documented that mechanical pressure causes nerve injuries, and that large diameter nerve fibers are more susceptible. Damage is usually attributed to ischemia or structural deformation. A number of studies have reported pressure effects on nerves, using different force levels and time periods, from tens to thousands of millimeters of mercury, and from several minutes to several weeks (Macgregor RJ, 1975; Lundborg G, 1983; Dahlin LB, 1989; Fern R, 1994; Ochoa J 1972; Powell HC, 1986, Gelberman RH, 1983). The nerves for the pressure stimulation in animal models are often surgically exposed (Dahlin LB, 1989; Fern R, 1994; Sarikcioglu L, 2007). However, our method uses a much shorter time period, two minutes, and direct application of pressure against intact skin. So far, we have not found any adverse side effects in our practice at 10 hospitals and universities including more than six hundred subjects. Furthermore, this level of acute skin pressure,11 - 20 kg (150 – 380 mm Hg) with each fist for two minutes, is not uncommon in daily activities, especially for people in sports or workers in heavy labor jobs. On the other hand, chronic pressure on nerves, even if by a very small amount of force, may cause severe nerve dysfunction as is seen in clinics. For example, chronic pressure on the sciatic nerve by internal tension of the obturator muscle, or by an anatomical abnormality of the piriformis muscle, could cause pain (Benson ER, 1999; Solheim LF, 1981; Mullin v, 1990; Meknas K, 2003). Surgery to relieve the muscle pressure resulted in immediate pain relief (Benson ER, 1999; Meknas K, 2003; Chen WS, 1994; Sayson SC, 1994).

The precise application of the pressure is important for successful pain relief. Applying the pressure using the palms or fists produces better results than the knuckles or finger tips; because, it is too easy to miss the sciatic nerve when using knuckles or finger tips. The pressure application time is for two minutes. However, the pressure application can be interrupted briefly when the practitioner needs to adjust his/her body for comfort. The rate of success decreased greatly, and the duration of pain relief declined proportionally when times shorter than 90 second were used for the press in our studies. For those patients who obtained pain relief from the method, 25% of patients obtained pain relief within 30 – 60 seconds of initiating the press; 54.7% patients by 60 – 90 seconds (He J, 2007). The rest needed pressure for a longer time for notable relief. A third important qualitative factor is the amount of pressure applied. Insufficient force lead to a failure of relief. The optimal force used for eastern Asian populations was established during our pilot studies as 11 - 20 kg from each fist. For western people, who generally have a larger body size, the suitable range of pressure will need further study to verify.

Our results showed that the two-minute sciatic nerve press produced significant relief from pain due to dental, renal, tumor and various other pathologies. The relief for various pathologies tested was achieved immediately, within or after the two minutes of pressure (He J, 2007; 2008a). In our clinical studies, despite slight variations in the pressure location and force applied, pain relief was consistently achieved in all test groups. Though a simple method, training helped practitioners to increase their success ratio. There were failures in our clinical practice. We found a higher failure rate in renal and emergency patients with 40% and 30% of patients respectively, experiencing no relief (He J, 2007; 2008a). Because of the limited sample size for our studies, we could not determine whether the failure was related to the disease's origin, or the severity of the baseline pain. Further systematic studies with larger numbers of patients would be needed to clarify this question.

Stimulation of peripheral nerves is proposed to elevate the pain threshold (Woolf CJ, 1980; Chung JM, 1984; Jorum E, 1988; Kawasaki M, 2002; Yao T, 1982; Salar G, 1981 and Hanai F. 2000). The sciatic nerve trunk, the largest and longest in the human body, originates in the lower spine as nerve roots exit the spinal cord. Large diameter nerves are more sensitive to pressure stimulation, because of greater deformation than thinner ones under a given pressure (Ochoa J, 1972; Macgregor RJ, 1975). So, this could be the reason why the sciatic nerve is so sensitive to pressure stimulation.

Intrinsic opioid release could partially explain the relief mechanism; however, opioid secretion takes time. Thus, opioid release may explain the relief of later time periods, dozens of minutes after application of pressure, but not the immediate relief during the first few minutes after pressure is applied. Gate Control Theory can explain the rapid relief of pain for some situations by this method (Melzack R,1965). According to this theory, stimulation of large-diameter afferent fibers can inhibit the transmission of nociceptive information from the dorsal horn to higher brain centers. This inhibition occurs rapidly, and the resulting analgesic effect is considered to be a short-lasting, segmental inhibition of pain. However, the theory cannot explain well, why pressure on the sciatic nerve can relieve pain throughout the body; nor, how the effect can continue for up to an hour.

The press stimulation by itself might cause pain, and such pain could activate a special form of descending pain inhibition called diffuse noxious inhibitory control (DNIC) (Hanai F, 2000; Melzack R, 1965; Cohen ML, 1992), the so called "pain inhibits pain", which can be rapid inhibition. However, our method uses the smoother, dorsal proximal phalangeal surface of the fist, or the palm to press on the leg, not the pointed knuckles or finger tips. Only a small amount of discomfort was reported by a few patients in our studies. Also, we used the same amount of pressure on the placebo patients as on the sciatic press patients, but, it produced much less pain relief. Again, significant pain relief with sciatic nerve pressure lasted for one hour, unlike the analgesia of DNIC which is extremely short-lasting, ceasing within a few minutes. For these reasons, it is not likely that analgesia by DNIC explains the relief achieved with the 2-min sciatic press method.

This method is general useful, and immediately effective. With this method, pain can be relieved immediately at home. However, this method works to achieve immediate and short-term pain relief, but does not cure diseases. Patients need to be encouraged to consult their doctors for proper diagnosis and therapy of their underlying diseases.

As a total new method, there are a lot of unknowns. Further studies of the sciatic press method await the outcome of those in other fields, some of which predicted findings have been included in our planning. Questions that need addressing include: Is the effectiveness of the method related to baseline pain level, or, to specific disease etiologies? Are there any possible side effects to two minutes of sciatic nerve pressure? What is the mechanism for immediate pain relief from various pathologies by this method? Are there any other clinical effects of this method?

This method is simple and convenient. Because of its simplicity, some doctors and patients only accepted the method after personally experiencing how well the method worked in our clinical studies. So, great effort is needed to overcome skepticism and disseminate information about the method as rapidly as possible to serve patients well.

Conclusion

The acute stimulation of sciatic nerve can produce immediate short-term relief of pain brought on by different diseases. Pain can be relieved at home with the 2 minute press. A new, simple, convenient and powerful method, it is not yet widely recognized. To properly benefit the most patients the soonest requires a lot more research to define its best uses and limitations, and a lot more advertisement to disseminate the news.

Authors' Contribution

Wei Zhao and Qiu Chen contributed equally to this paper. Jiman He was the primary investigator of the studies.

Acknowledgments

We thank: Jack R. Wands, MD of Brown University for his generous assistance with these studies, and Gail Donaldson, MD, of Buffalo, NY for her editorial assistance. We thank Xianrong Jiang, Hefei Teachers College, Pingniu Wei, BS, Biwen Lin, BS, Anqing Normal College, Bihua Zhao, Master, Anhui Normal University, and Xianzheng Qi, Hefei, Anhui province, for their assistance with the cold induced pain experiments. Thanks go to Hongmei Qian, Maanshan, Anhui province, China; Guojun Shi, Wuwei Count, Anhui province, China; Chen Taiyi, Affiliated Hospital of Luzhou, Luzhou, Sichuan Province, China; Zeyong Shao, Affiliated Hospital of Luzhou, Luzhou, Sichuan Province, China; zijian Liu, Tengnan Hospital, Zaozhuang Kuanye Company, Shandong Province, China; Mingxia Huang, Chuzou hospital, China; Sigang Yang, Tongling count hospital, Anhui province, China; Ming (Bing) Hu, Wuwei Yiyao Company, Wuwei count, China; Yu Baitao, Niubu hospital, Niubu, Wuwei count, Anhui Province, China; Jingsong Sun, Shenzhen Zhongyi Hospital, Guangdong province, China; Lin Liu, MD, and Yao Ma, BS, Maanshan People's Hospital, Anhui province, China, for their assistance with the clinical studies of this method.

References

Ahmad M, Goucke CR: Management strategies for the treatment of neuropathic pain in the elderly. *Drugs Aging*. 2002, 19(12):929-45.
Aker PD, Gross AR, Goldsmith CH, et al: Concservative management of mechanical neck pain: systematic overview and metaanalysis. *BMJ* 1996, 313:1291-6.

American Geriatrics Society. The management of chronic pain in older persons: AGS panel on chronic pain in older persons. *J. Am. Geriatr. Soc.* 1998 May; 46(5): 635-51.

Bassett FH III, Kirkpatrick JS, Engelhardt DL, Malone TR: Cryotherapy-induced nerve injury. *Am. J. Sports Med.* 1992, 20:516-518.

Benson ER, Schutzer SF: Posttraumatic piriformis syndrome: diagnosis and results of operative treatment. *J. Bone Joint Surg. Am.* 1999, 81(7):941-949.

Buonocore M, Mortara A, La Rovere MT, Casale R: Cardiovascular effects of TENS: heart rate variability and plethysmographic wave evaluation in a group of normal subjects. *Funct. Neurol.* 1992, 7(5):391-4.

Carroll D, Moore RA, McQuay HJ, Fairman F, Tramer M, Leijon G: Transcutaneous electrical nerve stimulation (TENS) for chronic pain. *Cochrane Database Syst. Rev.* 2001:CD003222.

Chen D, Philip M, Philip PA, Monga TN: Cardiac pacemaker inhibition by transcutaneous electrical stimulation. *Arch. Phys. Med .Rehabil.* 1990, 71(1): 27-30.

Chen WS: Bipartite piriformis muscle: an unusual cause of sciatic nerve entrapment. *Pain* 1994, 58(2):269-272.

Cherny NI, Foley KM: Current approaches to the management of cancer pain: a review. *Ann. Acad Med Singapore.* 1994, 23(2):139-59.

Cheuk DK, Yeung WF, Chung KF, Wong V: Acupuncture for insomnia. *Cochrane Database Syst. Rev.* 2007, 18(3): CD005472.

Chung JM, Lee KH, Hori Y, Endo K, Willis WD: Factors influencing peripheral nerve stimulation produced inhibition of primate spinothalamic tract cells. *Pain* 1984, 19(3):277-293.

Cohen ML, Arroyo JF, Champion GD, Browne CD: In search of the pathogenesis of refractory cervicobrachial pain syndrome. A deconstruction of the RSI phenomenon. *Med. J. Aust.* 1992, 156(6):432-436.

Dahlin LB, Shyu BC, Danielsen N, Andersson SA: Effects of nerve compression or ischaemia on conduction properties of myelinated and non-myelinated nerve fibres. An experimental study in the rabbit common peroneal nerve. *Acta Physiol. Scand.* 1989, 136(1):97-105.

Davis MP, Srivastava M: Demographics, assessment and management of pain in the elderly. *Drugs Aging* 2003, 20(1):23-57.

Deyo RA, Walsh NE, Martin DC, Schoenfeld LS, Ramamurthy S: A controlled trial of transcutaneous electrical nerve stimulation (TENS) and exercise for chronic low back pain. *N. Engl .J. Med.* 1990, 322(23):1627-34.

Driscoll CE: Pain management. *Prim Care.* 1987, 14(2):337-52.

Ernst E: Acupuncture--a critical analysis. *J. Intern. Med.* 2006, 259(2):125-137.

Ernst E, Fialka V. Ice freezes pain? A review of the clinical effectiveness of analgesic cold therapy. *J Pain Symptom Manage* 1994, 9(1):56-9.

Feine JS, Widmer CG, Lund JP: Physical therapy: a critique. *Oral Surg. Oral. Med. Oral Pathol Oral Radiol Endod.* 1997, 83(1): 123-7.

Fern R, Harrison PJ: The contribution of ischaemia and deformation to the conduction block generated by compression of the cat sciatic nerve. *Exp. Physiol.* 1994, 79(4):583-592.

Fisher S: Physical response to heat and cold. *Therapeutic Heat and Cold*. 2nd ed. Baltimore, Md. Waverly Press; 1965:126-129.

Forman WB: Opioid analgesic drugs in the elderly. *Clin. Geriatr. Med.* 1996, 12(3):489-500.

Fowler PD, Aspirin, paracetamol and non-steroidal anti-inflammatory drugs. A comparative review of side effects. *Med Toxicol Adverse Drug Exp*. 198, 2(5):338-66.

Gelberman RH, Szabo RM, Williamson RV, Dimick MP: Sensibility testing in peripheral-nerve compression syndromes. An experimental study in humans. *J. Bone Joint Surg. Am*. 1983, 65(5):632-638.

Golianu B, Krane E, Seybold J, Almgren C, Anand KJ: Non-pharmacological techniques for pain management in neonates. *Semin Perinatol*. 2007, 31(5):318-22.

Han JS: Acupuncture analgesia. *Pain*, 1985, 21(3): 307-10.

Hanai F: Effect of electrical stimulation of peripheral nerves on neuropathic pain. *Spine* 2000, 25(15):1886-1892.

He J, Wu B, Zhang W, Ten G: Immediate and short-term pain relief by acute sciatic nerve press: a randomized controlled trial. *BMC Anesthesiology*, 2007, 7:4.

He J, Wu B, Jiang X, Zhang F, Zhao T and Zhang W: A new analgesic method, two-minute sciatic nerve press, for immediate pain relief: a randomized trial. *BMC Anesthesiology*, 2008a, 8:1.

He J: Immediate relief of non-painful discomfort with an acute sciatic nerve press. AAPM meeting abstracts, *Pain Medicine*, 2008b, 9(1), 88-141.

Herman E, William R, Stratford P, Fargas-Babjak A, Trott M. A randomized controlled trial of transcutaneous electrical nerve stimulation (CODE-TRON) to determine its benefits in a rehabilitation program for acute occupational low back pain. *Spine*. 1994, 19:561-568.

Hersh EV, Moore PA, Ross GL: Over-the-counter analgesics and antipyretics: a critical assessment. *Clin. Ther*. 2000, 22(5):500-548.

Jorum E: The analgesic effect of peripheral nerve stimulation in various tests of nociception in rats. *Acta Physiol. Scand*. 1988, 133(2):131-138.

Kawasaki M, Ushida T, Tani T, Yamamoto H: Changes of wide dynamic range neuronal responses to mechanical cutaneous stimuli following acute compression of the rat sciatic nerve. *J. Orthop. Sci* .2002, 7(1):111-116.

Lundborg G, Myers R, Powell H: Nerve compression injury and increased endoneurial fluid pressure: a "miniature compartment syndrome". *J. Neurol. Neurosurg. Psychiatry* 1983, 46(12):1119-1124.

Luu M, Boureau F: Acupuncture in pain therapy: current concepts. *Ther. Umsch*. 1989, 46(8): 518-25.

Macgregor RJ, Sharpless SK, Luttges MW: A pressure vessel model for nerve compression. *J. Neurol. Sci*. 1975, 24(3):299-304.

Meknas K, Christensen A, Johansen O: The internal obturator muscle may cause sciatic pain. *Pain* 2003, 104(1-2):375-380.

Melzack R, Wall PD: Pain mechanisms: a new theory. *Science* 1965, 150(699):971-979.

Milne S, Welch V, Brosseau L, Saginur M, Shea B, Tugwell P, Wells G: Transcutaneous electrical nerve stimulation (TENS) for chronic low back pain. *Cochrane Database Syst Rev* 2001:CD003008.

Mullin V, de Rosayro M: Caudal steroid injection for treatment of piriformis syndrome. *Anesth Analg* 1990, 71(6):705-707.

Nadler SF: Nonpharmacologic management of pain. *J. Am. Osteopath. Assoc.* 2004, 104(Suppl 8):S6-12.

Ochoa J, Fowler TJ, Gilliatt RW: Anatomical changes in peripheral nerves compressed by a pneumatic tourniquet. *J.Anat.* 1972, 113(Pt 3):433-455.

Price DD: Psychological and neural mechanisms of pain. New York, Raven. 1988.

Portenoy RK, Lesage P: Management of cancer pain. Lancet, 1999, 353: 1695-700.

Powell HC, Myers RR: Pathology of experimental nerve compression. *Lab. Invest.* 1986, 55(1):91-100.

Rakel B, Barr JO: Physical modalities in chronic pain management. *Nurs. Clin. North Am.* 2003, 38(3):477-494.

Rusy LM, Weisman SJ: Complementary therapies for acute pediatric pain management. *Pediatr. Clin. North Am.* 2000, 47(3):589-599.

Salar G, Job I, Mingrino S, Bosio A: Trabucchi M. Effect of transcutaneous electrotherapy on CSF beta-endorphin content in patients without pain problems. *Pain.* 1981, 10:169-172

Sarikcioglu L, Yaba A, Tanriover G, Demirtop A, Demir N, Ozkan O: Effect of severe crush injury on axonal regeneration: a functional and ultrastructural study. *J. Reconstr. Microsurg.* 2007, 23(3):143-149.

Sayson SC, Ducey JP, Maybrey JB, Wesley RL, Vermilion D: Sciatic entrapment neuropathy associated with an anomalous piriformis muscle. *Pain* 1994, 59(1):149-152.

Solheim LF, Siewers P, Paus B: The piriformis muscle syndrome. Sciatic nerve entrapment treated with section of the piriformis muscle. *Acta Orthop. Scand.* 1981, 52(1):73-75.

Stiel D: Exploring the link between gastrointestinal complications and over-the-counter analgesics: current issues and considerations. *Am J Ther* 2000, 7(2):91-98.

Tan JC: Physical modalities. In: Tan JC, ed. *Practical Manual of Physical Medicine and Rehabilitation.* St Louis, Mo: Mosby; 1998: 133-155.

Titler MG, Rakel BA: Nonpharmacologic treatment of pain. *Crit. Care Nurs. Clin. North Am.* 2001, 13(2):221-32.

Trescot AM: Cryoanalgesia in interventional pain management. *Pain Physician* 2003, 6(3):345-360.

van Tulder MW, Koes BW, Bouter LM. Conservative treatment of acute and chronic nonspecific low back pain. *Spine.* 1997, 22:2128-56.

Woolf CJ, Mitchell D, Barrett GD: Antinociceptive effect of peripheral segmental electrical stimulation in the rat. *Pain* 1980, 8(2):237-252.

World health Organization: Technical Report Series. Cancer Pain Relief and Palliative Care. Geneva, World Health Organization, 1990.

Wright A, Sluka KA: Nonpharmacological treatments for musculoskeletal pain. *Clin. J. Pain.* 2001, 17(1):33-46.

Yao T, Andersson S, Thoren P: Long-lasting cardiovascular depressor response following sciatic stimulation in spontaneously hypertensive rats. Evidence for the involvement of central endorphin and serotonin systems. *Brain Res.* 1982, 244(2):295-303.

Ying KN, While A: Pain relief in osteoarthritis and rheumatoid arthritis: TENS. *Br. J. Community Nurs.* 2007, 12(8): 364-71.

Index

B

E

F

I

low back pain, 275, 276, 277
low birthweight, 266
low-income, 240
lumbar laminectomy, 201, 204
lumbar puncture, 255
lumen, 153, 157, 159
lung, 146, 164, 234
lung cancer, 146
lung disease, 234
lying, 271
lymph, 157
lymphadenopathy, 157
lymphocyte, 17
lymphoid, 152, 155, 156, 157
lymphoid hyperplasia, 155, 157
lysis, 164

M

macrophage, 172
magnesium, 203, 210
magnetic, 67, 77, 105, 112
magnetic resonance imaging (MRI), 67, 77
maintenance, 8, 11, 12, 20, 26, 33, 35, 44, 59, 57, 80, 81, 184, 197, 198, 200, 209
major depression, 2, 28, 31, 33, 37, 56, 63, 72
major depressive disorder, 48, 64, 66
malaise, 19
males, 78, 186
malignant, ix, 141, 142, 144, 145, 147, 164
management, vii, x, xii, 19, 21, 27, 30, 32, 45, 144, 159, 160, 163, 164, 171, 176, 178, 182, 187, 188, 190, 193, 196, 208, 209, 211, 216, 223, 224, 226, 227, 228, 234, 240, 244, 245, 247, 248, 249, 253, 259, 260, 262, 264, 274, 275, 277
management practices, 260
mandates, 239
manipulation, 78, 81, 163, 166, 179, 182
mapping, 161
market, 214
maternal care, xii, 231, 232, 233, 234, 237, 239, 241
matrix, 3, 81, 126, 130
McGill Pain Questionnaire, 79
meals, 184
measurement, 234, 255
measures, vii, viii, xiii, 1, 6, 26, 30, 35, 36, 82, 86, 165, 199, 201, 208, 224, 237, 242, 248, 249, 250, 251, 252, 254, 257, 259, 260, 261, 263

mechanical, x, xi, xiii, 142, 165, 195, 196, 197, 198, 200, 201, 204, 205, 206, 207, 208, 209, 214, 269, 271, 272, 274, 276
mechanical ventilation, 214
media, 106, 128, 220, 222
medial prefrontal cortex, 15
median, x, 15, 44, 152, 158, 175, 185, 187, 197, 198, 201, 257
mediation, 41, 64, 79, 243
mediators, 48, 197
Medicaid, 227
medication, 31, 41, 60, 83, 143, 168
medicine, vii, 76, 143, 176, 190, 194, 215
medline, 152
medulla, 51, 209
medulla oblongata, 51
melanoma, 144
memory, 6, 9, 18, 49, 72, 81
memory retrieval, 81
men, 85
menopause, 7
mental disorder, 36, 37
mental health, xii, 232, 233
mental state, 176
mercury, 272
mesencephalon, 4, 11, 18, 35, 39, 51, 66
mesocorticolimbic, 3, 5, 6, 7, 8, 10, 12, 21, 66, 72, 73
messenger RNA, 64, 72
meta analysis, 158
meta-analysis, 43, 82, 86, 160, 189, 194, 203, 265
metabolism, 38, 41, 43, 58, 64, 178
metabolite, 6
metabolites, 6, 41, 46, 55, 57, 144, 147
methane, 101
methanol, 107, 110, 114, 116, 118, 126, 133, 134
methylene, 106
methylene group, 106
mice, 4, 18, 19, 20, 22, 48, 50, 51, 52, 56, 64
microdialysis, 53, 54
microinjection, 49
midbrain, 60, 64, 87
midwives, 224, 229
migraine, 82, 87
military, 9
milk, 183, 235, 236, 237, 238
millennium, 216
mind-body, viii, 75, 83
Minnesota, 10
misleading, 21

N

O

P

T

W

Y

X